Handbook of Kidney Transplantation

Handbook of Kidney Transplantation

Editor: Alice Foster

AMERICAN
MEDICAL PUBLISHERS
www.americanmedicalpublishers.com

AMERICAN
MEDICAL PUBLISHERS
www.americanmedicalpublishers.com

Cataloging-in-publication Data

Handbook of kidney transplantation / edited by Alice Foster.
p. cm.
Includes bibliographical references and index.
ISBN 979-8-88740-148-5
1. Kidneys--Transplantation. 2. Kidneys--Disease--Diagnosis.
3. Kidneys--Diseases--Treatment. 4. Nephrology. I. Foster, Alice.
RD575 .H36 2023
617.461 059 2--dc23

American Medical Publishers,
41 Flatbush Avenue,
1st Floor, New York,
NY 11217, USA

ISBN 979-8-88740-148-5 (Hardback)

Contents

Preface

Every book is a source of knowledge and this one is no exception. The idea that led to the conceptualization of this book was the fact that the world is advancing rapidly; which makes it crucial to document the progress in every field. I am aware that a lot of data is already available, yet, there is a lot more to learn. Hence, I accepted the responsibility of editing this book and contributing my knowledge to the community.

A kidney transplant refers to a type of surgical procedure that involves implanting a healthy kidney from a deceased or living donor into a patient who is suffering from kidney dysfunction. It is the preferred treatment for kidney failure in contrast to lifelong dependence on dialysis. Kidney transplants are performed to benefit people suffering from end-stage renal failure or chronic kidney disease. Significant risks associated with kidney transplant surgery include a cancer or disease that can be transmitted through the donated kidney, rejection or failure of a donated kidney, etc. High blood pressure, bleeding, blood clots, and weight gain are examples of possible side effects of the kidney transplant procedure. This book unravels the recent studies on kidney transplantation and the latest advances in its clinical management. It will also provide interesting topics for research which interested readers can take up. This book will serve as a reference to a broad spectrum of readers.

While editing this book, I had multiple visions for it. Then I finally narrowed down to make every chapter a sole standing text explaining a particular topic, so that they can be used independently. However, the umbrella subject sinews them into a common theme. This makes the book a unique platform of knowledge.

I would like to give the major credit of this book to the experts from every corner of the world, who took the time to share their expertise with us. Also, I owe the completion of this book to the never-ending support of my family, who supported me throughout the project.

Editor

1

Ethical Controversies in Organ Transplantation

Ehtuish Ehtuish
Surgery Department Tripoli Central Hospital &
National Organ Transplantation Program
Libya

1. Introduction

Since the 1st successful kidney transplant in 1954 done between two identical twins [Merrill etal 1958] organ transplantation has become a life-saving procedure for many disease conditions hitherto considered incurable. Clinical organ transplantation has been recognized as one of the most gripping medical advances of the century as it provides a way of giving the gift of life to patients with terminal failure of vital organs, which requires the participation of other fellow human beings and of society by donating organs from deceased or living individuals [Ehtuish etal 2006 & Hariharan etal 2000]. The gap between the demand for organ transplantation and the supply of donor organs is growing [The economist 2008].The waiting list of the United Network for Organ Sharing has grown from 21,975 names in 2000 to 32,722 in 2008 Fig. (1).

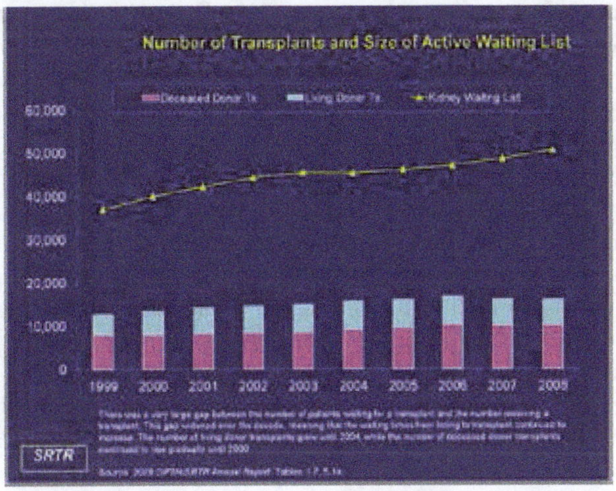

Fig. 1. The gap between the demand for organ transplantation and the supply of donor organs (UNOS) publications

The scarcity of organs has dire consequences. And an average of 19 people dies each day waiting for a transplant that never comes [United Network for Organ Sharing (UNOS) 1999]. The World Health Organization WHO global observatory showed that in 2009 about 100,900 people receive a lifesaving organ transplant, representing only less than 10% of the global needs Fig. (2). the entire issue has raised serious ethical concerns and the debate over

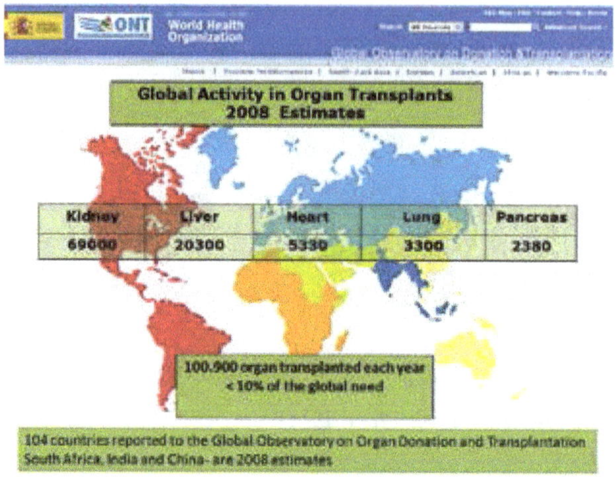

Fig. 2. Number of Transplants done worldwide WHO publication

them rages unabated. As further advances are made in such areas as cloning [Savules etal 1999], the ethical debate should grow more intense. The increasing incidence of vital organ failure and the inadequate supply of organs, especially from cadavers, have created a wide gap between organ supply and organ demand, which has resulted in very long waiting times to receive an organ as well as an increasing number of deaths while waiting. These events have raised many ethical, moral and societal issues regarding supply, the methods of organ allocation, and the use of living donors including minors. It has also led to the practice of organ sale by entrepreneurs for financial gains in some parts of the world through exploitation of the poor, for the benefit of the wealthy the ethical questions are complicated by an outgoing debate over the definitions of certain key terms such as life, death, human, and body. One example is the definition of brain death [Delmonico etal 1973]. People have been confused over the issue because of the highly public cases of people recovering from comas even after many years. The distinction between the idea of brain death and coma becomes a matter that must be clearly defined. A family that is asked to donate body organs from dead relative on the basis of brain death must be confident that there is no hope of recovering. Other ethical issues of organ donation are considered bioethical an important one is the idea of cloning. The technology that would allow the cloning of genetically matched clones for the purpose of body harvesting another issue is known as xenotransplantation which involves the harvesting of certain compatible animal organs for use in humans. A whole new plethora of ethical issues surround this idea due to fear from animals and the diseases might transmitted form them, or to protect them, even animal rights groups have joined in these debates. There is no question that body donation and organ donation will remain a hot topic for many years to come. Organ transplantation in general, and kidney transplants in particular, are fraught with ethical issues and dilemmas worldwide, about which there is ongoing debate, especially because of the shortage of organs The ethical questions associated with transplantation are many [Abouna 2008]. Is the human body a commodity? How should decisions be made about who should receive scarce organs? Who should pay for transplants? Should someone who has received one organ transplant be given a second transplant? Or should people who have not had a transplant be given priority over those who have already had one? Should one person receive several organs or should several people each receive one? Should one person have a second transplant when the first one fail or should a different person be given a first chance at new organ? Should people who have young children be given an organ transplant over a single person? Should young people be given an organ transplant over an elderly person? Should age and whether or not a person has children even matter? Should organs be given to people who have abused their bodies (smoking and drinking etc,) or only to people whose organs are damaged by disease? Should hands or other appendages, which are not essential to life, be transplanted? Who can "donate" the organs of people who cannot give informed consent to the process? Should money now spent on transplantation be put to other uses? Is it possible to prevent the coercion of some donors? Should suicidal individuals be given an organ transplant? What if they attempted suicide in the past but are not currently contemplating suicide? Should people who can't afford expensive anti-rejection drugs be passed over for a transplant? Should people who don't have Insurance and can't pay for a transplant be allowed to go on the National waiting list? Should condemned prisoners receive organ transplants? What if they are serving a life sentence without parole? Should country lawmakers be involved in transplantation? When should courts be involved in these questions?

The questions go on and on; the answers are never simple. Knowing that there are more people who need organs than there are organs available, how would you answer these questions? Are your answers based on a belief of equal access or maximum benefit distribution?

2. What is organ transplantation?

An organ transplant is a surgical operation involves removing of an organ from one person (donor) and transferring it to another (recipient), keeping the native organs like Kidneys or removing them like Livers and Hearts. The need to obtain informed consent from both persons (and their surrogate decision-makers) is compulsory. This is in keeping with the ethical principle of respect for persons and is expressed in many ethical guidelines today.

3. Important milestones in the history of organ transplantation

- 1950 – 1954 The first successful kidney transplant. A kidney is taken from one identical brother and transplanted in another, where it worked for 8 years.
- 1960 - 1962 The first successful cadaveric transplant used deceased donor kidney. The kidney worked for almost 2 years.
- 1966 First successful liver transplant. The liver worked for over one year.
- 1967 First successful heart transplant. The heart worked for 2 1/2 weeks.
- 1980 – 1981 First successful heart-lung transplant. The organs worked for 5 years.
- 1982 First artificial heart transplant.
- 1983 Cyclosporine, an immunosuppressant drug, was approved by the FDA.
- 1986 A baboon heart was transplanted into Baby Faye and worked for 20days.
- 1989 The first successful living-related liver transplant.
- 1990 – 1996 The first "split liver" transplant was performed where one cadaveric liver was split into several pieces to transplant into more than one person.
- 2000 First culture of human embryonic stem cells.

4. Types of organ donors

The sources of organs for transplantation, i.e., living donor (related and nonrelated), cadaveric donor, and brain-dead patients. In countries where transplantation is well established, organs are sourced from living and cadaveric donors using different strategies, i.e., an opt-in (explicit consent), opt-out (presumed consent), and donation after brain death, donation after controlled cardiac death, and extended criteria for deceased donors.

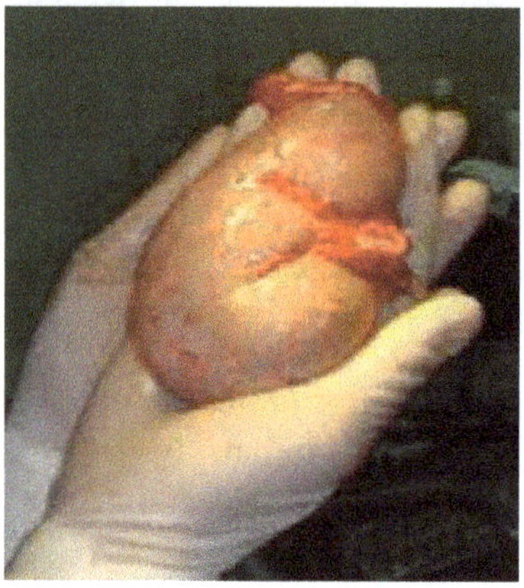

Gift of Life

4.1 Living organ donation

Four categories of donation by living persons can be distinguished: **Living Related Organ Donation "blood or emotional"**: directed donation to a loved one; **Altruistic Organ Donation:** non-directed donation, in which the donor gives an organ to the general pool to be transplanted into the recipient at the top of the waiting list; **Living Non-Related Organ Donation:** directed donation to a stranger, whereby donors choose to give to a specific person with whom they have no prior emotional connection; and **Cross donation** where a living donor wants to donate to his blood or emotional relative an organ but blood groups does not match, there is a complete mismatch or cross matching is positive. Two families or more can cross donate if matches exist. Each type of donation prompts distinct ethical concerns. Living Related Organ Donation is presumed to be the most ethical form of organ donation [Spittal A 1997]. One can argue that the psychological and non-specific benefits to the donor are real, particularly when a close relative is returned to normal health. There can, however, be no doubt that the physical consequences of living donation are entirely detrimental to the donor. Motives behind the 1st degree living renal donation are understandable and one may assume that the living donation between relatives carries the same altruistic motives. In related organ donation, the donor saves the life and attains the wellbeing of its immediate relative by accepting a physical injury and debilitation to itself. While many related donors fall neatly into this altruistic categorization, unfortunately, there are many examples where the related donors have attained physical, emotional or financial toll from the recipient. With directed donation to loved ones or friends, worries arise about the intense pressure that can be put on people to donate, leading those who are reluctant to do so to feel coerced. In these cases, transplantation programs are typically willing to identify a plausible medical excuse, so that the person can bow out gracefully. Equally important, however, are situations in which people feel compelled to donate regardless of the consequences to themselves. In cases like these, simply obtaining the informed consent of the relative is insufficient; physicians are obligated to prevent people from making potentially life-threatening sacrifices unless the chance of success is proportionately large. Non directed donation raises different ethical concerns. The radical altruism that motivates a person to make a potentially life threatening sacrifice for a stranger calls for careful scrutiny [Garwood etal 2007].

Transplantation teams have an obligation to assess potential donors in all these dimensions and prohibit donations that arouse serious concern. Directed donation to stranger raises similar ethical questions with a few additional wrinkles. This type of donation usually occurs when a patient advertises for an organ publicly, on television or billboards or over the Internet. Such advertising is not illegal, but it has been strongly discouraged by the transplantation community. Two central objections are that the practice is unfair and that it threatens the view that an organ is a "gift of life," not a commodity to be bought and sold. Some argue that just as we have a right to donate to the charities of our choice, so should we be able to choose to whom to give our organs. In practice, however, this means that those who have the most compelling stories and the means to advertise their plight tend to be the ones who get the organs – rather than those most in need. This strikes some ethicists as unfair. Unlike monetary gifts, they argue, organ transplantation requires the involvement of social structures and institutions, such as transplantation teams and hospitals. Hence, the argument goes, these donations are legitimately subject to societal requirements of fairness, and transplantation centers should refuse to permit the allocation of organs on the basis of anything but morally relevant criteria [Hull etal 1997].

The most ethically problematic cases are those in which the recipient is chosen on the basis of race, religion, or ethnic group [Epstein 2007]. A person with organ damage or organ failure may look for a living donor to donate an organ, allowing the patient to bypass the national waiting pool to receive a cadaveric organ.

4.1.1 Directed versus anonymous donation

Currently there is some debate whether altruistic donation should be anonymous or the donor should choose the recipient that he wishes to donate the organ to [Epstein etal 2009]. Donation could be criticized ethically that it unfairly favors some potential recipients by allowing them to jump to the top of
the waiting list; however, many transplant surgeons and ethicists believe that this is a very special kind of advantage when a good Samaritan donates one of his organs to a friend or colleague who is on the waiting list. For this not only helps the recipient, but actually also helps those who are on the waiting list who will move up the ladder and will have a better chance of having a cadaveric organ.

4.1.2 Benefits to living donation [Abouna 1998]

- The operation can be pre-arranged so, the hot and cold ischemia will be minimized which will have a good impact on the transplantation outcome.
- There are often better matches between donors and recipients with living donation, because many donors are genetically related to the recipient.
- Psychological benefits for both the donors and recipients.

Not everyone encourages the practice of living donation for all people.

4.1.3 Drawbacks of living donation [Landolt etal 2001]

- Health consequences: Pain, discomfort, infection, bleeding and potential future health complications.
- Psychological consequences: Family pressure, guilt or resentment.
- Pressure: Family members may feel pressured to donate when they have a sick family member or loved one.
- No donor advocate: While the patients have advocates, like the transplant surgeon or medical team (who are there to advise the patient and work in favor of his or her best interests) donors do not have such an advocate and can be faced with an overwhelming and complicated process with no one to turn to for guidance or advice.

A few medical and ethical professionals argue that living donation is inappropriate under any circumstances and should not only be discouraged but abandoned all together because of the risk and dangers associated with donating organs.

WHO publications

Other critics seek to discourage living donation because they think extending life through costly and physically taxing medical procedures is not the purpose of health systems. Although there are some who object to the practice of living donation, this potential source of organs is currently a major focus as a way to reduce the shortage of organs. Increasing the number of living donors could occur through a variety of strategies from education and civic duty promotion to the sale and purchase of organs Fig. (3).

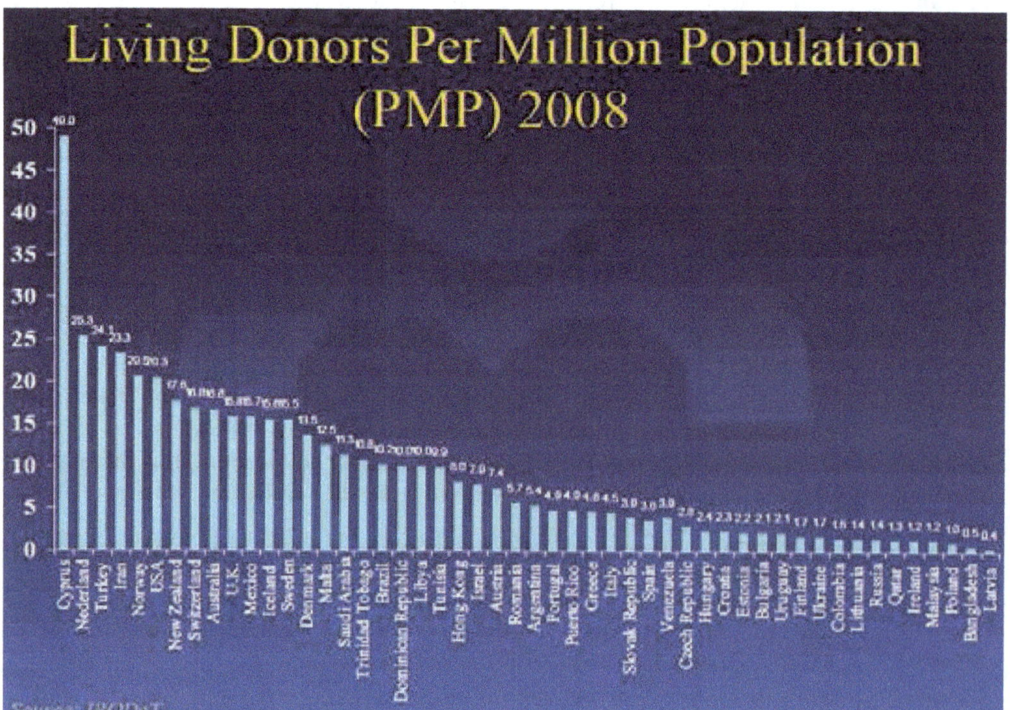

Fig. 3. International Registry of Organ Donation

4.1.4 Justification of transplantation from living donors

Living related donation, emotional related or altruistic are very justifiable on humanistic grounds and they are ethically and medically acceptable, providing that donor evaluation both medical and psychological is carried out in accordance with accepted protocols and that a fully informed consent is given by the donor. Also, the rate of donor complications after kidney donation is extremely small. The reported mortality rate after kidney donation is 1 in 10,000 [Delmonico etal2007].

On the side of the donor, there are many psychological and spiritual benefits, and most donors express an increased sense of pride and satisfaction and the joy of giving a gift of life to a relative, a friend or to another fellow human being. Another justification is that the success rate of living donor kidney transplantation is considerably higher than that of cadavers [Hunsicker 1999]. The expected patient survival rate and graft function at 5 years in 2007 is 99 and 96%, respectively, with living donors and 96 and 91% with cadaver donors, which is much better than 1998 statistics and that is most probably due to the recent introduction of more effective immunosuppression medications Fig. (4a&b).

In living donor transplantation it must be shown that the benefits to both donor and recipient outweigh the risks associated with donation and transplantation.

Unadjusted 1-Year Graft and Patient Survival by Organ (1998 and 2007)

Graft Survival	Year of Transplant 1998	2007	% Change	P-Value
Kidney: deceased donor graft survival	89%	91%	3%	<0.0001
Kidney: living donor graft survival	95%	97%	2%	<0.0001
Pancreas transplant alone	78%	76%	-1%	0.8341
Pancreas after kidney	72%	82%	10%	0.0302
Kidney-pancreas: kidney	91%	93%	2%	0.1355
Kidney-pancreas: pancreas	83%	86%	4%	0.0392
Liver: deceased donor graft survival	80%	86%	6%	<0.0001
Liver: living donor graft survival	70%	87%	16%	0.0022
Intestine	50%	75%	25%	0.0004
Heart	85%	88%	3%	0.0006
Lung	75%	80%	5%	0.0115
Heart-lung	54%	90%	36%	0.0001

Patient Survival	Year of Transplant 1998	2007	% Change	P-Value
Kidney: deceased donor patient survival	95%	96%	1%	0.0055
Kidney: living donor patient survival	98%	99%	1%	0.0015
Pancreas transplant alone	98%	98%	0%	0.9320
Pancreas after kidney	94%	97%	3%	0.2472
Kidney-pancreas	94%	97%	3%	0.0093
Liver: deceased donor patient survival	86%	89%	3%	<0.0001
Liver: living donor patient survival	80%	91%	11%	0.0173
Intestine	67%	78%	11%	0.0995
Heart	86%	89%	3%	0.0006
Lung	77%	82%	6%	0.0016
Heart-lung	57%	90%	34%	0.0003

SRTR

Source: *2009 OPTN/SRTR Annual Report*, Table 1.11b, 1.12b.

Fig. 4a. Patient & Graft survival (UNOS Published Reports)

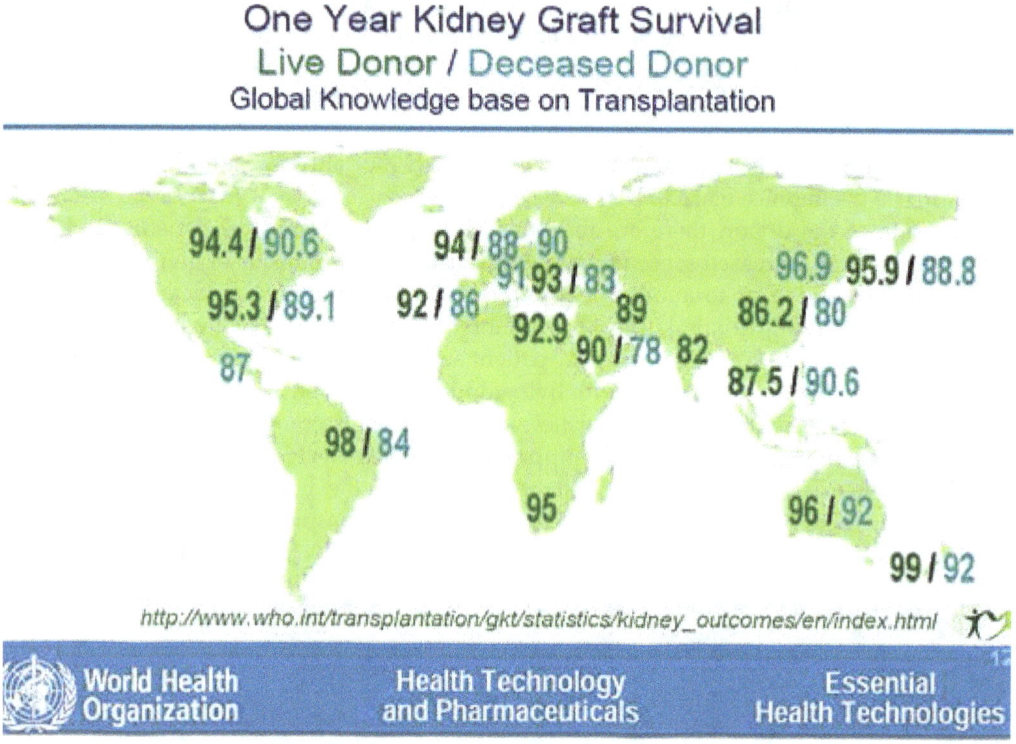

Fig. 4b. Patient & Graft survival (WHO Published Reports)

4.1.5 The decision to donate organs within the family

Many decisions to be living donors will be made within a family context - whether blood relations or less commonly, spouses, or in-laws - and involve the needs of specific members of that family. Very often, in living donation, there will be a host of pressures and family complexities to take into account. These may affect the extent to which a decision to donate or not to donate is genuinely free. Understanding some of these complexities and family dynamics can assist greatly in reaching a decision that is genuinely voluntary. It is important to distinguish between different kinds of pressure that a person faced with the decision about living donation may feel Avoidable pressures or Unavoidable pressures [Spital A 1996]. The decision to be a living donor should be based on adequate information and understanding, an informed decision is one based on information relevant to the making of that decision. Of course, in assisting a potential donor to make his or her decision about donation, doctors have an ethical and legal duty to warn about material risks in a treatment [Danovitch 2007]. Material risks are those that most people would want to know and also those that would be significant for a particular individual. It follows that a donor, before deciding about donation, should ask the appropriate medical practitioner to disclose the risks of the intended procedure and of its short and long term effects.

4.1.6 Psychological issues in live donation

This includes information and understanding about possible emotional and psychological consequences of making a decision one way or the other, for the potential recipient, the potential donor, the relationship between these two people, and for other family members. These questions can only be answered within the context of understanding a particular family and/or the particular individuals involved whatever the outcome, certain issues may take some time to resolve.

Tissue typing and other medical checks may identify only one suitable donor in a family, which can lead to great pressure being put on that person. There may be more than one suitable donor and in these cases there can be complex pressures again as a choice is made between these people. As examples of such pressures, focus may fall on one of the suitable people for various reasons, perhaps without sufficient thought. In other cases there may be one person who is extremely eager to donate and so perhaps too willing to overlook possible difficulties that may be encountered. Often, such very willing people may need even more careful counseling to ensure that their decision is sound.

Living donation offers the recipient immediate hope. Because the results are generally favorable, the mood of the recipient, family and donor are usually optimistic. Against this background, other issues need to be considered [Jarvis 1995]:

Chances of survival of recipient:

It is argued by some that it is preferable to donate to recipients who are not critically ill, because choosing recipients with higher chances of survival better balances the risk to the donor. In addition, when such recipients are chosen, there is less need to make a decision under pressure and the additional time allows thorough medical and psychological evaluation of the proposed donor.

Changes in donor/recipient relationship:

The exceptional nature of what has happened and what both the donor and recipient have shared may be mutually enhancing. After a donation, there is often increased contact between a donor and the recipient where they are known to each other. Our experience suggests that reaction to being identified as a donor is very positive [Mathieson 1999].

Feeling if the transplant fails:

If the donation does fail, the donor may have feelings of guilt or inadequacy or feelings of anger, sadness, or that the donated organs or tissues have been wasted, and that the discomforts he or she has suffered have been made for nothing.

Feelings of 'ownership' towards the recipient:

Living donors can feel closer to recipients and have expressed attitudes of ownership about the state of health and activities of the recipient. They may feel that they have a right to ensure that the recipient is taking good care of his or her health and therefore of the donated organ or tissue. Conversely, the recipient may identify with the donor and feel that part of the donor is living in them. Ultimately such feelings may not be in the best interest of either party.

Recipient feelings of guilt if the donation has harmful effects on the donor:

A recipient may feel guilty and responsible if the donor suffers from his or her donation.

Consequences of not donating:

A decision not to donate can have a major impact on relationships within a family. The recipient's illness is often life-threatening and death may occur before or after transplantation. It is therefore important that the family, including prospective donors, do not have unrealistic expectations for the recipient nor underestimate the difficulties for the donor. A decision not to donate might be entirely appropriate for the individual, but still have profound effects on family relationships if the proposed recipient dies. It is very important to consider whether such factors amount to undue pressure on a potential donor

4.2 Deceased organ donation

Organs for transplantation which obtained from living donors unfortunately, have so far been unable to keep up with demand. As a result, there are a large and steadily increasing number of potential recipients awaiting transplantation, some of whom will die before an organ can be found. This scarcity of organs for transplantation can only be met from the cadavers Fig. (5). Cadaveric source is beneficial in another way that it provides multi-organ donation. To utilize cadaveric organs effectively, it needs legal formalities and most of the countries have passed cadaveric law [Alashek, Ehtuish etal 2009].

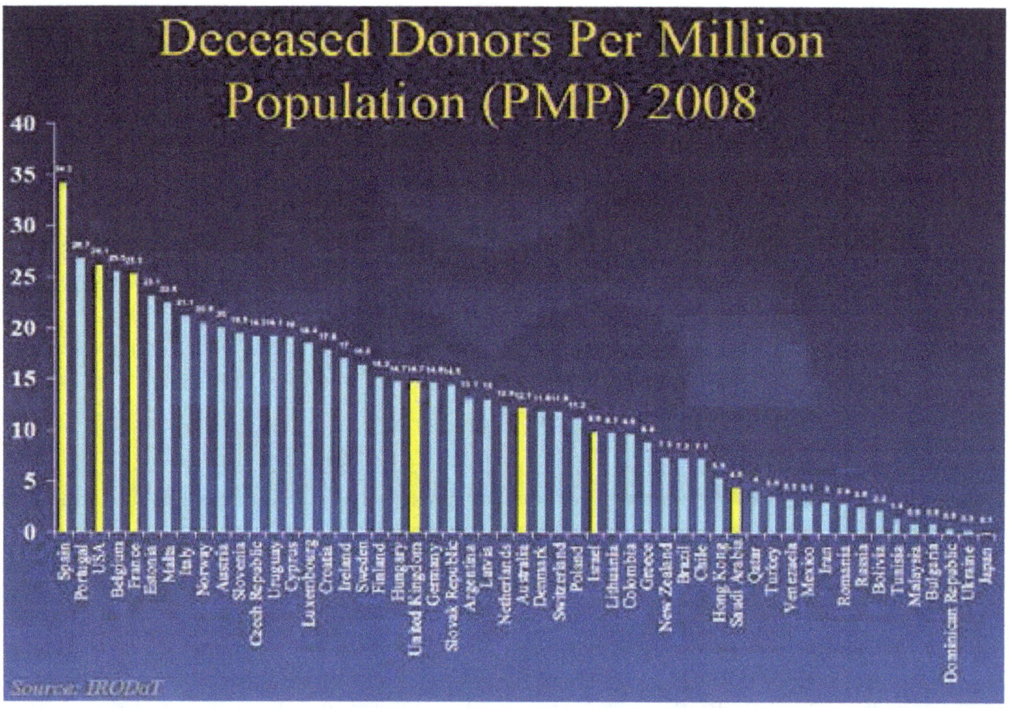

Fig. 5. International Registry of Organ Donation WHO Publications

4.2.1 Strategies to promote cadaveric organ donations and self sufficiency

a. Education

Educational efforts focus on increasing the number of people who consent to be an organ donor before they die. And educating families when they are considering giving consent for their deceased loved one's organs. Social responsibility and the idea of "the gift of life" should be popularized

b. Mandated choice

Under this strategy, every individual would have to indicate his wishes regarding organ transplantation, perhaps on driver's licenses. When a person dies, the hospital must comply with their written wishes regardless of what their family may want. The positive aspect of this strategy is that it strongly enforces the concept of individual autonomy of the organ donor. A mandated choice policy would require an enormous level of trust in the medical system. People must be able to trust their health care providers to care for them no matter what their organ donation wishes

c. Presumed consent

This method of procuring organs is in fact the policy of many European nations. In countries with presumed consent, their citizens' organs are taken after they die, unless a person specifically requests to not donate while still living. Advocates of a presumed consent approach might say that it is every person's civic duty to donate their organs once they no longer need them (i.e. after death) to those who do. People against presumed consent would argue that to implement this policy, the general public would have to be educated and well-informed about organ donation, which would be difficult to adequately achieve. Doubters of the presumed consent approach might also argue that requiring people to opt out of donating their organs requires them to take action and this might unfairly burden some people. The countries having presumed consent principles like Spain and Canada shows higher donation rate 40-50 per million population [Miranda etal 1998 & Rithalia etal 2009].

d. Incentives

Incentives take many forms [Beier etal 2008]. Some of the most frequently debated incentive strategies are:

1. Give assistance to families of a donor with funeral costs
2. Donate to a charity in the deceased person's name if organs are donated
3. Offer recognition and gratitude incentives like a plaque or memorial
4. Provide financial or payment incentives

One of the most highly debated incentives would give donating families assistance with burial or funeral costs for their loved one this could be an attractive incentive for many families.

Proponents say that since the person will be dead and unable to receive the recognition, that this would not be a coercive action. Some ethicists believe that many of the incentives above, while not attached directly to cash money, are still coercive and unfair. They believe that some people will be swayed to donate, in spite of their better judgment, if an incentive is attractive enough. They further argue that a gesture may seem small and a mere token to one person, but others might interpret it quite differently. A final anti-incentives argument offered by some ethicists discourages the practice of incentivizing organ donation [Jasper etal 1999]. They believe that society should instead re-culture its thinking to embrace a communitarian spirit of giving and altruism where people actively want to donate their organs

4.2.2 Maximizing donation form deceased donors

In order to maximize the donation from deceased donors it is important to consider the following:

- Legal and organizational framework

- Coordinating authority over health system
- Citizen's understanding: donation in school curriculum
- Ongoing reality and momentum in media
- Adaptation of relevant models (Spain) in emerging countries

4.3 Minors and children as donors

It is another issue that needs considerate discussion. Living donors provide the best outcome for children undergoing renal transplantation. Most of these donors are parents. When parents are unable to donate, siblings are often considered. But what if the siblings are also children? Should they be permitted to donate? They are below 18 years of age and not able to consent and they might be pushed or convinced to donate. And what about those who are mentally subnormal and their families wants to use them as donors?

Sometimes there are reports that children have been kidnapped, only to re- appear later lacking one kidney, or that they simply disappear and are subsequently killed to have all their transplantable organs removed for profit. However, the issue is covered in a broader sense by more general provisions. There are endless rumors surrounding this area. Members of various organizations who travel in the suspected countries say that the trafficking in children who are sold for transplantation is well known, but it is too difficult and very dangerous to catch the people involved [Spital A 1997],

4.4 Executed prisoners as donors

Several authors and ethicists have recently commented on the current practice in some countries of the use of organs from executed prisoners. While all societies strongly condemn the arbitrary use of taking organs from executed prisoners, which is a common practice in some countries, where organs are taken and given to various institutions for transplantation or even sold to other countries. It is suggested that it will be ethically permissible to allow a prisoner on death row to donate an organ to a relative or a friend. [Miller 1999].

One argument in favor of taking organs from prisoners, who are put to death, is that it is the execution that is ethically unsound and not the organ removal. Indeed, in light of the severe organ shortage, some ethicists could make the argument that to not use the organs for transplantation is wasteful. Some ethicist, put forth the argument that obtaining organs from condemned prisoners is allowable if the prisoner or their next of kin consents to donation, as long as organ donation is not the means by which the prisoner is killed because that violates the principle that a cadaveric donor be dead prior to donation. Some could argue that organ retrieval from executed prisoners is morally justifiable only if a "presumed consent" donation practice was in place. Many, if not most, bioethicists consider taking organs from condemned prisoners a morally objectionable practice. And immoral [Cameron etal 1999].

4.5 Alternative organ sources

Some potential non-traditional sources of organs are:

4.5.1 Animal organs – "xenotransplantation"

Animals are a potential source of donated organs. Experiments with baboon hearts and pig liver transplants have received extensive media attention in the past. One cautionary argument in opposition to the use of animal organs concerns the possibility of transferring animal bacteria and viruses to humans. Some argue that xenotransplantation is the only potential way of addressing this shortage. As immunological barriers to xenotransplantation are better understood, those hurdles are being addressed through genetic engineering of donor animals and the development of new drugs therapies [Starzl etal 1964 & Grant etal 2001]. The focus of ethical attention has changed from the moral correctness of using animals for research/therapy to an increasingly appreciated danger of the establishment and spread of xenozoonses in recipients, their contacts and the general public. There are a number of reasons for not using subhuman primates for xenotransplantation, including their closeness to humans, the likelihood of passing on infections, their availability (gorillas, chimpanzees), their slow breeding and the expense of breeding them under specified pathogen free conditions. The pig, although domesticated and familiar, is too distant to evoke the same feeling as we have for primates, has the correct size organs, is probably less likely to pass infections, breeds rapidly and is not endangered; moreover, millions of them are eaten every year. Although drawing ethical conclusions is difficult at the stage of knowledge and debate, it seems acceptable to manipulate pigs genetically and to proceed to using their organs for xenotransplantation trials when infection control measures and the scientific base justify it [Bukler etal 1999 & Sim etal 1999]. The use of pigs in Muslim countries would be more controversial and disruptive although it is acceptable by Islamic religion in case of a real need and when there is no alternative [Rahman 1998]. In this case the question of informed consent is likely to be ambiguous and awkward. It might end up more of a binding legal contract than consent, as we understand it now. Xenotransplantation is also unlikely to cost less than or significantly alleviate the shortage of cadaveric organs in the short term. The international dimension of the risk of infection is becoming obvious, but there has so far been no effort to convene an international forum to agree on universally acceptable guidelines However, before xenotransplantation can be fully implemented, both the scientific/medical communities and the general public must seriously consider and attempt to resolve many complex ethical, social and economic issues that it presents [Platt 1999].

4.5.2 Artificial organs

Artificial organs are yet another potential option.

The ethical issues involved in artificial organs often revert to questions about the cost and effectiveness of artificial organs. People who receive artificial organ transplants might require further transplanting if there is a problem with the device.

4.5.3 Organs from fetuses

The ethics of using tissues and organs from fetuses have been a matter of enormous discussion. Aborted fetuses are a proposed source of organs. Debates address whether it is morally appropriate to use organs from a fetus aborted late in a pregnancy for transplantation that could save the life of another infant. Many people believe that this practice would encourage late-term abortions, which some individuals and groups find morally objectionable. Another objection comes from people who fear that encouraging the use of aborted fetal organs would encourage "organ farming," or the practice of conceiving a child with the intention of aborting it for its organs[Golmakani etal 2005]., but the use of spontaneously aborted fetus or anencephalic newborn could be encouraged. Although there is ethical debate concerning the possible use of organs of anencephalic babies for transplant. Some have argued that because of the absence of neocortex these are 'nonpersons 'and are 'brain-dead' and thus, such infants should be available for organ donation if this is the wish of the parents. However, as brain stem function is present in these infants, the 'whole of the brain' or 'brain stem' requirement for certification of brain death precludes removal of organs until cardiorespiratory death occurs.

4.5.4 Stem cells –"The future"

Stem cells are cells that can specialize into many different cells found in the human body. Researchers have great hopes that stem cells can one day be used to grow entire organs, or at least groups of specialized cells [Bartholomew etal 2001 & Eradini 2002]. Some of the very recent developments in transplantation over the past decade have been the use of stem cells from bone marrow, cord blood, and from fetal and adult tissue, including somatic cells and neural cells. These cells have the great potential for differentiation and proliferation into other types of body cells including neuronal, hepatic, hemopoietic and muscular and thus help many patients with organ failure after their transplantation into the patients. These stem cells have also been shown to induce immunological tolerance and chimerism when they are transplanted into recipients of vital organ grafts and their rejection of a transplanted organ such as bone marrow, kidney, heart, liver, is prevented [Fandrich 2002]. A new hope is emerging now with the possibility of preserving the architecture of an organ i.e. preserving capsule, vascular structures and draining system and removing the destroyed or fibrosed cells and replace them with new cell mass produced by stem cells like removing all non-functioning Hepatocytes and replacing them with a new Hepatocyte cell mass, The ethical objections concerning stem cells have focused primarily on their source. While stem cells can be found in the adult human body, the seemingly most potent stem cells come from the first few cells of a human embryo. When the stem cells are removed, the embryo is destroyed. Some people find this practice morally objectionable and would like to put a stop to research and medical procedures that destroy human embryos in the process.

5. Life & death

With the development of mechanical ventilators, new drugs, and other forms of treatment, it became possible to artificially maintain circulatory and respiratory functions, even after the brain had stopped functioning. In the past four decades many countries amended their death statutes to include a definition of death by the complete and irreversible cessation of all brain functions. Since that time almost all cadaveric organs have been recovered from patients who have been declared "brain dead." Veatch has never been comfortable with the term "brain death," preferring instead "brain-oriented definition of death." Since the 1970s he has argued that the entire brain does not have to be dead for the individual as a whole to be dead. Instead, he advocates a "'higher-brain-oriented definition' of death—in other words, one is dead when there is irreversible loss of all 'higher' brain functions" he further proposes creating a new definition of death law that incorporates the notion that one need only have an irreversible loss of consciousness as opposed to an irreversible loss of all brain functions [Veatch 2008]. Veatch's proposal is clearly controversial. It suggests a violation of an ethical boundary most clinicians are currently unwilling to cross. Perhaps he is correct that such a change is inevitable and that the "definition of death at the conceptual level is a religious/philosophical/social policy choice rather than a question of medical science" .There was clear leadership from individuals such as pioneering transplant surgeon, Dr. David Hume; Dr. Hume wrote "there is only one definition of death, irreversible brain damage. Cessation of heart beat does not constitute death unless it has caused irreversible brain damage there must be no spontaneous respirations" [Delmonico 2010]. These observations were later corroborated by Dr. William Sweet published in the New England of Medicine when he wrote "it is clear that a person is not dead unless his brain is dead [Sweet 1978]. The time-honored criteria of stoppage of heart beat in circulation are long enough for the brain to die". Dr. Sam Shemie has clarified the paradigm for donation and death by emphasizing on the "required absence of circulation" and by underscoring the vital functions of the brain as an essential criterion of life [Shemie 2007]. "Where the extracorporeal machines of transplantation can support or replace the function of organs such as the heart, lung, liver or kidney, the brain is the only organ that cannot be supported by medical technology". On the other hand Byrne and others have rejected brain death as constituting death of the person contending the "cessation of the entire brain function, whether irreversible or not, is not necessarily linked to total destruction of the brain or the death of the person". Byrne, apparently, bases his opinion regarding death as philosophically constituting a separation of the soul from the body [Byrne 1979]. However, applying that personal philosophy to the diagnosis of death defies a legal and medical standard, and an ethical and practical sensibility. No one knows when the soul may separate from the body at the time of death. However, the legal and medical definition of death is clear in terms of neurological and circulatory function. It becomes unethical to impose futile clinical treatments to a comatose individual, if the function of the entire brain is irreversibly lost. What would opponents of the brain death determination do with a patient on a ventilator with such a clinical condition have them maintained indefinitely in such a state? To propose the brain death criteria as constituting death was the central issue that confronted the Harvard Committee in 1967 [Ad Hoc 1968]. No one knows when the soul separates from the body, but a precise time of death must be specified for obvious legal, medical and social reasons, so that futile treatment can be concluded (without further obligation or responsibility to provide resuscitative or supportive technologies) and proper disposition of the body with burial and estate and property transfer, etc can be exercised. For many years, Truog has also objected to the determination of death by neurologic evaluation and by circulatory function. He wrote in the New England Journal of Medicine that "arguments about why these patients should be considered dead have never been fully convincing [Truog 1997]. The definition of brain death requires a complete absence of all functions of the entire brain yet many of these patients retaining essential neurologic function, such as regulated secretion of hypothalamic hormones". The rebuttal to this assertion has been given by Shemie [Shemie etal 2006] who claimed that "the release of antidiuretic hormone (ADH) from the hypothalamus is not considered to be essential neurologic function. Brain death is determined by an absence of consciousness, receptivity and responsiveness, spontaneous movement, spontaneous breathing and absence of brainstem reflexes". Brain death does not require every brain cell to be nonviable but the criteria require an irreversible loss of neurologic function of a patient interminably supported by a mechanical respirator. For Truog and others however, these patients are not considered dead because they indeed can be supported indefinitely beyond the acute phase of their illness. It is well known however that despite the irreversible loss of brain function the remainder of the body can be maintained by mechanical support; for example, even by patients who become brain-dead during pregnancy yet successfully have their fetuses brought to term. The clinical condition still constitutes the death of the mother and a viable fetus buys continued mechanical support until birth. Again in the New England Journal of

Medicine. Truog and Veatch [Veatch 2008 &Truog etal 2008 & Life 9 November 1962] have asserted the donation after cardiac death (DCD) is not acceptable; that is, the recovery of organs after the determination of death by circulatory and respiratory criteria. Troug suggests that recovery of the heart following DCD is "paradoxical" because the hearts of patients who have been declared dead on the basis of the irreversible loss of cardiac function have in fact been transplanted and successfully functioned in the chest of another". Veatch is similarly not convinced that the donor is dead and stated that "if someone is pronounced dead on the basis of irreversible loss of heart function, after all. It would not be possible for heart function to be restored in another body. Both Veatch and Truog misinterpret the uniform declaration of death act UDDA which precisely stated that it applies to an individual who had sustained irreversible cessation of circulatory and respiratory functions. It is not a matter of the cessation of heartbeat or cardiac function per se but an irreversible cessation of circulation in the donor. The consequence of the absence of circulation is upon the function of the brain results in an irreversible loss or neurologic function - the UDDA definition of death [Ad Hoc committee 1968 & President Commission 1981 & Delmonico etal 1999].

Bernat has written that circulation - not heartbeat - is the critical function that must be lost using circulatory-respiratory tests to determine death [Bernat 2008]. For example, we do not declare patients dead who are on heart lung machines during cardiac surgery, on ECMO awaiting heart transplantation (even if they never receive a heart), or carrying artificial hearts because, despite absence of heartbeat, their circulation remains continuously maintained. That is why the death standard requires absence of circulation. "Whether the asystolic heart is subsequently left alone, removed and not restarted or removed and restarted in another patient is irrelevant to the circulatory status of the just-declared dead patient [Norton 1992]. Removing and restarting the heart elsewhere simply has no impact on the previous death determination because that patient remains permanently without circulation in exactly the same way as if the non-beating had been left in place". And as an everyday example after slaughtering the rooster it jumps higher and stronger as never than done in its life, this movement doesn't indicate that he is still alive and it continues bleeding strongly indicating that the heart is still functioning, and on the opposite side the heart beating may stop spontaneously, known as cardiac arrest and attempts of rescue continue, in many cases the restitution succeed. The heart start beating again and life gets back to its normal state, moreover doctors can stop the heart for hours during the operation of the open heart, however the blood circulation does not stop, not even for seconds, therefore the heart beating does not mean life and the stoppage of heart beating does not necessarily mean death. Irreversible loss of consciousness may be due to partial or total brain injury [Shewmon 1998]. For the determination of brain death, irreversible coma must be due to injury to the brain so severe as to cause loss of brain functions

Death is when blood stop reaching the brain causing a permanent harm to the brain and leading to a permanent loss of all its functions including the brainstem functions and to diagnose death it is necessary to prove the cessation of the functions of the brain, and then brain commences disintegration and its known that many cells from a dead person remain alive after the declaration of his death. Therefore we find that the muscular cells responds to electrical stimulations and some cells within the liver continue transforming the glucose to glycogen, so cells do not die all at once, however they differ in their timing of death and perish after death of the person. We can extend the life of these cells if they are put in saline solution, especially with the flow by means of a pump hence allowing the use of organs and cell of the dead person for another patient needing them, the death is a process and not an event.

Brain death can be defined as follows: When the brain is damaged, and its activities completely cease, brain death is present, even if it is possible for the patient to be kept breathing and his heart is beating with artificial respiration and medications; even if the heart and liver are functioning that is not live it is just artificial. The consideration of legality of brain death as "true death" was first considered in the early 1960's; with the 1968 Harvard report becoming the "standard" definition of brain death. the majority of countries and international professional associations have accepted it.

5.1 Islamic opinion

The majority of Muslim jurisprudents consider organ transplantation to be permissible on the basis of principles that needs of the living outweigh those of the dead. Saving a life is of paramount value in Islam as the following verse from the Quran illustrates "And if any one sustains life, it would be as if he sustained the life of all mankind" [Ebrahim 1995 & Ebrahim 1998 & Van Bommel 1999 & Al Faqih 1991]. The Islamic jurisprudence Assembly Council in its meeting in Saudi Arabia on Feb 6-11, 1988 ratified resolution number 26.1.41 declared the following fatwa the permissibility of proxy consent: "Transplantation of an organ of the dead to a living human being whose life or essential function of the body would rely on the donated organ is allowed, provided that the dead (before his death) or his heirs permit it. Shiite scholars have made similar rulings. The majority of Shiite jurisprudents confirm organ transplantation especially when human life is at stake.[Moqaddam 2000 & Ghods etal 2006 & Zargooshi 2008].

Ordinarily, the dead have a right in Islam to the sanctity and wholeness of their body, but as we have already noted, the need to save a life overrides this injunction as it has a prima facie importance in the mundane affairs of mankind. While saving a life is of paramount importance in Islam, the family of the deceased must consent and there are in no way obliged to consent to organ donation even if it involves the death of another person who is alive but gravely ill. It has been reasoned that the "ownership" of organs, like that of property, is relative and subjective because God is the ultimate "owner" of the universe having created it. Therefore, it would be permissible to donate them because God had placed great value on saving a life.

5.2 Church opinion

In the address of pope John Paul II to the Transplantation Congress in Rome in 2000, regarding the determination of death, he said ..."it is helpful to recall that the death of the person is a single event, consisting in the total disintegration of the unitary and integrated whole that is the personal self". And that "it is a well-known fact that for some time certain scientific approaches to ascertaining death have shifted the emphasis from the traditional cardio respiratory signs to the so-called neurological criterion. Specifically, this consists in establishing, according to clearly determined parameters commonly held by the international scientific community, the complete and irreversible cessation of all brain activity (in the cerebrum, cerebellum and brain stem). This is then considered the sign that the individual organism has lost its integrative capacity" [Abouna 1984 & Pope John Paul II 2000].

6. Brain death is death

6.1 Misuse of terminology

Patients who fulfill the brain function criterion for death are commonly said to be 'brain dead'. This term, unfortunately, suggests that there are two ways of being dead, being 'brain dead' and being 'really dead'. The term 'brain death' is also used, incorrectly, in other contexts to describe much lesser degrees of neurological dysfunction than it strictly implies. This misuse of the term is to be found in the medical and related professions as much as in the general public. It has lead to confusion surrounding the idea of a brain function criterion and its relation to 'brain death'. It may be that it is too late to reclaim the term for its legitimate use. Whenever it is used, it is important that it is sufficiently qualified to ensure that its meaning is clear, and professional medical bodies may have a role to play in encouraging correct application of the term.

6.2 Explaining brain function criterion to the family of the deceased donors

Even apart from confusion over the use of the term 'brain death' it can be very difficult for families to fully understand the reality of death based on a brain function criterion. To casual observation, patients fulfilling the brain function criterion for death appear to be sleeping rather than dead. The skin is warm. The chest rises and falls with mechanical ventilation. The heart and the kidneys continue to function. There are even reports that pregnancy may be maintained in patients fulfilling the brain function criterion for death. This ambiguity is reflected in the way medical and paramedical staff relates to the beating-heart cadaver in the period before organ donation. Nurses will often talk to such a cadaver as they carry out their nursing care as if the body retained the ability to hear. Acceptance of death by the brain function criterion in the context of organ donation asks much more of a family than does the same diagnosis with a view to cessation of treatment. Community education programs might go part way in helping families understand the issues involved. Detailed explanations with appropriate written material should be provided. Practitioners dealing with families should be trained in the process of explaining the brain function criterion and in grief counseling in general. Families should be provided with the opportunity to ask relevant questions and to have their questions answered in a genuinely sympathetic environment. Sufficient time should be provided to ensure that families really understand the brain function criterion before the issue of organ donation is broached. Families should then be allowed whatever time and assistance are necessary to make a decision concerning organ donation and then to deal with the particular grieving problems over the ensuing days and weeks. They should be offered the opportunity to view the body after the retrieval process has occurred when it has the appearance of being dead [Shemie etal 2006 & Delmonico etal 1999 & Norton 1992].

6.3 Deciding to donate or not to donate organs after death

The main reason why people may consider donating organs is because of the very great benefit that this can bring to others. Organ transplantation may be a lifesaving treatment for patients with liver or heart disease, and it may be the only hope of treatment there is. For kidney patients, having a transplant can mean being able to cease, and this can bring a great improvement in health and lifestyle. For instance, it may enable a kidney patient to return to the workforce, or to work longer hours, and it can even mean that a woman can now have a baby. The transplantation of a cornea can give someone back his or her sight [Ehtuish etal 2006 & Abouna 1998 & Hunsicker 1999 & Alashek etal 2009 & Cohen etal 1995].

Transplantation is generally a very successful procedure. The success rates of transplantations vary, but in all cases these have increased considerably since transplantation first began (Fig. 4b). It can be difficult in medical science to predict which procedures will become more successful and eventually routine. However, kidney transplantation is now considered to be accepted medical treatment and this is likely to happen in other areas of transplantation. Some people decide not to donate organs because they are not confident that donation would be in accordance with their dead relative's wishes. Some people think that transplantation is a very costly procedure from which relatively few people benefit. If you believe that your family may gain some comfort from donation, this may be a reason to consider it for yourself. On the other hand, if you feel that your family may be upset about donation, you may decide against it. This shows the importance of discussing donation with your family. You need also to bear in mind that the people who donate organs are mostly those who have died suddenly and unexpectedly and they are often quite young. For the families of these patients, death may be especially traumatic. When deciding about donation for yourself before death, you may begin by thinking of how you would feel if you were in the position of needing lifesaving organ or tissue transplantation. In making your decision, you also may feel, for instance, that you no longer need your body, and would like to feel that you had done something to help others. Or you may feel that it is important that your body remains intact for burial or cremation. If you belong to a religious faith, you may want to consider how organ donation and transplantation is understood from that religious point of view. Indeed you may wish to consult a religious advisor on the appropriateness of organ donation in your particular circumstances.

6.4 Making a decision when a relative has died

Deciding about organ donation on behalf of a loved relative who has just died may be a very difficult decision to make. Often the relative's death will have been the result of a traumatic event such as a car accident or a head injury. This makes the death an especially sad one for family and friends, means that people are asked to make a serious decision at a difficult, stressful and emotional time. You may feel shocked, bewildered, angry, and numb [Norton 1992]. But, for practical reasons, if organ donation is to occur, it must take place within a certain time period: so there will be only a limited time in which to make this decision. The difficult circumstances in which the decision has to be made make it all the more important that you are well-informed and that you feel confident that you have considered the matter as fully as you wish. Families are greatly assisted in their decision-making at a time of crisis if they have previously discussed organ and tissue donation and the wishes of individuals are known. There are three scenarios that need to be considered: (1) Your relative dies having made known his or her wish to donate organs after death: in this case the family is consulted in order to clarify what the person's wishes were in relation to organ donation and to see whether the family has any objections to the deceased's wishes being acted on. Donation will not proceed in the face of objection from families. If you know that your relative wished to donate his or her organs and/or tissues, this may provide you with a substantial reason for you to consent to the request for donation. Islamic religion respect the intestate and wishes of the person before he died and the relatives are obliged to implement the intestate that is clear in many verses in Quran. (2) Your relative dies having made known to you his or her wish not to donate organs: in this case, made this known to hospital staff and organ donation will not be discussed further. (3) Your relative dies and either had no views about organ donation (as in the case of a young child) or had not made his or her views known to you: in this case the hospital authorities will consult the family to find out whether anything is known about the deceased person's wishes and/or to find out whether the family will consent to donation on behalf of their deceased relative. One thing that you may like to do in this situation is to make a judgment based on your knowledge of that person. What was his or her attitude to transplantation: had he or she ever shown any sign of being in favor or against it? What were his or her beliefs and feelings about the body and about how it should be treated after death? Was he or she the kind of person who would want to help others? Would he or she have been likely to have discussed organ donation with someone outside the family? It is professional practice not to pressure people in any way. The decision that you have to make is not a purely rational or 'head' decision but also an emotional or 'heart' decision. You may need time to come to terms a little more with the emotional significance of events, may be to accept that your relative really is dead. You may wish for time to imagine how you may feel afterwards, whatever decision you make; and how others in your family may feel. You may feel you need time alone, or time with just your family [Evans 1993 & Courtney etal 2009].

6.5 Some key questions you might consider in case of organ donation

Do I think that donating organs and/or tissues for transplantation (or other purposes) is a worthwhile cause? How would I feel if I needed a transplanted organ? How does organ donation fit with my religious, spiritual and moral beliefs? How would I feel if a friend or relative needed an organ? What do my other family members think about organ donation? Have I made my wishes about organ donation known to my family? If I decide I want to donate organs, how will this affect my family? Am I satisfied that I understand the concept of 'brain death' as a way of determining death? Do I feel that I could trust the medical staff involved if I were ever in a situation to be a potential organ donor? How do I think of my body after death? Are there some organs I would like to donate, and not others? Will my family try to carry out my wishes? Will counseling be available for my family if they need it? Am I satisfied that respect will be shown to my body? Are there other people I would like to consult? [Miranda etal 1998 & Jasper etal 1999 & Cameron etal 1999 & Cohen etal 1995]

7. Entry of patients to transplantation programs

Decision-making becomes necessary at two stages of the process of organ and tissue allocation. The first stage deals with those considerations which should be taken into account in deciding on the identity of the individual patients to whom offers of transplants are to be made. Decisions of this type, by reason of the technical details involved, will remain a responsibility of medical personnel. Entry to, and exclusion from, a transplantation program both raise ethical issues.

Entry to a program is offered following assessment of patients by the program personnel. Exclusion criteria include age restrictions, abnormalities in other organ systems, previous history of malignant disease and other medical considerations. In making decisions about which patients are to be admitted to a program, there is merit in more than one medical practitioner being involved.

The second stage of decision-making relates to whether an individual chooses to become a transplant recipient. This is a decision to be made by the patients in the light of advice received from their medical attendants and consultation with their families. Acceptance of the offer requires an informed decision on the part of a patient and/or their family. Prior to this decision, a patient should receive a full description of what is entailed in being in the program, what procedures can be expected and their possible risks and benefits. On the other hand, if a patient is excluded from a transplantation program, he or she is entitled to know why? [Turcotte etal 1989].

In an attempt to ensure that transplanted kidneys have the best outcome possible for individual patients, concurrent medical conditions that introduce a potential risk following transplantation should be managed before acceptance on to the waiting list, If a pre-existing condition is likely to be affected adversely by the ongoing immunosuppression required after transplantation (for example, immunosuppression increases the risk of recurrence of cancer and of persistence of chronic infection) a patient may be excluded from transplantation in his or her own interest. Though some may think it is unfair to deny a patient the opportunity to receive a transplanted kidney because of renal disease which could recur in the graft, others might consider it unreasonable to inflict repeated transplantation when there is a high risk of rejection. In rare circumstances, the kidney allocation system may be suspended to provide an organ for transplantation to a critically ill patient. To ensure fairness in allocation, the selection criteria and weighting of different criteria are subject to repeated review by personnel from all institutions involved in renal transplantation.

7.1 Factors influencing entry to, and ranking in, a transplantation program

a. The patient sickness.
b. The patient most likely to benefit based on medical or other criteria.
c. The length of the patient on the waiting list.
d. All patients on the waiting list should have an equal chance.
e. The patient's importance for the well-being of others, for example previous organ donors.
f. The patients who have previously had one or more transplants.
g. Capacity of the patient to pay.

8. Allocation of kidneys

The allocation of kidneys occurs under circumstances not paralleled in the case of other organs because candidates for transplantation are drawn exclusively from patients already within a dialysis program. This introduces the difficulty that, whereas selection to receive a kidney is determined by clearly defined and promulgated criteria that are uniformly applicable nationally, selection to enter dialysis programs is affected by a variety of sets of guidelines. In some cases uniform criteria for entry to dialysis are being formulated. However, in other instances, individual clinics have their own guidelines, not all of which are readily available. This lack of transparency precludes ethical assessment of the procedures employed and this should occasion concern: it is an ethical issue in itself. As kidneys can be preserved safely by simple cold storage for at least twenty-four hours, the results of a blood T-cell cross match and tissue matching can be available before transplantation is undertaken. Because of the length of waiting lists, several potential recipients are commonly equally well matched with each presenting donor. Allocation of kidneys should be organized on a national basis so that recipients with the closest tissue matching with the donor are selected to receive the organs. This provides the best chance of success. Currently, kidneys are raised by allocation of transplant resources allocated to potential recipients according to the best available tissue match. If there are no suitably matched potential recipients on the national waiting list, the length of time on dialysis usually determines the recipient. Factors such as recipient age, period on dialysis, pre-sensitization to tissue antigens, presence of diabetes mellitus and the previous receipt of a transplant are likely to be taken into account.

The concept of distributive justice - how to fairly divide resources - arises around organ transplantation. Distributive justice theory states that there is not one "right" way to distribute organs, but rather many ways a person could justify giving an organ to one Particular individual over someone else. Equal access criteria include [UNOS 2001]:

- Length of time waiting (i.e. first come, first served)
- Age (i.e. younger to younger, older to older or youngest to oldest)
- Organ type, blood type and organ size
- Distance from the donor to the patient
- Level of medical urgency

Equal access supporters believe that organ transplantation is a valuable medical procedure and worth offering to those who need it. They also argue that because the procedure is worthy, everyone should be able to access it equally.

Successful transplants are measured by the number of life years gained. Life years are the number of years that a person will live with a successful organ transplant that they would not have lived otherwise. This philosophy allows organ procurement organizations to take into account several things when distributing organs that the equal access philosophy does not - like giving a second organ transplant to someone who's already had one or factoring in the probability of a successful medical outcome.

Three primary arguments oppose using the maximum benefit distribution criteria. First, predicting medical success is difficult because a successful outcome can vary. Is success the number of years a patient lives after a transplant? Or is success the number of years a transplanted organ functions? Is success the level of rehabilitation and quality of life the patient experiences afterward? These questions pose challenges to those attempting to allocate organs using medical success prediction criteria. The second argument against maximum benefit distribution is that distributing organs in this way could leave the door open for bias, lying, favoritism and other unfair practices more so than other forms of distribution due to the subjective nature of these criteria. Third, some ethicists argue against using age and maximizing life years as criteria for distributing organs because it devalues the remaining life of an older person awaiting a transplant. Regardless of how old someone is, if that person does not receive a transplant they will still be losing "the rest of his or her life," which is valuable to everyone.

9. Organ trafficking

Organs trading

The transfer, traveling, hosting, receiving living or deceased persons, or their organs, through threat, by force or any other forms of oppression or kidnapping or fraud, or deceit, or misuse of power or position, mis-receipt by a third party of money or subsidies submitted to oppress the contingent donor and use him as an organ donor.

Commercialization of organs

It is the policy or conduct by which the organ is dealt with as if it is a trade goods, including their purchase, sale or use for material gain.

Travel for organs transplantation

It is the travel of organs, donors, recipients or professionals of organs transplantation over the international borders for purpose of organs transplantation.

9.1 Methods and means used for organ trafficking and transplant tourism

The donor, recipient and surgeon may be of the same country. The agreement may be done before they get to the surgeon. The donor and recipient may travel to the country of the surgeon. The patient may travel to the donor country and vice-versa. The donor may be from one country, the patient from another country and the surgeon from third country, and all may travel to a fourth country to perform the transplantation
[Bramstedt 2007] Fig (6a&b). This needs organizers and coordinators, until the matter arrived to the existence of organized gangs aiming for benefit and do not care of the donor or the patient. They are standing on extortion principle and earning profits on the account of poor people and those in need. The matter arrived to even stealing organs, yet to kidnap children and women and even men in order to get their organs for selling them to whom pays more [Fasting etal 1998].

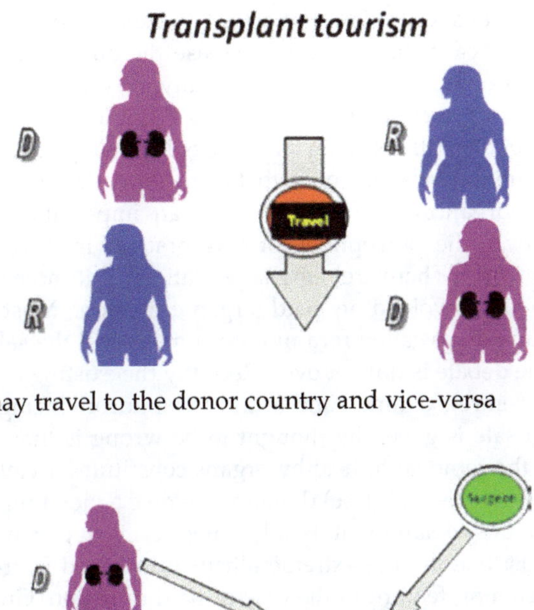

Fig. 6a. The patient may travel to the donor country and vice-versa

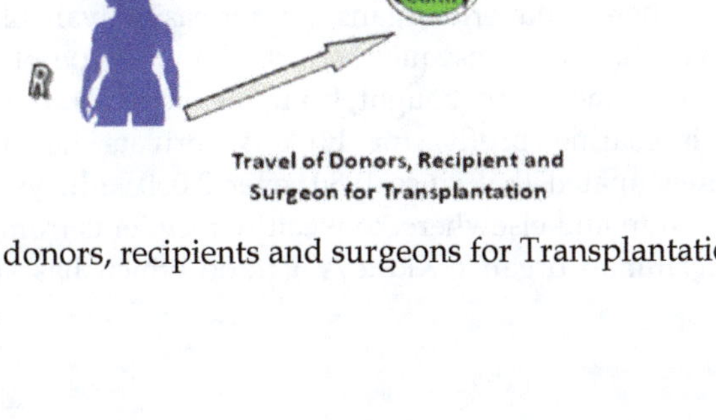

Fig. 6b. The travel of donors, recipients and surgeons for Transplantation

9.2 Organ sale

Paying people to donate their kidneys is one of the most contentious ethical issues being debated at the moment. The most common arguments against this practice include:

- Donor safety
- Unfair appeal of financial incentives to the economically disadvantaged
- Turning the body into a money-making tool "commodity'
- Wealthy people would be able to access more readily

The idea of nonfinancial incentives may be rising in popularity as a way to entice people to donate their organs. Financial incentives aimed at encouraging living donation have received much attention from bioethicists lately. Most experts argue that buying and selling human organs is an immoral and disrespectful practice [Daar 1998]. The moral objection raised most is that selling organs will appeal to the socioeconomically disadvantaged (poor, uneducated people) and these groups will be unfairly pressured to sell their organs by the promise of money. This pressure could also cause people to overlook the possible drawbacks in favor of cash incentives. On the other hand, wealthy people would have unfair access to organs due to their financial situations. It has been noticed that almost all of the people sold their kidneys to pay off debts and those will still had debt some time later but they will have a deterioration in their health status after donation and most of them would not recommend to others that they sell kidneys. Arguments that favor the buying and selling of human organs are scarce, but a few do exist. One of them is that payments aren't necessarily a bad idea if they work to increase the number of donated organs. The position contends that donating an organ is a relatively small burden compared to the enormous benefit reaped by recipients. Some argues that buying and selling organs is not morally objectionable, but that the system as it exists is inadequate to provide appropriate safeguards. This critique extends not only to the medical system, but also to legal and religious safeguarding organizations as well. It is an important ethical issue in organ transplantation. Whatever the perceptions of this practice in developed countries, it is widespread across the world. There are regional variations in its acceptance and practice. In France it is crime to get involved in paid organ donation. Most of the international organizations and forums have called fora moratorium against the sale of organs [Budiani-Saberi etal 2008] but the debate is not yet over. Recently the existing arguments against paid organ donation have been re-examined and found to be unconvincing. It is argued that the real reason why organ sale is generally thought to be wrong is that (a) bodily integrity is highly valued and (b) the removal of healthy organs constitutes a violation of this integrity [Wilkinson etal 1996]. Both sale and (free) donation involve a violation of bodily integrity. In case of free donation the violation of bodily integrity is typically outweighed by the presence of other goods: mainly, the extreme altruism involved in free donation. There is usually no such outweighing feature in the case of paid donation. Given this, the idea that we value bodily integrity can help to account for the perceived moral difference between sale and free donation. International trade in human organs, particularly in the developing countries of the world where cadaveric organs are not easily available and where there is marked disparity in wealth. As a consequence, a deplorable type of medical practice has emerged, where human kidneys are bought from the poor for transplantation into the wealthy clientele with soaring profits for brokers, private hospitals and physicians [Danovitch 2008]. It is estimated that since 1980, over 2,000 kidneys are sold annually in India, Iraq, Philippines, Iran and elsewhere. to wealthy recipients from the Middle East, the Far East and Europe. Human organ ("Kidneys") trade which has shifted from India to

Pakistan [Noorani 2008 & Naqvi etal 2007 &Delmonico 2007]. Media, in particular had gone to the extent of labeling it as shifting of "Kidney Bazar", "Bombay Bazar" from India to Karachi, Lahore and Islamabad [Naqvi etal 2008 & Sajjad etal 2008 & Beasley etal 2000 & Amerling 2001]. Fig (7).

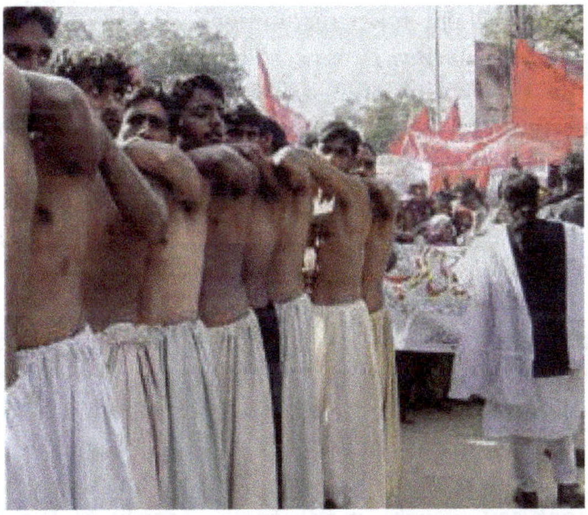

Fig. 7. Kidney bazar

The drawback is that physical harm comes to one person for the benefit of another. However, this is considered an acceptable side effect because of the rule of choosing between the lesser of two maladies, i.e. one person dies and one lives, or, two people live, both with physical deformities. It is not surprising, therefore, that this practice of trading in human organs has alarmed the medical profession, the public and many governments and it has rightly been condemned by all major religions, and by most transplant societies. Organ sale has serious negative impact on all aspects and on everyone involved in the process of transplantation, including the donor, the recipient, the local transplant program, the medical profession and the moral and ethical values of the society. Most ethicists believe that organ sale is an affront not only to altruism, but also to basic human dignity as opposed to a utilitarian approach to the important issue of transplantation for the following main reasons: (a) Organ sale promotes coercion and exploitation of the poor. (b) It promotes poor quality of care to the donor and particularly to the recipient as a result of poor standards of donor selection and inadequate screening for transmissible disease. (c) It benefits ruthless entrepreneurs, greedy doctors who care for their egos and financial gain. It is also against the patient's right for autonomy. It is contrary to accepted moral and ethical beliefs of most societies, including the major religions of Islam, Christianity, and Judaism. It diminishes the current benefit of altruistic donation by living donors and the families of cadaveric donors. It makes human organs a commodity for profit and sale thus inviting corruption and an unjust and unfair system of organ access and distribution and it predisposes to criminal tendencies of selling, kidnapping or killing children and women for organ sale, which has been reported [Spital 1997 & Danovitch etal 2006]. Some proponents of organ sale claim that well-controlled organ purchase does have several major advantages: by making more organs available it can reduce the waiting time for organs, reduce the number of deaths among waiting list patients as well as reduce the overall cost of treatment of patients with end-stage kidney disease. Some professionals in the transplant community believe that it will be much more productive as well as protective from sale of organs by vendors, at least in the developing countries where cadaver organs are not available, if the practice of organ sale is regulated by an independent organization. They argue that the feeling of repugnance of organ sale for the rich and the healthy should not justify removing the only hope for the destitute and dying. Cameron and Hoffenberg [Cameron etal 1999 & Ghods etal 2006 & Friedman 2006 & Laurance 2008] have recommended that organs be paid for through nationally established organ sharing networks to ensure the quality of care received by donors and to promote the equity of distribution which will involve the ethical and medical problems that exist with organ sale. Radcliffe-Richards et al. [Radcliffe etal 1998] have emphasized that current exploitation of donors and lack of informed consent through organ purchase are due to poverty and lack of education, which do not justify banning organ sale. They suggest that a national organization be established to regulate the sale of organs or provide educational and appropriate consultation to patients to enable them to have informed consent and even a 'guardian' for the donor. Also this organization will regulate and control organ vending, proper selection, payment of fees and provision of necessary care which will prevent the current exploitation, the risk of removing organs, both for the donor and the recipient, and provide screening and counseling, together with reliable payment and financial incentives [Friedman E 2006 & Friedman Al 2006 & Surman etal 2008]. They believe that this will not affect cadaveric donation, since payment can also be made to the family of the deceased. Some have proposed a market for organ donation or sale. The proponents of this model propose a legitimate governmental or nonprofit nongovernmental organization to take charge for the responsibility of compensating the donor, without any direct contact between donors and recipients. This would eliminate profit-seeking middlemen and organ brokers. While in certain instances, this practice has led to elimination of the waiting list [Matas 2008], evidence for negative impact of kidney donation for the donors have been reported. The best is to avoid people and their organs of being a commodity in the market weather it is an open black market or an organized and controlled market. In addition to direct payment, various other forms of compensation such as life and health insurance, medal of honor, reimbursement for travel expenses, compensation for time out of work, or a tax credit have been proposed. The potential problem with this model is that if it is not well organized, it will open the door to an organ market, where the organs are sold to the highest bidder, benefiting the rich and disadvantaging the poor [Chapman 2008 & Godlee 2008 & Thomas 2000]. Concern has also been raised that this will reduce altruistic kidney donation and discourage deceased multi-organ donation. However, some believe that it does not preclude increased donation, and others have shown that it has not inhibited the establishment of deceased donor transplantation programs. Opponents to any form of compensation and an organ market cite the concern that the poor will be viewed as mere providers of spare parts and will live with fewer organs, adding to this their list of disadvantages. According to this viewpoint, the market will be driven by poverty and the poor will be a disadvantage compared to the ealthier, feeling a disproportionately higher pressure to sell their organs Fig (8). On a global scale this could translate into people from rich nations travelling to poor countries to buy organs. There is the concern that the market could potentially lead to demeaning bodies to "articles of trade". Degrading human relationships, and particularly damaging the altruistic bond. There is also the concern about the occasional coercion of a spouse by an addicted spouse into selling an organ to pay for the addiction.

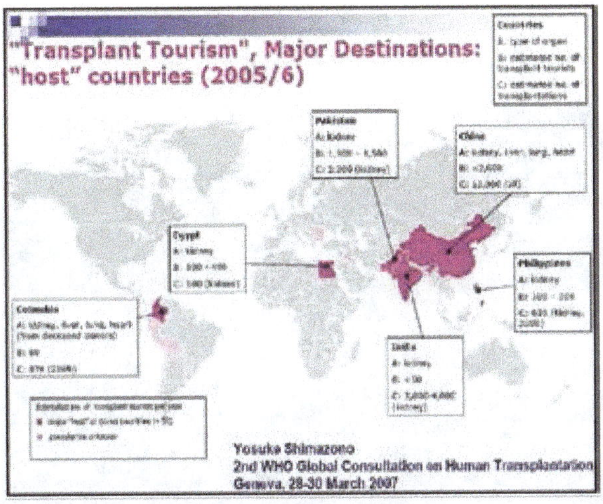

Fig. 8. Major destination host countries WHO publications

With related donor transplantation, altruism is the expected driving force; however, regarding unrelated donors, several valid question have been raised. Why should the unrelated donors not be at least partially rewarded for their donation? Why should they be expected to undergo the surgery and live with one less organ for the rest of their lives? Are the other parties involved (physicians, surgeons, nurses, etc,) providing their services only altruistically? Why should the only individuals sacrificing their bodies not be appropriately acknowledged? Although current laws in most countries and guidelines by WHO and professional societies prohibit the sales of organs, it has been debated that provision of financial incentive seems not only fair, but may also encourage donation and subsequently benefit the patients on the waiting list [Novelli etal 2007 & Satel etal 2008 & Kranenburg etal 2008]. The main opponents of providing financial incentives have voiced concern over "devaluing" the body to a mere commodity and the potential for commercialization. Some would argue that the body is a property and, in fact, the most valuable commodity that an individual possesses. They would contend that the owner of this property has a right to sell part of it for his/her better good.

There is little doubt that commercialization of organ donation is fraught with drawbacks, dangers and potential immoral consequences. On the other hand, it is clear that efforts to increase the rate of organ donation through education have failed and sole moral incentives have not worked [Delmonico etal 2008 & Colakgin etal 1998 & Prasad etal 2006]. Organs are currently limited by supply, and in the hope of expanding the available organs, it seems prudent to provide incentives not only to encourage donation, but also in order to express appreciation. In the process, we should be cognizant of the fact that we might be sacrificing some good for the sake of other potentially more meritorious goods, weighing the ethical and morals risks of one against the other. The obligation of society is to establish safeguards to protect all parties involved, as well as the humane inter-relationship between donor and recipient. In this regard, the method of acknowledging the good deeds of donors is of paramount importance.

It is clear that we need to look for feasible, ethical alternatives to the current model. This is not limited to whether or not donors should be compensated. Now that living unrelated transplant (LURT) has become an ever increasing reality Fig (9). Society and the transplant community should devise safeguards to scrutinize the process [Matas 2007 & Chapman 2008 & Godlee 2008 & Novelli etal 2007 & Satel etal 2008 &Kranenburg etal 2008 & Leung 2006].

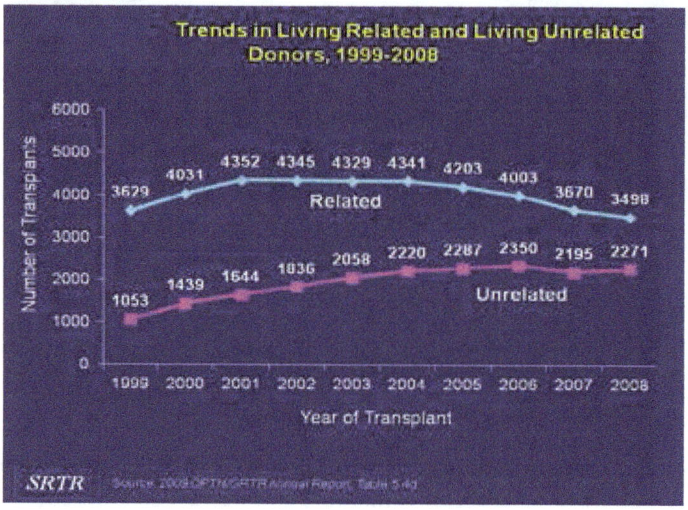

Fig. 9. Trends in living related and living unrelated donors UNOS publications

10. The struggle against international organ trafficking

The antimarket campaign could change things. To be able to do so, however, it needs to embrace a strategy combining new discursive and practical elements.
The campaign against transplant commercialism could be coherent and possibly successful only if it explained that the suffering-preventing capacity of a kidney disease-free and poverty-free world is considerably greater than that of any regulated market in organs [Danovitch etal 2008 & Turner 2008].

10.1 WHO guiding principles for cell, tissue and organ transplantation

WHO has condemned the commercialization of organs in several occasions, starting from the decision of the General assembly No. 40.13 in year 1987 and No. 42.5 in year 1989, and requested the countries to consolidate efforts to implement the decision, then the decision No. 44.25 for the year 1991 which has adopted the first draft of the WHO guiding principles regarding the human cells, tissues and organs transplantation, and which has contoured the methodological and ethical standard framework.
Among the most important recommendations issued by the general assembly, are those issued in its fifty-seventh session (decision 57.18) in may 2004, where the organization has required from the member countries the necessity of existence of an actual supervision on the organ transplantation, and promotion of both living and deceased donation, and to take the necessary measures to protect the poorest and exposed to the organs transplantation tourism. In year 2008, the guiding principles of the WHO have been updated regarding the human cells, tissues and organs transplantation [WHO 2008]. They were adopted by the executive council in its session held in November 2008 these guidelines are.

- Consent for deceased donation
- No conflict between physicians determining death

- Deceased but also live consenting donors
- Minors and incompetent persons be protected
- No sale or purchase
- Promotion of donation no advertising nor brokering
- Physician responsibility on origin of transplant
- Justifiable professional fees
- Allocation rules
- Quality safety efficacy of procedures and transplants
- Transparency and anonymity

10.2 International consultation for the organization of organ transplantation

A group of meetings were held by the WHO joined number of scientists and international and national organizations in order study the challenges facing human cells, tissues and organ transplantation. Open consultations were done in Karachi, Geneva and Madrid, different experts were invited The purpose of all such consultations is to determine the problem about such a matter and also to extract preparatory ideas in order to make them implemented and to encourage countries to have national or regional strategies for self sufficiency by promoting both living and deceased donation and to cooperate towards organ trafficking free world. They urge the need for an international binding treaty to regulate transplantation and to combat organ trafficking [Carmi 1996]. Fig (10)

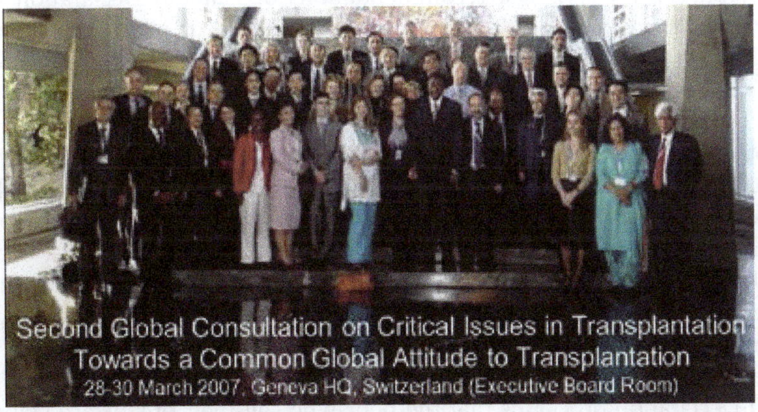
Second Global Consultation on Critical Issues in Transplantation
Towards a Common Global Attitude to Transplantation
28-30 March 2007, Geneva HQ, Switzerland (Executive Board Room)

Fig. 10.

10.3 Amsterdam forum on the care of the kidney donor: Data and medical Guidelines

Kidney and transplant surgeons met in Amsterdam. The Netherland, from April 1-4, 2004 for the international forum on the care of the live kidney donor. Forum participants included over 100 experts and leaders in Transplantation representing more than 40 countries from around the world. The Forum analyzed the sentinel events associated with live kidney donation; the data emphasized the extremely low Operative mortality rates and the long-term safety of this procedure. Forum participants affirmed the necessity for live donors to receive complete medical and psychosocial evaluation prior to donation. A great detail of discussion focused on prevention of transmissible infectious diseases through live kidney transplantation [Delmonico etal 2007].

10.4 Lisbon conference for the care of kidney transplantation recipients in February 2006

An international conference about the care of the kidney transplantation recipients, held in Lisbon, Portugal, February 2nd-4th 2006, with the cooperation between the WHO and different international and national societies of organs transplantation. The conference has joined more than 100 experts and leaders in organ transplantation. It represents more than 40 countries from all over the world. The conference aimed to determine the main issues and to set recommendations to improve the outcome of kidney transplantation all over the world [The Consensus Statement of the Amsterdam Forum 2004].

10.5 Asian campaign against organs commercialization

A meeting was held in Taipei - January 2008, About the immoral and unfair practices related to the organs transplantation in Asia by local citizens and by others from other areas. The recommendation of the Asian campaign stressed the importance of collective measures against organ trafficking [Bagheri 2005].

10.6 Istanbul declaration

An international summit was held in Istanbul on May 2nd 2008, joining more than 150 representatives for medical professional, governmental and non governmental organizations, and transplant societies from 78 countries and 20 international organizations, The meeting was organized by The Transplantation Society (TTS) and the International Society of Nephrology (ISN). The recommendations of Istanbul Declaration have added very important dimensions to the international standards of organ transplantation and emphasized the encouragement of living and deceased donation and stressed on the living donors care and to view their act as a championship as they are sharing in the Gift of life and the necessity to evaluate the donors medically and psychologically before and after donation [Steering Committee of the Istanbul Summit 2008]. The declaration was centered on Organ commercialism, which targets vulnerable populations (such as illiterate and impoverished persons, undocumented immigrants, prisoners, and political or economic refugees) in resource-poor countries, has been condemned by international bodies such as the World Health Organization for decades. Yet in recent years, as a consequence of the increasing ease of Internet communication and the willingness of patients in rich countries to travel and purchase organs, organ trafficking and transplant tourism have grown into global problems.

The Istanbul Declaration proclaims that the poor who sell their organs are being exploited, whether by richer people within their own countries or by transplant tourists from abroad. Moreover, transplant tourists risk physical harm by unregulated and illegal transplantation. Participants in the Istanbul Summit concluded that transplant commercialism, which targets the vulnerable, transplant tourism, and organ trafficking should be prohibited. And they also urged their fellow transplant professionals, individually and through their organizations, to put an end to these unethical activities and foster safe, accountable practices that meet the needs of transplant recipients while protecting donors.

Countries from which transplant tourists originate, as well as those to which they travel to obtain transplants, are just beginning to address their respective responsibilities to protect their people from exploitation and to develop national self-sufficiency in organ donation. The Declaration should reinforce the resolve of governments and international organizations to develop laws and guidelines to bring an end to wrongful practices. "The legacy of transplantation is threatened by organ trafficking and transplant tourism. The Declaration of Istanbul aims to combat these activities and to preserve the nobility of organ donation. The success of transplantation as a life-saving treatment does not require—nor justify—victimizing the world's poor as the source of organs for the rich" [Epstein 2008]

10.7 Madrid conference March 23th-25th, 2010

A conference was held in Madrid. It has concentrated about the self-sufficiency of organs for each country or region. The conference has recommended the necessity to set national plans and strategies to promote the donation of organs from deceased and living persons, arriving to the self-sufficiency and to fight, struggle and limit organ trafficking and transplant tourism.

10.8 Global leadership symposium on organs donation

During the period May 10th-13th, 2010, the global leadership symposium on organs donation was held in California. It was attended by a lot of workers in the promotion of organs donation and a number of the international experts in the organs donation and transplantation and ethicists from several countries to more support the organs donation and fight organ trafficking.

11. References

Abouna GM: Recent Pronouncements by Two Major Religions on Organ Transplantation: Current Status of Clinical Organ Transplantation. The Hague, Nijhoff, 1984, pp XI-XII.

Abouna GM: Kidney transplantation from live donors: Benefits, possible risks and dilemmas. *J Kuwait Med Assoc* 1998; 30:89–92

Abouna GM. Organ shortage crisis: problems and possible solutions. *Transplant* Proc 2008; 40:34-38

Ad Hoc Committee. A definition of irreversible coma: report of the Ad Hoc. Committee of the Harvard Medical School to Examine the Definition of Brain death. *JAMA* 1968; 205: 337-40

Alashek WA, Ehtuish EF, Elhabashi A, Emberish W, Mishra A: Reasons for Unwillingness of Libyans to Donate Organs after Death. *LIBYANJOURNAL OF MEDICINE*, VOL 4, NO 3 2009

Al-Faqih SR: The influence of Islamic views on public attitudes towards kidney transplant donation in a Saudi Arabian community. Public Health, 1991; 105(2): 161-65.

Amerling R: A market for living organs revisited. Transplant News Issues 2001; 2:S16–S17.

Bagheri A. "Organ Transplantation Laws in Asian Countries: A Comparative Study," Transplantation Proceedings 37, no. 10 (December 2005): 4159-4162

Bartholomew A, Sher D, Sosler S, Stock W, Lazda V, Koshy M, Devine S, van Besien K:Stem cell transplantation eliminates allo-antibody in a highly sensitized patient. *Transplantation* 2001;72:1653–1655.

Beasley Cl, Cherry MJ: Body parts and the market place: insights from Thomistic philosophy. Christ Bioethics, 2000; 6(2): 17193.

Beier UH, Hidalgo G, John E. Financial incentives to promote prolonged renal graft survival: potential for patients and public health. Med Hypotheses 2008; 70:218-220.

Bernat JL. The Boundaries of organ donation after circulatory death. N Engl J Med 2008:359" 669-71

Bramstedt KA, Xu J. Checklist: passport, plane ticket, organ transplant. Am J Transplant 2007; 7:1698-1701.

Budiani-Saberi DA, Delmonico FL. Organ trafficking and transplant tourism: a commentary on the global realities. Am J Transplant 2008; 8:925-92

Bukler L, Cooper DK: Xenotransplant: *State of the art. Front Biosci* 1999;4:416.

Byrne PA, O'Reilly S. Quay PM. Brain Death an opposing viewpoint. *JAMA* 1979; 242:1985-90

Cameron JS, Hoffenberg R: Ethics of organ transplantation reconsidered: Paid organ donation and the use of executed prisoners as donors. Kidney Int 1999; 55:724–732.

Carmi A: Organ transplantation in the mirror of the recent world- wide legislation. Med Law, 1996; 15: 341-9

Chapman J. Should we pay donors to increase the supply of organs for transplantation? No.BMJ 2008; 336:1343.

Cohen B, D'Amaro J: Some contemporary ethical consideration related to organ transplantation. Transpl Int 1995;8:238–243.

Colakgin M, Yenicesu M, Akpolat T, et al: Nonrelated living donor kidney transplantation: Medical & ethical aspects. Nephron, 1998; 79: 447-51

Courtney AE, Maxwell AP. The challenge of doing what is right in renal transplantation: Balancing equity and utility. *Nephron Clin Pract.* 2009;111:62–6778.

Daar AS: Paid organ donation-the grey basket concept. J Med Ethics, 1998; 24: 365-8

Danovitch GM, Leichtman AB. Kidney vending: the 'Trojan horse' of organ transplantation. Clin J Am Soc. Nephrol 2006 1: 1133-1135

Danovitch GM. The doctor/patient relationship in living donor kidney transplantation. Curr Opin Nephrol Hypertens 2007; 16:503-505.

Danovitch GM. Who cares? A lesson from Pakistan on the health of living donors. Am J Transplant 2008; 8:1-2.

Danovitch GM, Delmonico FL. The prohibition of kidney sales and organ markets should remain. Curr Opin Organ Transplant 2008;.

Delmonico FL, Radolph JG. Death: a concept in transition. *Pediatrics* 1973;51:234-9

Delmonico FL, Murray JE.A medical defense of brain death.Ethics & Medics1999;224:1-268.

Delmonico FL, Dew MA Living donor kidney transplantation in a global environment. Kidney Int. 2007 Apr;71(7):608-14. Epub 2007 Feb 7

Delmonico FL. The Pakistani revelation. Transplant Int 2007; 20:924-925.

Delmonico FL, Danovitch GM. Regulated market for organs is unattainable. Minn Med 2008; 91:6.2

Delmonico FL. The concept of Death and Deceased organ donation. *Int J OrgTransplantation Med.*, 2010; 1(1): 15-20.

Ebrahim AF: Organ transplantation: contemporary Sunni Muslim, legal and ethical perspectives. Bioethics, 1995; 9(3-4): 291-302.

Ebrahim AF: Islamic jurisprudence and the end of human life. Med Law, 1998; 17(2): 189-

Ehtuish EF, Abouna GM, Shebani AH, Abdulmola TS, Shawesh TZ. Kidney transplantation in Libya: a North African and Middle Eastern perspective Exp Clin Transplant. 2006 Jun;4(1):425-8

Epstein M. The ethics of poverty and the poverty of ethics: the case of Palestinian prisoners in Israel seeking to sell their kidneys in order to feed their children. *J Med Ethics* 2007; 33:473-474.

Epstein M. The Declaration of Istanbul on Organ Trafficking and Transplant Tourism: an important international achievement with one disturbing loophole. BMJ 2008.

Epstein M, Danovitch G. Is altruistic-directed living unrelated organ donation a legal fiction? Nephrol Dial Transplant 2009; 24:357-360.

Eradini S:Stem cells for all seasons ? Experimental and clinical issues. *JR Soc Med* 2002;95:5–8.

Evans RW: Organ transplantation and the inevitable debate as to what constitutes basic health care benefit. Clin Transpl 1993:359- 391.

Fandrich F: Pre-implantation stage stem cells induce allogeneic graft acceptance with host conditioning. *Nat Med* 2002;8:171.46.

Fasting U, Christensen J and Glending S: Children sold for transplant: Medical & legal aspects. Amnesty International-Danish Working Group for children. Nurs Ethics, 1998; 5: 518-

Friedman AL. Payment for living organ donation should be legalized. BMJ 2006; 333:746-748.

Friedman E, Friedman AL. Payment for donor kidneys: pros and cons. Kidney Int 2006; 69:960-2.

Garwood P. Dilemma over live-donor transplantation. Bull World Health Organ 2007; 85:1

Ghods AJ, Savaj S. Iranian model of paid and regulated living-unrelated kidney donation. *Clin J Am Soc Nephrol.* 2006;1:1136–1145.

Godlee F. Is it time to pilot paying for organs? BMJ 2008; 336.

Golmakani MM, Niknam MH, Hedayat KM. Transplantation ethics from the Islamic point of view. *Med Sci Monit.* 2005;11:105–109.

Grant D, Mendicino M, Levy G: Xenotransplantation: Just around the corner? Surgery 2001;129:243–247

Hariharan S, Johnson CP, Bresnahan BA, Taranto SE, McIntosh MJ, Stablein D. Improved graft survival after renal transplantation in the United States, 1988 to 1996. *N Engl J Med.* 2000;342:605–612.

Hull AR & Rosenthal JT: Living kidney donation: A survey of professional attitudes & practices. *Am J Kidney Dis*, 1997; 30: 549-57

Hunsicker LG: Survival advantage for renal transplantation. N Engl J Med 1999; 341:1762–1763.

Jarvis R: Join the club: A modest proposal to increase availability of donor organs. J Med Ethics 1995;21:199–204

Jasper JD, Nickerson CA, Hershey JC Asch DA: The public's attitudes toward incentives for organ donation. Transplant Proc, 1999; 31(5): 2181-84.

Kranenburg L, Schram A, Zuidema W, *et al.* Public survey of financial incentives for kidney donation. Nephrol Dial Transplant 2008; 23:1039-1042.

Landolt MA, Henderson SJ, Barrable WM, Greenwood SD, McDonald MF, Soos JG, Landsberg DN: Living anonymous kidney donation: What does the public think? *Transplantation* 2001; 71:1690–169

Laurance J. Surgeon: organ trade should be legalized. The Independent 13 June 2008.

Leung G. Fun, sun, get a surgery done! The growing trend of transplant tourism. Issues Berkeley Med J 2006; 13:7-8.. BMJ 2008; 336:1377.

Life, They decide who lives, who dies: Medical miracle puts a moral burden on a small committee." Life, 9 November 1962,102

Matas AJ. A gift of life deserves compensation: how to increase living kidney donation with realistic incentives. Cato Institute Policy Analysis 2007; 604:15.

Matas AJ. Should we pay donors to increase the supply of organs for transplantation? Yes. BMJ 2008; 336:1342.

Mathieson PW, Jolliffe D, Jolliffe R, Dudley CR, Hamilton K & Lear PA: The spouse as a kidney donor: Ethically sound. Nephrol Dial Transplant, 1999; 14: 46-8

Merrill JP, Murray JE, Harrison JH, Guild WR: Successful homotransplantations of human kidneys between identical twins. *Am J Surg* 1958; 148:343

Miller DB: Ethics of paid organ donation and the use of executed prisoners as donors. Kidney Int 1999; 55:733–737.

Miranda B and Matesanz R: International issues in transplantation. Setting the scene & flagging the most urgent & controversial issues. Ann N Y Acad Sci, 1998; 862: 129-43

Moqaddam A: Organ transplant not a non-religious act in Iran any more. Tehran Times, 2000 27 September.

Naqvi SAA, Ali B, Mazhar F, *et al.* A socioeconomic survey of kidney vendors in Pakistan. Transplant Int 2007; 20:934-939.

Naqvi SAA, Rizvi SAH, Zafar MN, *et al.* Health status and renal function evaluation of kidney vendors: a report from Pakistan. Am J Transplant 2008; 8:1444-1450.

Noorani MA. Commercial transplantation in Pakistan. BMJ 2008; 336:1378.

Norton DL: Clinical application of brain death protocol. J Neurosci Nurs 1992;24:354–35883.

Novelli G, Rossi M, Poli L, *et al.* Is legalizing the organ market possible? Transplant Proc 2007; 39:1743-1745.

Platt JL: Genetic engineering for xenotransplantation. Transplant Proc 1999;3:1488.

Pope John Paul II. Address to International Congress on Transplants. August 29,2000. (available from http://www.cin.org/pope/organ- transplant-cloning.html)

Prasad GV, Shukla A, Huang M, *et al.* Outcomes of commercial renal transplantation: a Canadian experience. Transplantation 2006; 82:1130-1135

President's Commission for the Study of Ethical Problems in Medicine and Biomedical and Behavioral Research. *Defining Death: A report on medical legal, and ethical issues in the determination of death.* Washington, DC: The Commission; 1981.

Radcliffe-Richards J, Daar AS, Guttmann RD, Hoffenberg R, Kennedy I, Lock M, Sells RA, Tilney N: The case for allowing kidney sales. Lancet 1998;351:1950 -1952.

Rahman F: Haealth and medicine in the Islamic tradition: change and identity. Chicago, IL: ABC International Group, 1998.

Rithalia A, McDaid C, Suekarran S, Norman G, Myers L, Sowden A. A systematic review of presumed consent systems for deceased organ donation. *Health Technol Assess.* 2009;13:1–95.

Sajjad I, Baines LS, Patel P, *et al.* Commercialization of kidney transplants: a systematic review of outcomes in recipients and donors. Am J Nephrol 2008; 28:744-754.23.

Satel S, Hakim N. 'What's wrong with selling kidneys?' International Herald Tribune 20 June 2008

Savules J: Should we clone human beings? Cloning as a source of tissue for transplantation. *J Med Ethics*, 1999; 25: 87-956

Shemie SD, Baker AJ, Knoll G, et al. National recommendations for donation after cardiocirculatory death in Canada: Donation after cardiocirculatory death in Canada. *Can Med Assoc J*. 2006;175:S1..

Shemie SD. Clarifying the paradigm for the ethics of donation and transplantation: was "dead" really so clear before organ donation? *Philos Ethics Humanit Med* 2007;2:18

Shewmon DA. Chronic "brain death": meta-analysis and conceptual consequences. Neurology 1998;51:1538-45.

Sim KH, Marinov A & Levy GA: Xenotransplantation: A potential solution to the critical organ donor shortage. Can J Gastroentrol, 1999; 13: 311-8

Spital A: Do US transplant centers encourage emotionally related kidney donation? Transplantation, 1996; 61: 374-7

Spital A: Should children ever donate kidneys? *Views of US transplant centers. Transplantation*, 1997; 64: 232-6

Spital A: Ethical & policy issues in altruistic living & cadaveric organ donation. *Clin Transplant*, 1997; 11: 77-78.

Starzl T, et al: Renal transplantation from baboon to man: Experience with six cases. Transplantation 1964;2:752.

Steering Committee of the Istanbul Summit. Organ trafficking and transplant tourism and commercialism: the Declaration of Istanbul. Lancet 2008; 372:5-

Surman OS, Saidi R, Purtilo R, *et al*. The market of human organs: a window into a poorly understood global business. Transplant Proc 2008; 40:491-493.

Sweet WH. Brain death. *N Engl J Med* 1978;299:410-2

The Consensus Statement of the Amsterdam Forum on the care of the live kidney donor. Transplantation 2004; 78: 491-492.

The Definition of Irreversible Coma: Report of ad hoc Committee of Harvard Medical School of Definition of Brain Death. JAMA 1968;205: 337

The Economist The gap between supply and demand. 11-17 October 2008:85- 87

Thomas C: Living donor receives leave benefits. Transplant Chronicle 2000;7:4.

Truog RD. Is it time to abandon brain death? Hastings Cent Rep 1997;27:29-37

Truog RD Miller FG. The dead donor rule and organ transplantation. *N Engl J Med* 2008;359:674-5

Turcotte JT, Benjamin M, Caplan AL: Patient selection criteria in organ transplantation: The critical questions. Transplant Proc 1989;21: 3377–3445.

Turner L. Let's wave goodbye to ' transplant tourism' BMJ 2008; 36:1377

United Network for Organ Sharing (UNOS): Annual Report,1999.

United Network for Organ Sharing (UNOS): Policy of Organ Distribution. June 2001

Van Bommel A: Medical ethics from the Muslim perspective. Acta Neurochir Suppl (Wien), 1999; 74: 17-277.

Veatch RM. Donating hearts after cardiac death - reversing the irreversible. N *Engl J Med* 2008;359:672-3

WHO. WHO guiding principles on human cell, tissue and organ transplantation. EB123/5 2008:1-8. Another document that reaffirms the principles of the international campaign against transplant commercialism and global transplant commercialism in particular.

Wilkinson S & Garrad E; Bodily integrity & the sale of human organs. J Med Ethics, Lancet, 1996; 22: 334-9

Zargooshi J. Iran's commercial renal transplantation program: results and complications. In: Weimar W, Boss MA, Busschbach JJ, editors. Organ transplantation: ethical, legal and psychosocial aspects. Lengerich: Pabst Science Publishers; 2008. pp. 80-94

2

Anaesthesia for Kidney Transplantation

Yasser Haggag and Imran Ahmad
Guy's and St Thomas NHS Foundation Trust UK

1. Introduction

Kidney transplantation improves the quality of life and the long-term survival of end-stage renal failure (ESRF) patients compared to those on dialysis (1). It has also been shown to be a more economic option than both haemodialysis and peritoneal dialysis (2)

With the increasing incidence of organ failure, the demand for organ transplantation has increased, resulting in longer waiting lists and increased waiting list deaths.

Recently, live organ donation has helped to relieve the shortage of deceased donor grafting. Living donor kidney transplantation offers recipients the best hope for long-term rehabilitation and its advantages are indisputable.

This chapter looks at the anaesthetic principles and management of kidney transplantation, the most frequently performed organ transplantation.

2. Preoperative assessment

Hypertension and diabetes mellitus (DM) are the two most common causes of ESRF

Hypertension should be assessed thoroughly in terms of severity, antihypertensive medications and cardiovascular complications. Hypertension associated with renal failure is usually treated with ACE inhibitors or angiotensin II receptors antagonists. (3)

A target blood pressure of 140/90 or less is usually associated with decreased incidence of left ventricular hypertrophy. (4)

Type 1 DM is usually associated with impaired renal function and can lead to the development of severe nephropathy and ESRF. Diabetic patients have increased cardiovascular risk of peripheral vascular disease. (5)

There are few other medical problems associated with advanced kidney diseases, such as:

- Endocrine abnormalities such as hyperparathyroidism
- increased calcium and phosphate serum levels.
- Dyslipidaemia
- Autoimmune diseases as vasculitis – Systemic Lupus Erythematosus (SLE)

3. Medical history

The preoperative visit plays an important role to alleviate patient's anxiety, especially for patients who have been suffering from a life-long kidney problem and anticipating to undergo a procedure that would change their life style completely.

The importance of such a visit to the anaesthetist cannot be over-emphasised, many of these patients have had general anaesthesia in the past, so useful information may be found from previous anaesthesia charts.

The aetiology of a failing kidney cannot be clearly identified every time, but it is important to be aware of the cause if this has been identified, as this may have other implications to the anaesthetic management. The associated morbidity, whether it is the cause of the renal failure or as a consequence of it, has to be sought very clearly.

The duration of renal failure and the requirement of any renal replacement therapy (RRT), either peritoneal dialysis (PD) or haemodialysis (HD) must also be noted. The longer the duration of renal failure, the more likely there will be implications to the anaesthetic management, for example the patient may have required numerous central venous cannulations in the past, resulting in stenosed or thrombosed central veins or they have had numerous arterio-venous (AV) fistulas which make intravenous access difficult.

It is useful to be aware of the patient's 'dry weight' as this will allow estimation of the preoperative fluid status. The frequency of dialysis per week should be asked and the last dialysis session the patient received must also be noted. Ideally this should be as close to surgery as possible. This will ensure optimised fluid balance (although the patient may be under filled after a session) and electrolyte balance, most importantly the potassium and urea levels. A higher potassium plasma concentration can be accepted in this group of patients, but always try to achieve a normal range.

If the patient is due a dialysis session or has elevated electrolyte levels and appears fluid overloaded, then this patient must undergo haemodialysis prior to general anaesthesia and surgery.

The normal daily fluid intake and daily volume of any native urine output (if present) should also be noted, this will act as a further guided to fluid management intra-operatively.

Prior to anaesthesia, the presence of any AV fistulas should be clearly marked and labelled to avoid cannulation and BP measurements.

A history of previous dialysis line or central line insertions into the internal jugular or subclavian veins should also be sought; this may have implications on the insertion of central lines for monitoring during the kidney transplantation. Long term dialysis lines or numerous central lines can cause stenosis and thrombosis of the central veins.

Exercise tolerance can give an indication of the severity of the condition and its associated problems, it is also a useful guide to the general health of the patient.

4. Examination

Routine examination includes vital signs and the state of hydration. Is the patient dry after recent dialysis or fluid overloaded?

Some patients presenting for renal transplant might have associated rare medical conditions that require thorough examination, conditions like Prune Belly syndrome and VATER association (please see later).

Particular attention should be made to the cardiovascular system, including blood pressure control and clinical signs of left ventricular hypertrophy (LVH).

Assessment of the respiratory system will determine further management of the patients following their surgery, if they have associated respiratory disease then they may require post-operative non-invasive ventilation or prolonged intubation and ventilation.

Airway assessment will determine the management of the patient's airway following induction of anaesthesia, but these patients should always be intubated and ventilated for a renal transplant. Patients with DM may have associated difficult airways so appropriate equipment and techniques for managing the difficult airway must be available.

5. Investigations

Routine investigations such as full blood count (FBC) and kidney function particularly serum creatinine and blood urea nitrogen (BUN) and creatinine clearance.

Serum potassium should to be within the normal levels; usually less than 5.5 mmol/L. A further cycle on dialysis may be required if raised. Also note the bicarbonate and base excess.

Lots of important information can be obtained from the electrocardiogram (ECG), such as left ventricular hypertrophy, ischaemic heart disease or ECG changes associated with electrolyte imbalances, especially hyperkalaemia.

If the patient has a significant history of cardiovascular disease with associated ECG changes, then further assessment maybe required, such as an echocardiogram, radioactive isotope scan or even angiography. Patients with ESRF as a result of DM, may have undiagnosed cardiovascular disease, so particular care should be taken in these patients.

All patients undergoing renal transplant should at least have blood group and saved, blood should be made available if there is a high risk of bleeding.

6. Anaesthetic technique

Normally patients are not prescribed pre-medications prior to induction of anaesthesia, unless strongly indicated. Temazepam can be given orally 10 - 20 mg the night before and/or the morning of surgery in particularly anxious patients. Rantidine, metoclopramide or sodium citrate orally may also be given if the patient has reflux disease.

Induction of anaesthesia always takes place with the routine monitors ECG, non-invasive blood pressure and oxygen saturation monitoring. In patients with associated cardiovascular disease, invasive blood pressure monitoring should be considered, to ensure close monitoring of the blood pressure.

Haemodynamic stability should be maintained throughout the period of the operation with special attention to depressing the vasopressor response to intubation.

Fluctuations of the blood pressure should be within 20% of the baseline reading, this can be achieved by dampening surgical stimulation with the use of opioids.

Intraoperative opioids can be achieved via repeated boluses of Fentanyl or continuous infusion of Remifentanil, as target controlled infusion (TCI) between 4 to 6 ng/mL.

Atracurium (0.5 mg/Kg) is the muscle relaxant of choice in renal failure, it undergoes Hofmann degradation mainly and ester hydrolysis to a lesser extent.

Other muscle relaxants can be used, including all non-depolarizing muscle relaxants, but care must be taken with large or repeated doses as accumulation may result in a prolonged neuromuscular block.

The only depolarizing muscle relaxant in clinical use (suxamethonium) can be used as long as serum potassium levels are less than 5 mmol/L.

After induction of anaesthesia a central line should be inserted, ideally with ultrasound guidance, this allows monitoring of central venous pressure and the infusion of inotropes if necessary. The preferred site of insertion should be the internal jugular vein, be careful with the subclavian approach, particularly if on the fistula side as the vein may be arterialised and bleed profusely.

Immediately following induction of anaesthesia prophylactic dose of antibiotic should be given, this can vary depending on local protocol, commonly used are:
Amikacin 5 mg/Kg or gentamicin 3 mg/Kg
Co-amoxiclav dose 1.2 g can be given as well
Transplant surgery requires the administration of 'goodies', to reduce the incidence of organ rejection and to help functioning of the transplanted kidney. These are usually administered prior to revascularization and vary from centre to centre. Commonly used drugs are furosemide, mannitol, methylprednisolone (which should given as a slow intravenous infusion over half an hour, if given as a bolus it causes marked vasodilatation and may cause pronounced hypotension).

7. Maintenance of anaesthesia

All inhalational agents can be used safely, with the exception of enflurane (which is hardly being used in clinical practice nowadays)
Total intravenous anaesthesia (TIVA) is successfully being used with propofol and remifentanil to maintain GA.
The use of nitrous oxide is not associated with any ill effects, having said that, there is a trend among anaesthetists to avoid the use of N_2O in patients even with a normal kidney function.
The combination of Desflurane and Remifentanil infusion ensures smooth anaesthesia and a quick response to the challenging heart rate and blood pressure control throughout the procedure. This is in addition to smooth and rapid recovery.
Fentanyl can be given cautiously towards the end of the procedure in multiple small doses of 50 - 100 mcg; the total dose is titrated according to patient's response to pain while recovering from general anaesthesia.

8. Intraoperative monitors

Core Temp should ideally be measured via a nasopharyngeal probe, attention should be paid to keep the patient's temperature within the normal range. Hypothermia delays drug metabolism and is associated with increased incidence of postoperative complications namely chest infection and bleeding diathesis
Central venous pressure (CVP) alone can be a misleading guide to fluid requirements throughout the operation.
Oesophageal Doppler can be used to guide fluid management intraoperatively
Arterial blood gas testing (pH , PaO_2 , $PaCO_2$, bicarbonate, lactate, haemoglobin, potassium, sodium and blood glucose) is helpful if an arterial line has been placed, alternatively a venous sample could be used.
Serum potassium can go either way. Hypokalaemia should not be treated unless K is less than 3.0 mmol/L. Where as hyperkalaemia should be dealt with if K levels is 6.0 mmol/L or more. Calcium gluconate is the drug of choice in this case, as opposed to the traditional dextrose-insulin regimen.
Neuromuscular blockade monitor, an additional dose of muscle relaxants has to be judged carefully. Adequate reversal of the neuro-muscular function is extremely important before planning extubation at the end of the procedure.
Bi-spectral index (BIS) monitor can be used to assess depth of anaesthesia.

9. Fluid management

Transplant procedures are routinely short duration, minimal blood loss and preserved capillary permeability.

Patients undergoing renal transplant operations are usually receiving haemodialysis and their intravascular filling status should be monitored closely. The risk of hypovolaemia and under-filling can impair the perfusion to the transplanted kidney, whereas hypervolaemia from overzealous infusion of intravenous fluids can adversely affect myocardial contractility, especially for patients with pre-existing coronary artery disease (CAD) and impaired left ventricular function.

Even fluid balance and maintenance of the eu-volaemic status is strongly advisable

Type of intravenous fluid is of great importance, as the use of 0.9% sodium chloride is thought to be the standard fluid to be used in transplants patients, but the use of other crystalloid fluids such as Hartmann's solution (Lactated Ringer's) was used safely as long as serum potassium levels are monitored closely. (6)

Colloids could also be used safely in these procedures as long as its use does not exceed 15 mL/Kg.

Careful monitoring of the filling status of the patient is paramount, the use of central venous pressure (CVP) as the sole indicator or in combination with other monitors such as oesophageal doppler is advised. (7)

Immediate urine output can be seen in 90% of live kidney donation and up to 50% of cadaveric donation. Appropriate fluid management is the single most important factor to determine good urine output following the transplant.

It has been clearly demonstrated that it is more important than other pharmacological agents such as dopamine or the use of mannitol and colloids

Blood transfusion is better avoided in transplant procedures as the activation of autoimmune system may induce early rejection of the graft.

Renal failure patients are always anaemic, and it is quite safe to keep their haemoglobin levels as low as 7.0 g/dL in the perioperative period as long as continuous haemoglobin monitoring is available. It is a compromise between a low haemocrit that helps flow to the new kidney and the oxygen carrying capacity and delivery of oxygen to the tissues

10. Low Dose Dopamine (LDD)

Dopamine exerts its effect - at this low dose - mainly via peripheral dopaminergic receptors (renal) rather than its effect via the adrenergic receptors (cardiovascular) (8)

Few studies have shown that dopamine infusion at a rate of up to 2.5 mcg/Kg/min. would increase both urine output and creatinine clearance (9)

Other studies have questioned the value of dopamine infusion following graft of denervated kidney as evidenced by Doppler examination of renal blood flow (10), (11). The rational behind the use of dopamine – in the first 12 hr postoperatively - is mainly to ensure arteriolar vasodilatation and increase the renal perfusion pressure and to prevent acute tubular necrosis (ATN). There is no clear benefit from infusing or withholding dopamine, it is usually left to individual institution guidelines and protocols.

If the patient's blood pressure is thought to be high enough to grant satisfactory renal blood flow and ensure adequate reperfusion of the graft, then here is no need to initiate a dopamine infusion.

It is important to maintain adequate mean arterial pressure and central venous pressure prior to the release of the clamps once the donor kidney has been transplanted. This will ensure good blood flow to the kidney. The target values are dependant on the patient's normal mean arterial pressures.

11. Postoperative management

The postoperative fluid management is an important part of maintaining adequate renal perfusion. Various regimes are available. One commonly used is, crystalloid 50mls/hr plus previous hour's urine output. The urine output should be closely monitored and liase closely with the surgeons, especially if the patient remains anuric.
Local anaesthesia wound infiltration with L-Bupivacaine (2 mg/Kg) by the surgeons at the end of surgery, may help reduce post-operative pain.
Fentanyl patient controlled analgesia (PCA) is the standard pain control method
Bolus dose 10 to 20 mcg with 5 minutes lock out interval and no background infusion, but if high doses of opiates are anticipated or required a background infusions can be established, with careful monitoring.
Morphine can be used for postoperative pain control following transplant procedures; care must be exercised as accumulation of its metabolite morphine-6 glucuronide (M-6-G) may occur (12)

12. Regional anaesthesia

The use of epidural for renal transplant surgery is rare and controversial; the main reason is that uraemic patients tend to have a tendency to develop coagulopathy.
Few recent studies have shown that it is a safe technique to use as long as prothrombin time (PT) is normal and the patient should have heparin-free dialysis sessions before epidural placement.
Epidural can be used as the sole anaesthetic technique or in combination with GA.
Both techniques were found to have similar encouraging results with respect to early graft function. The level of insertion is usually low thoracic to high lumbar (T12 - L1 or L1 - L2). Local anaesthetic infusion of Levo-Bupivacaine or Ropivacaine can be used safely. (13) Facilities to continuously monitor the neurological status of the patient, and to pick early signs of epidural haematoma should be readily available. (14)

13. DVT Prophylaxis

Intraoperatively TEDS elastic stockings and flowtron boots should be routinely used. Unfractionated Heparin 5000 iu twice daily subcutaneously should be prescribed post-operatively. LMWH are to be avoided, as their metabolic end products are execreted via the kidney and can adversely affect the renal function

14. Conclusion

Kidney transplantation is the only definitive modality of treating ESRF
Patients undergoing transplant procedures present many challenges to the anaesthetist.
Success of transplant is all-dependent on thorough preoperative, close intraoperative monitoring and appropriate fluid management.

The anaesthetic technique plays an important role to ensure the immediate success of the graft. (15)

15. Prune Belly syndrome

This is a congenital abnormality mostly occurring in boys, with an incidence of 1 in 30,000 live births, it is of unknown aetiology and has three characteristic features: underdevelopment of the abdominal muscles, undescended testis and abnormalities of the urinary tract (most commonly hydronephrosis and vesico-ureteric reflux). Mortality is as much as 50% before the age of 2 years, depending on the type and severity of the abnormalities. 25-30% of patients develop chronic renal failure, often requiring renal transplantation. This group of patients has several features which could pose problems for the anaesthetist, so anaesthetic management must focus on airway, pulmonary and renal systems. Micrognathia, pulmonary hypoplasia and urinary tract abnormailities should all be evasluated prior to anaesthesia.

16. VATER association

This arises from abnormalities in mesodermal differentiation and is an acronym for Vertebral abnormality, Anal atresia, Trachoe-oesophageal fistula with oEsophageal atresia and Renal dysplasia. Renal failure is a common, there is also an increased frequency of mental retardation and these patients may also have cardiac anomalies such as ASD, VSD and dextrocardia. Anaesthesia for this group of patients must focus on the cardiovascular, respiratory and renal systems.

17. Anaesthesia for Hand-assisted Laparoscopic Donor Nephrectomy

Hand-Assisted laparoscopic donor nephrectomy (HALDN) is a fairly novel technique to harvest the kidney from a live donor.

It is minimally invasive technique compared to the standard open surgical approach.

The donor is a healthy individual, who is usually related to the recipient. He/she can be either ASA grade 1 or 2 (i.e. with a mild systemic illness that does not affect his physiological reserves).

The conduct of anaesthesia in such cases is not different from any other laparoscopic procedure.

The airway should be secured with a re-enforced endotracheal tube.

Position of the patient is the lateral decubitus, with the operating table broken in the middle

The patient should be securely strapped to the table firmly in order to prevent any change to his position during the operation.

Careful positioning needs extra-padding to protect nerves and bony prominences, the upper arm has to be kept in neutral position on an arm support.

18. References

Wolfe RA, Ashby VB, Milford EL, Ojo AO, Ettenger RE, Agodoa LY et al. Comparison of mortality in all patients on dialysis, patients on dialysis awaiting transplantation, and recipients of a first cadaveric transplant. N Engl J Med 1999; 341:1725-30.

Karlberg I, Nyberg G. Cost-effectiveness studies of renal transplantation. Int J Technol Assess Health Care 1995; 11: 611-622.

Heart Outcomes Prevention Evaluation (HOPE) Study Investigators. Effects of an angiotensin -converting enzyme inhibitor, ramipril, on cardiovascular events in high-risk patients. N Engl J Med 2000; 342: 145–53.

Foley RN, Parfrey PS, Harnett JD, Kent GM, Murray DC, Barre PE. Impact of hypertension on cardiomyopathy, morbidity and mortality in end-stage renal disease. Kidney Int 1996; 49: 1379–85.

Norio K, Makisalo H, Isoniemi H, Groop Ph, Pere P, Lidgren L. Are diabetic patients in danger at renal transplantation? An invasive perioperative study. Eur J Anaesthesiol 2000; 17: 729–36.

Hadimioglu N, Saadawy I, Saglam T, Ertug Z, Dinckan A. The effect of different crystalloid solutions on acid-base bal3ance and early kidney function after kidney transplantation. Anesth Analg 2008;107:264-9.3

De Gasperi A, Narcisi S, Mazza E, Bettinelli L, Pavani M, Perrone L et al. Perioperative fluid management in kidney transplantation: is volume overload still mandatory for graft function? Transplant Proc 2006;38:807-9.

Grundmann R, Kindler J, Meider G, Stowe H, Sieberth HG, Pichlmaier H. Dopamine treatment of human cadaver kidney graft recipients: a prospectively randomized trial. Klin Wochenschr 1982; 60:193-7.

Carmellini M, Romagnoli J, Giulianotti PC, Pietrabissa A, Di Stefano R, Rindi P et al. Dopamine lowers the incidence of delayed graft function in transplanted kidney patients treated with cyclosporine A. Transplant Proc 1994; 26:2626-9.

Kadieva VS, Friedman L, Margolius LP, Jackson SA, Morrell DF. The effect of dopamine on graft function in patients undergoing renal transplantation. Anesth Analg 1993; 76: 362-5.

Sandberg J,Tyden G, Groth CG. Low-dose dopamine infusion following cadaveric renal transplantation: no effect on the incidence of ATN. Transplant Proc 1992; 24:357.

Smith I, Walley G, Bridgman S. Omitting fentanyl reduces nausea and vomiting, without increasing pain, after sevoflurane for day surgery. Eur J Anaesthesiol 2008; 25: 790–913. Hammouda GE, Yahya R, Atallah MM (1996) Plasma bupivacaine concentrations following epidural administration in kidney transplant recipients. Reg Anesth 21:308–311

Akpek AE, Kayhan Z, Kaya H, Candan S, Haberal M (1999) Epidural anesthesia for renal transplantation: a preliminary report. Transplant Proc 31:3149–3150

Evans M, Pounder D (1988) Anaesthesia and perioperative management for renal transplantation. In: Farman JV (ed) Trans- plant surgery: anesthesia and perioperative care. Elsevier Science, Netherlands, pp 289–318

3

The History of Kidney Transplantation: Past, Present and Future (with Special References to the Belgian History)

Squifflet Jean-Paul
University of Liege
Belgium

1. Introduction

The history of kidney transplantation is thought to have originated at the early beginning of the previous century with several attempts of Xenografting, and experimental works on vascular sutures (Küss & Bourget, 1992)[1]. But it really started more than 60 years ago with first attempts of deceased donor transplantation (DCD) and the first successful kidney transplantation of homozygote twins in Boston (Toledo-Pereyra et al, 2008)[2]. Belgian surgeons contributed to that field of medicine by performing in the early sixties the first ever organ procurement on a brain dead heart beating donor (DBD) (June 1963) (Squifflet, 2003)[3]. Later on, in the eighties, they published a first series of living unrelated donor (LURD) transplantations, as well as ABO-Incompatible living donor (ABO-Inc LD) transplantations. With the advent of Cyclosporine A, and later other calcineurin inhibitors such as Tacrolimus, with the advent of more potent immunosuppressive drugs (IS), the gap between the number of renal transplant candidates and the number of transplanted recipients was and is continuously increasing in Belgium and most countries. It opened the search for other sources of organs such as donors after cardiac death (DCD) defined with the Maastricht conference and the extended criteria donors (ECD) compared to standard criteria donors (SCD). In Belgium another source of DCD was identified after the promulgation in 2002 of a law on euthanasia. The Belgian example and all its historical measures could help others to fight against organ shortage and its consequences, organ trafficking, commercialization and tourism.

2. The prehistory of transplantation

Already in old civilizations, the Egyptians, the Greeks, the Romans, were dreaming and expecting morphological changes in the structure and behavior of the human body. Old mythologies with their sculptures and art offer many examples such as gods, heroes, sirens, tritons, centaurs which are "prefiguration" of the xenotransplantation era (Küss & Bourget, 1992)[1].

The real transplantation story started with Saints COSMAS and DAMIAN during the fourth century: the extraordinary influence of these physicians extended far beyond the Middle Ages and even into modern times (Squifflet, 2003)[4]. After learning the medical art, these legendary early Christian brothers were said to have earned so much grace through the

Holy Spirit that they were able to banish all diseases from man and beast. Therefore, in the fourth century, they transplanted a Moor's leg to their Sacristan (Fig. 1). In Rome, the healing brothers were venerated, but they were also martyred under Diocletian (Fig. 2) and subsequently canonized. Today, they are acknowledged as the patron Saints of Surgery.

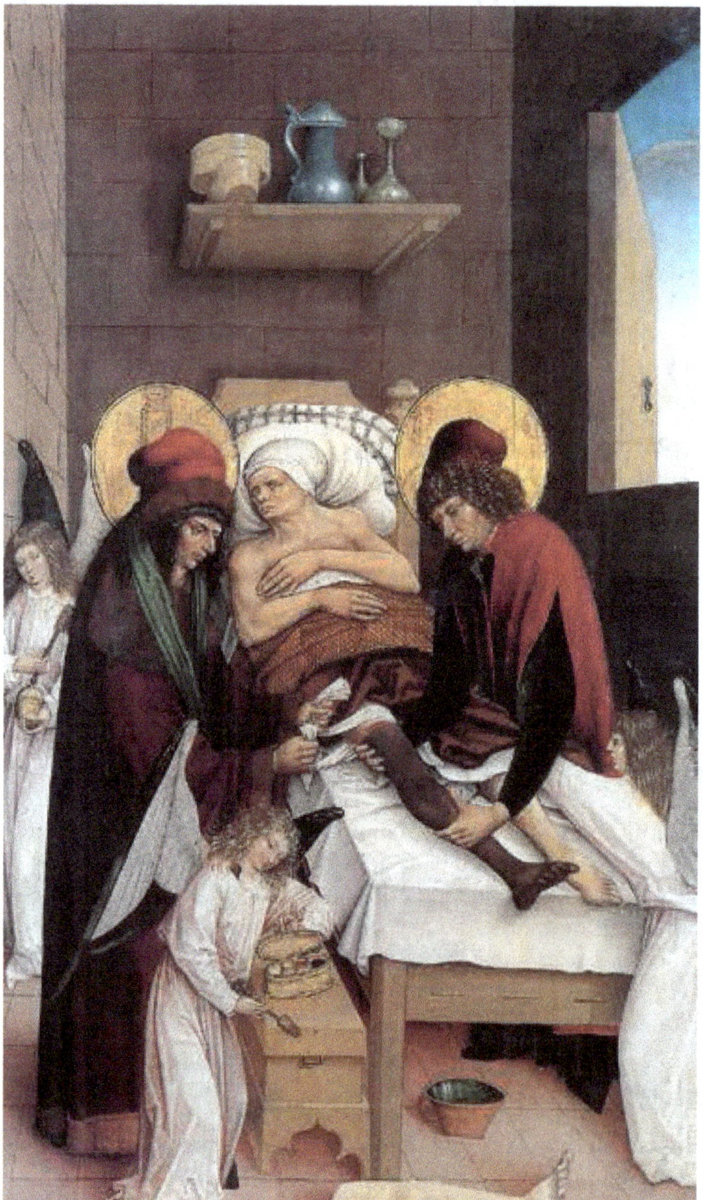

Oil on wood. Wüttembergisches Landesmuseum, Stuttgart, Germany.
Fig. 1. Transplantation of the Moor's leg by the brothers Cosmas and Damian.

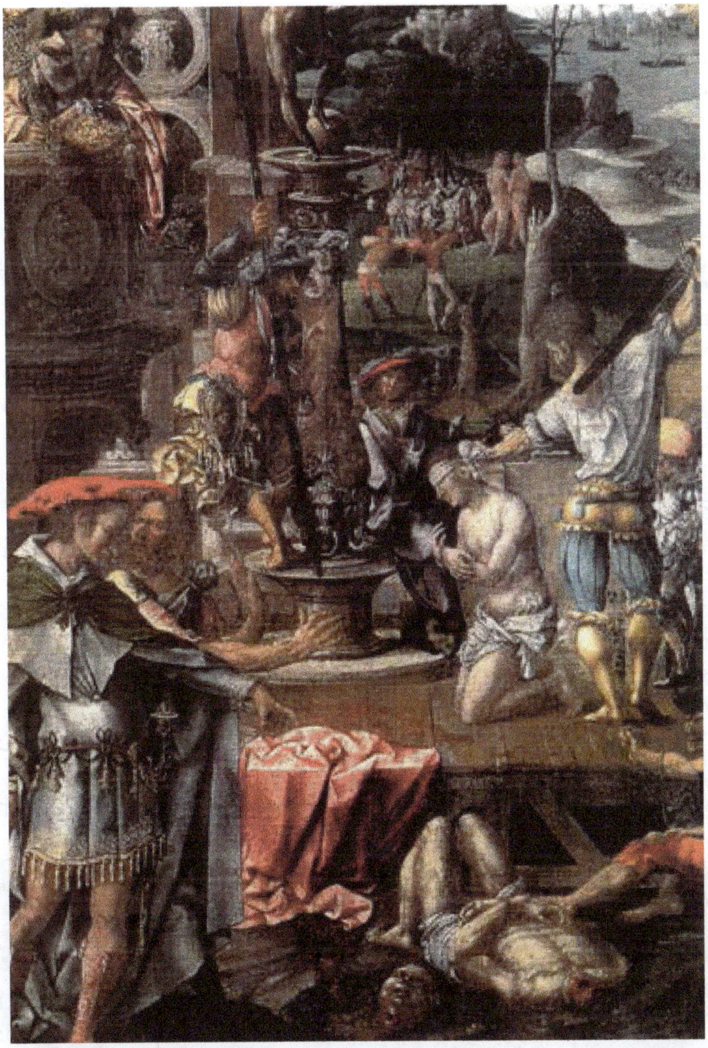

Sint-Jacobskerk, Brugge, Belgium.
Fig. 2. Lancelot Blondeel'stritych on canvas. The martyrdom of the twin brothers Cosmas and Damian.

At the beginning of the twentieth century (Table 1), the kidney became the pilot organ in the field of transplantation development with Emerich Ullmann (Vienna, Austria, 1902) who successfully transplanted a dog kidney into the animal neck. In parallel, the Lyon School with Mathieu Jaboulay described the circular suture of the arteries, a first step towards transplanting in 1906 a pig kidney and shortly after, a goat kidney in the inner elbow of end-stage renal failure patients. Both kidneys rapidly thrombosed, while Mathieu Jaboulay was erroneously blaming his suture technique!

An indelible mark on the pages of the transplantation history was made by one of Jaboulay's pupil, Alexis Carrel who immigrated to the United States and got, later on, the 1912 Nobel price. For vascular sutures, he moved to another technique, the so-called "triangulation" while using and exchanging dog legs in order to prove its efficiency (Fig. 3). Even if the procedure was effective for vascular anastomosis and organ revascularization, Carrel mis-recognized that transplanted organ allografts were not permanently accepted. Indeed he did not recognize the immunological reaction and the existence of the immune system. Nevertheless, his surgical technique for vascular suturing is still valid and persists today, with several modifications introduced for microsurgery like the eccentric biangulation technique proposed by Cobett in the Sixties (Fig. 4) (Squifflet et al. 1993)[5].

Year	Author	Dicovery or application
1902	Ullmann	Dog kidney into the neck
1902	Carrel	Developed vascular anastomotic techniques
1906	Jaboulay	Pig and goat kidneys to the elbow
1909	Unger	En bloc Maccacus kidneys
1912	Carrel	Nobel price
1928	Voronoff	Testis transplantation
1936	Voronoy	First deceased donor kidney transplantation
1951	Küss	Free kidneys from guillotined donors transplanted with surgical techniques still in use today
1952	Hamburger	First use of living related donor kidney (mother to son)
1954	Hume Murray Merril	First transplantation of identical twin kidney (+ first post-transplant pregnancy) (+ TBI: total body irradiation)
1962	Hamburger	Successful transplantations of two living related but non-twin kidney allografts (TBI-Steroids)
1962	Küss	Successful transplantations of two non-related kidney Allografts (TBI-Steroids-6-Mercaptopurine)
1962	to 1964 Remtsma Starzl Hume	Xenograft period: 5 en-bloc kidneys from chimpanzees 6 baboon kidneys and 1 liver 1 baboon kidney (54 Liters of urine)
1963	Starzl	First three attempts at orthotopic liver transplantation in humans 25/27 successful renal transplantations with 6-MP
1966	Kelly Lillehei Barnard	First human pancreas transplantation at the University of Minnesota
1967		First transplantation of a human heart in Cape Town

Table 1. A timeline in organ transplantation.

In 1909, Ernst Unger used en-bloc Macaccus kidneys in humans which rapidly failed, due to the unknown hyperacute vascular rejection. By contrast, the success of dog autografts at the Mayo Clinic in Rochester helped the transplant physicians to suspect the rejection phenomena; it was also the open door for human kidney homografting.

In 1928, Serge Voronoff at the Collège de France in Paris, who was well-known for his monkey to human testis transplantations, was ready to transplant a young girl with renal tuberculosis. The candidate for the organ donation was a murderer condemned to be beheaded, but willing to offer his organs after death. Unfortunately, the Prosecutor of the Republic took a wrong decision and opposed his veto. That's why, only 5 years later, in 1933, another Russian Surgeon, Voronoy, underwent in Kherson, the first ever renal

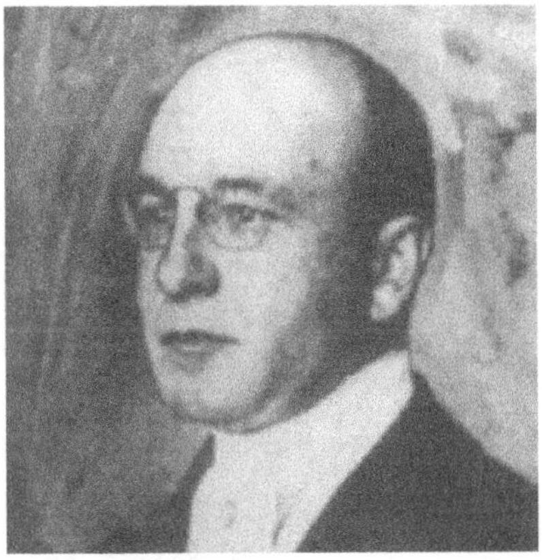

a.

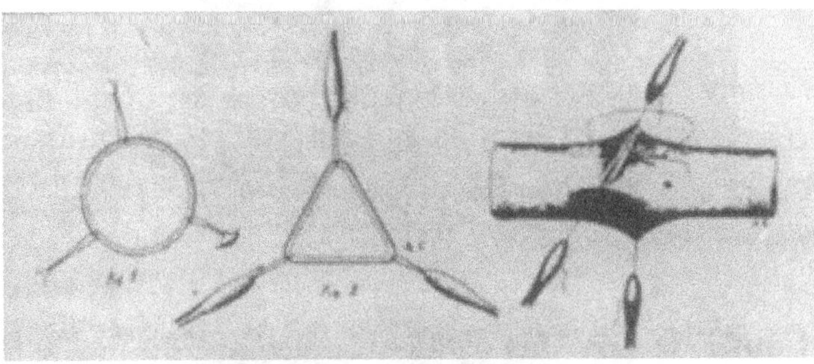

b.

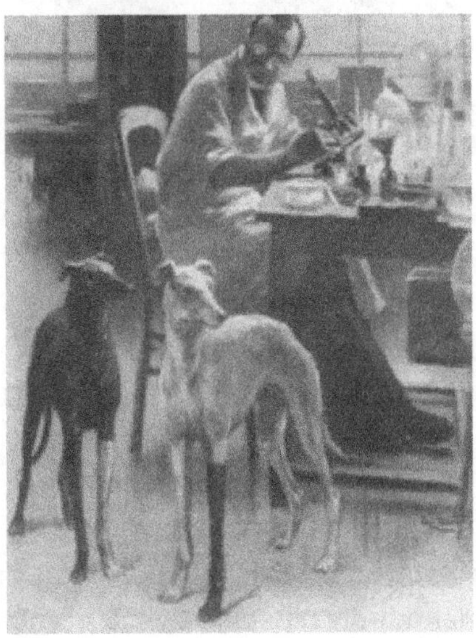

c.

Fig. 3. Alexis Carrel (a) and his surgical technique of vascular sutures (b) exchanging dog legs to prove its efficiency (c). (Küss & Bourget, 1992)[1].

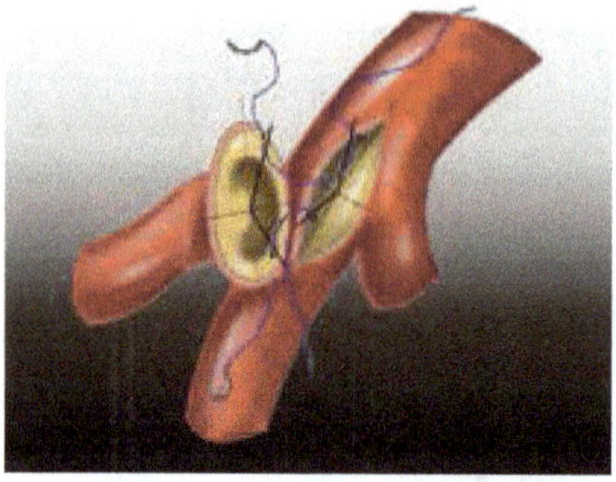

a.

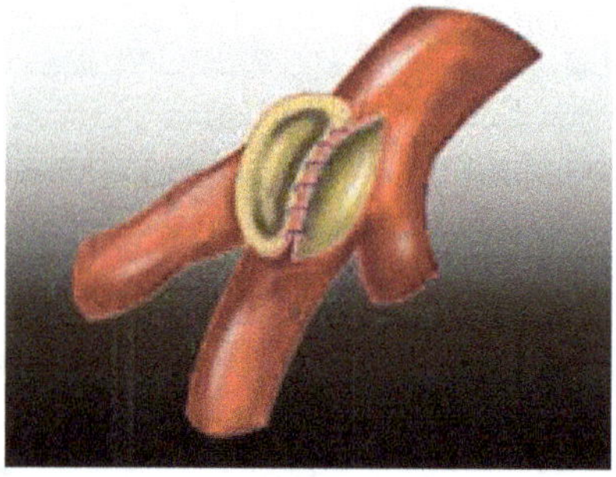

b.

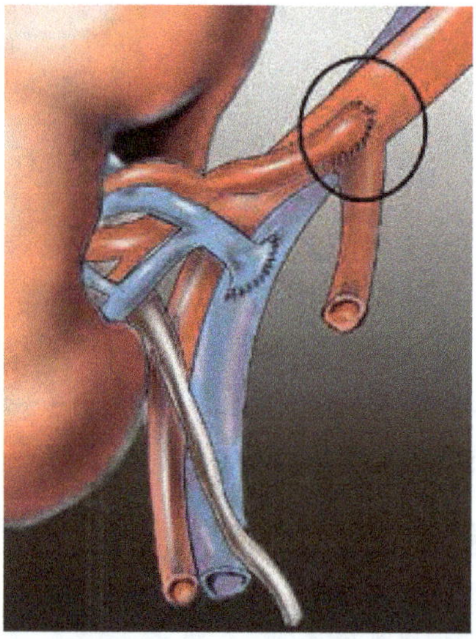

c.

a: two stitches are place on both sides at 1 hour and 11 hour, at 5 hour and 7 hour, in order to correctly tackle the posterior ridge of the vessels, while opening the anterior wall.
b: the posterior running suture is placed from the inside.
c: the anterior running suture.
(Meurisse M., drawings).
Fig. 4. The eccentric biangulation technique for end-to-side vascular anastomosis

homotransplantation in human using a kidney from a deceased–brain trauma, 60-years-old donor (DCD) (Blood group B). The recipient was a 26-years-old woman (Blood group O), who was dying from acute renal failure due to mercury intoxication. The kidney was placed into the groin (Fig. 5). Despite the ABO incompatibility, the urine output remained on 5 ml per hour until PO day 2 while the recipient died on PO day 4 with no vascular thrombosis of graft vessels.

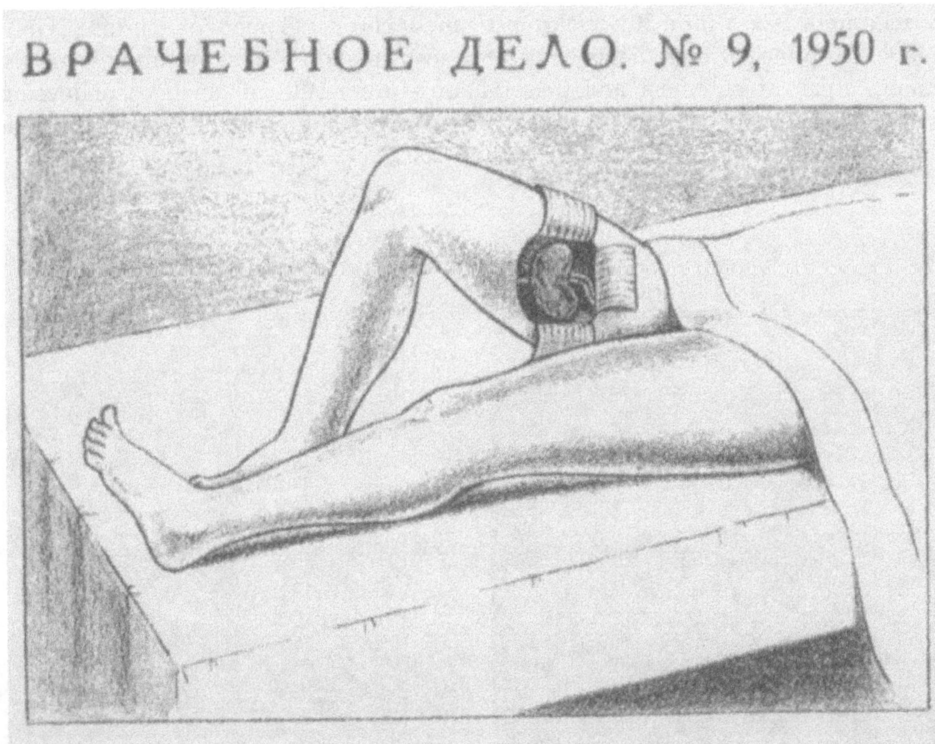

(Küss & Bourget, 1992)[1].

Fig. 5. First renal homotransplantation by Voronoy in 1933. Implantation in the groin of the recipient.

Later on, David Hume in Boston (1947) and Lawler in Chicago (1950), using again DCD kidney did not encounter better success; they used the Voronoy surgical technique for implantation. In 1951, a further and definitive step was taken in the surgical technique of kidney transplantation, by the French School in Paris. Dubost, Œconomos, Servelle and Rougeulle were using kidneys procured in guillotined murderers; Küss, Teinturier and Millez, used also the Matson kidney (nephrectomy of a normal kidney for ventriculo-peritoneal shunt placement to treat hydrocephalia). All kidneys were implanted with the French technique: in the right iliac fossa with vascular anastomosis on the iliac vessels (Fig. 6). That technique was used at the Necker Hospital in Paris on Christmas Eve 1952, to transplant Marius Renard with his mother kidney (Fig. 7). Marius had a single kidney, which had to be removed following a trauma (ladder fall). The mother kidney functioned well without any IS therapy during 3 weeks until rejection occurred, followed by recipient death.

The procedure developed by Küss and the other French surgeons is currently widely used: it inspired Joseph E. Murray, John Merril and their associates at the Peter Bent Brigham Hospital in Boston with their identical monozygotic twin transplantation, which was first attempted two days before Christmas 1954. The US surgeons proved without any IS agents that living renal transplantation could be safely performed for either the recipient who survived eight years, but also, for the donor (Fig. 8) who recently died at the age of 79 years (Murray, 2011)[6]. Following that attempt, other 19 twin transplantations were successfully performed until 1956 with a 30% recurrence rate of chronic glomerulonephritis (CGN). At that time, the principal ingredients of organ transplantation - immunosuppression, tissue matching, organ procurement and preservation - were still unknown or undeveloped. Therefore, the failure of all other types of grafts, usually resulting in the death of the patient, left little room for optimism (Groth & Longmire, 2000)[7].

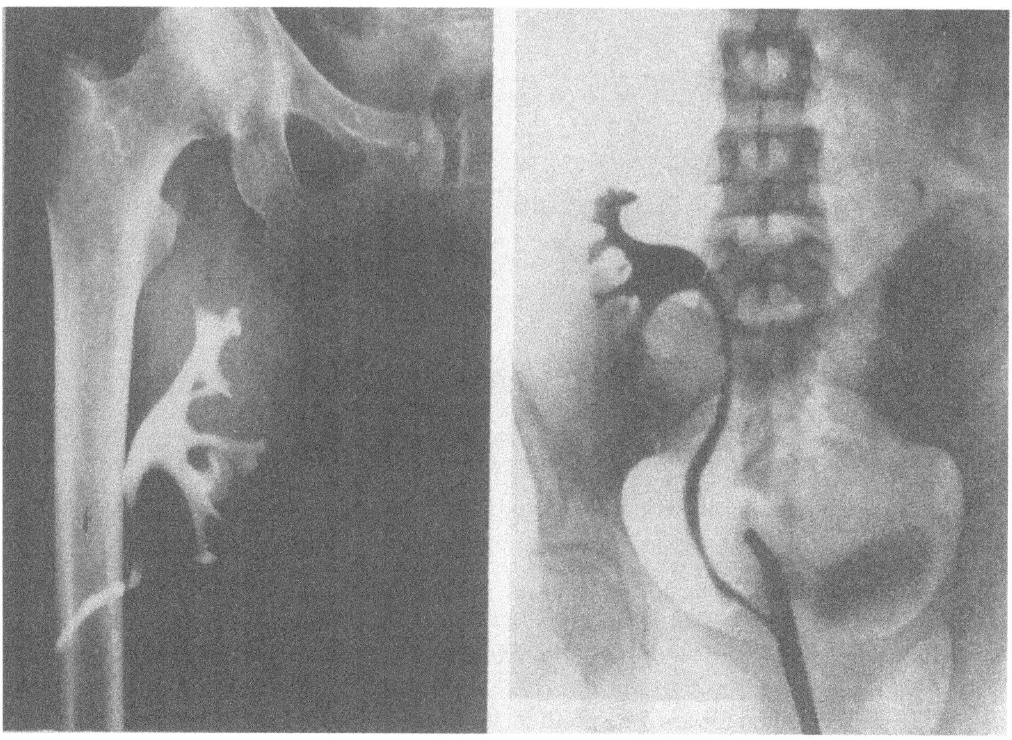

a. b.

(Küss & Bourget, 1992)[1].

Fig. 6. Surgical techniques for kidneys implantation. a. The groin technique (Voronoy). b. The French technique

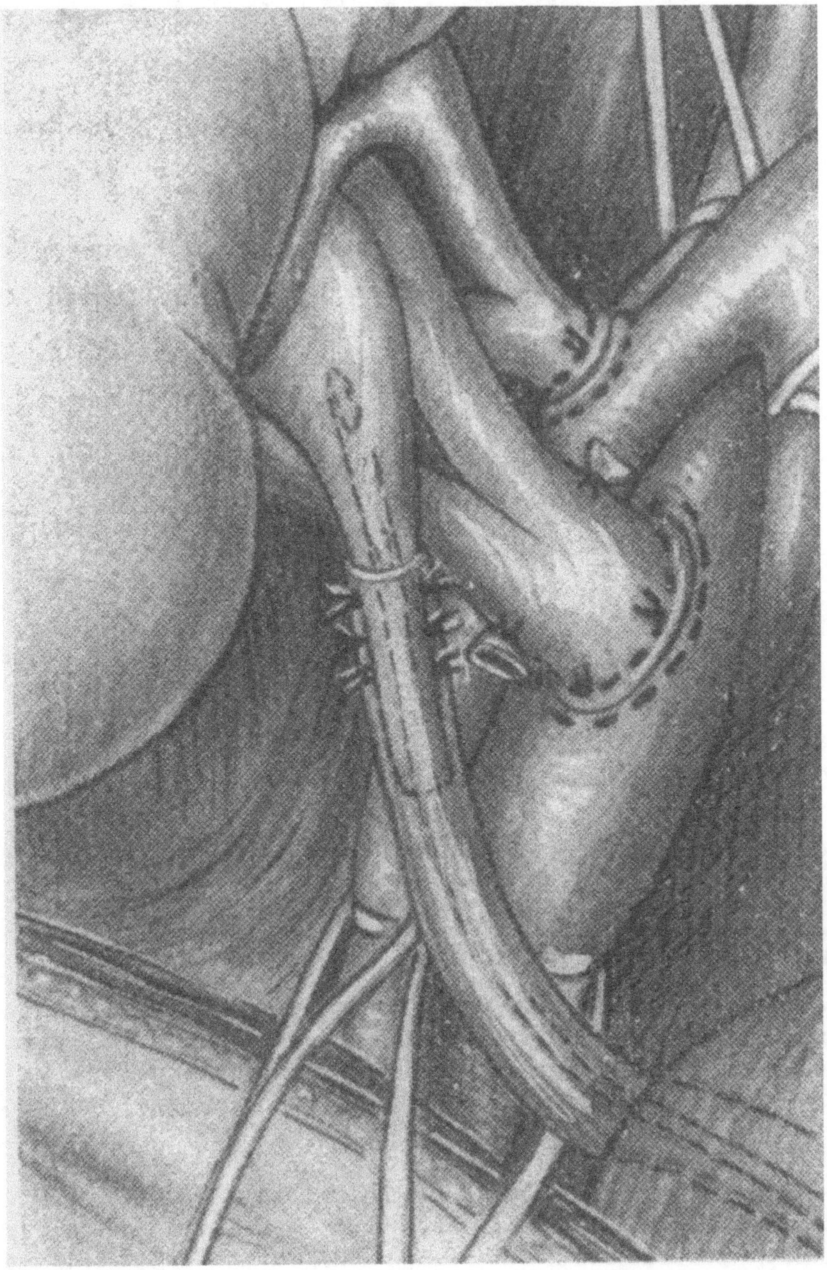

(Küss & Bourget, 1992)[1].

Fig. 7. The French technique used for transplanting Mr. Marius Renard at Necker Hospital (1952).

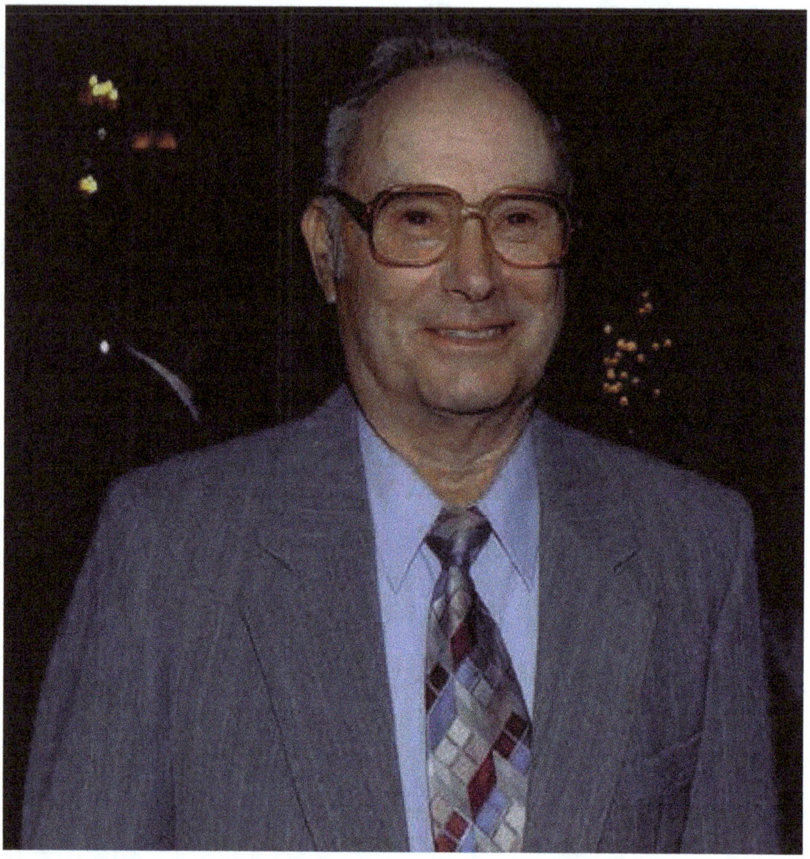

Fig. 8. Ronald Lee Herrick: first living donor for his twin brother, in December 1954 (Murray, 2011)[6].

3. Organ procurement and preservation

The sudden arrival of clinical kidney transplantation during 1962-1963 was so unexpected that little collateral research on the preservation of organs had been done. Kidney transplantation was accomplished at first with total body hypothermia of living volunteer kidney donors using methods developed by cardiac surgeons for open heart operations. In the experimental laboratory, Lillehei et al. simply immersed excised intestine and pancreas in iced saline before its autotransplantation. Thus the principle of hypothermia was understood at an early time, although not efficiently applied (Squifflet et al., 2008)[9].

Today, intravascular cooling is the first step in the preservation of all whole organ grafts. The practice was introduced in 1963 of infusing chilled lactated Ringer's or low-molecular-weight dextran solutions into the renal artery of kidney grafts immediately after their removal. By late 1981, however, it had become obvious that pancreas, liver and thoracic organ transplant procedures were going to be widely used. Methods of multiple organ procurement were required by which the kidneys, pancreas, liver, heart and lungs or various combinations of these organs could be removed without jeopardizing any of the individual organs (Squifflet et al., 1990)[10]. With these methods, all organs to be transplanted are cooled in situ, rapidly removed in a bloodless field, and dissected on a back table (Fig.

9). Fluids of differing osmotic, oncotic, and electrolyte composition are infused into the allografts before placing them in a refrigerated container. The solution described by Collins et al. or modifications of it (Eurocollins®) were used for almost two decades. Renal allograft preservation was feasible for 1 to 2 days, long enough to allow tissue matching and sharing of organs over a wide geographic area (Squifflet et al., 1981)[8]. The introduction of the University of Wisconsin (UW) solution to pancreas, firstly, and then, liver transplantation in 1988 by Belzer, Jamieson and Kalayoglu was the first major development in static preservation since the Collins solution. The superiority of the UW solution for preservation of kidneys and other organs was promptly demonstrated and confirmed in clinical trials.

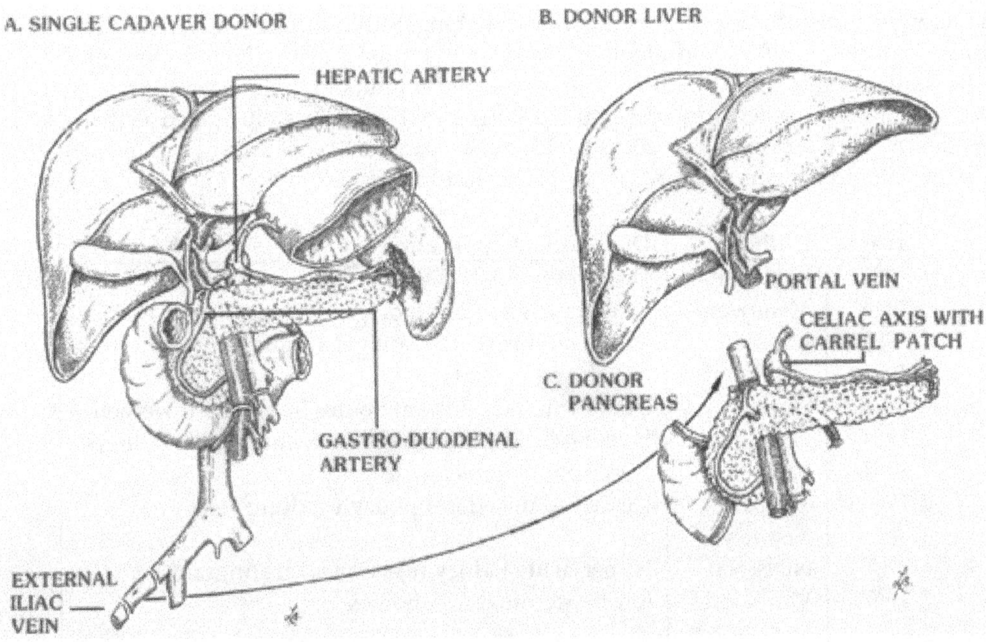

Fig. 9. Maneuvers for en-bloc removal of a whole pancreas and a liver from a cadaver donor with normal vascular anatomy. The gastroduodenal artery must be divided so that the common and proper hepatic arteries can remain in continuity and be retained with the liver. The portal vein is divided just superior to the entrance of the splenic vein. Then, the pancreatic portion is lengthened by an iliac vein graft. The celiac and superior mesenteric arteries can remain with the pancreas with a Carrel aortic patch (Squifflet et al., 1990)[10].

The ex-vivo perfusion technique also permitted good preservation of kidney or liver allografts. However, the complexity of the method precluded its general use. Thus, it was firstly abandoned in most European kidney transplant centers. A renewal of interest in the perfusion technique resulted from the lack of brain-dead cadaveric donors and the search for other sources such as the non-heart beating donors, or extended criteria donors (ECD). In these types of DCD kidneys, agonic ischemic damages are happening. They could be evaluated by a period of re-conditioning on machine perfusion prior to implantation (Moers et al., 2009)[11].

4. The concept of immunosuppression and need for pharmacological agents in transplantation

After Medawar's demonstration in 1944 that rejection was an immunological event, a logical and inevitable question was how to protect the organ allograft by weakening the immune system (Table 2).

Firstly Owen, Medawar and Billingham discovered the phenomena of neonatal tolerance, demonstrating that it was possible to prevent immune responses to allo-antigens. Secondly, works by Dausset and others (Payne, Van Rood, Bodmer, Amos, Ceppellini, Terasaki, Bach and Batchelor) defined what allo-antigens were, namely the major histocompatibility complex (MHC), which in humans is called HLA. Finally, an explosion of information about how the immune system works and further studies on the MHC have led to the concept of tissue typing, histocompatibility and cross-matching. Studies in the early 1960s defined the function of lymphocytes and identified separate roles for T cells (cellular immunity) and B cells (humoral immunity). The T cell receptor and immunoglobulins were discovered, and the role of HLA proteins in presenting antigens to T cells was elucidated (Turka, 2001)[12] (Halloran & Gourishankar, 2001)[13]. Thus, to interfere with that complex reaction, pharmacological agents were introduced for controlling rejection.

Year	Author	Discovery or application
1901	Landsteiner	Discovery of ABO blood groups
1944	Medawar	Rejection as an immunological event
1952	Dausset	Discovered first HLA antigens using antiserum from
1958	Van Rood	transfused patients
1964	Starzl	Demonstrated HLA antibodies in pregnant women
1964	Terasaki	Hyper-acute rejection of ABO-incompatible kidneys
1964	Bach	Description of microcytoxicity test
1966	Terasaki	Described mixed lymphocyte culture test
	Kissmeyer-	
	Nielsen	Hyper-acute kidney rejection with antigraft
1967	Van Rood	lymphocytotoxic antibodies
		First international organ exchange organization
		(Eurotransplant)

Table 2. A timeline in tissue matching and transplant immunology.

Based upon the demonstration in 1950 that inflammatory diseases could be treated by adrenal steroids, it was natural to apply glucocorticoids to prevent or reserve the severe inflammation of graft rejection.

By the late 1950s, the first attempts to use whole body irradiation to prolong transplant survival were also reported (Halloran & Gourishankar, 2001)[13]. But the real IS options that would allow for successful cadaveric transplantation emerged at the end of the 1950s. During that period, Elion and Hitchings developed 6-mercapto-purine (6-MP) and azathioprine (AZA) (Table 3). By the early 1960s, the practice of using glucocorticoids in conjunction with AZA had been initiated with high-dose steroid used to reverse rejection. The first application of antilymphocyte globulin (ALG) took place in the 1960s. Efforts at immune cell depletion included thoracic duct drainage, irradiation, thymectomy and splenectomy.

In 1963, during a first International Transplantation Congress in Washington, 244 renal allografts were reported. Among them, 28 identical twin transplants. Starlz reported also the first three attempts at orthotopic liver transplantation in humans as well as 25 over 27 successful renal transplantations using 6-MP (Table 1).

With the emerging IS therapy, it was also a period in which attempts of xenografting took place and quickly abandoned.

By the late 1970s, the centers that had access to ALG were reporting improved survival rates in kidney transplantation. However, many patients experienced severe steroid side effects. Graft survival remained poor and only kidney transplants were performed in significant numbers with good success (Squifflet et al. 1981)[8].

The discovery of cyclosporine (CsA) and its first clinical use in 1978 changed transplantation. Results also improved with widespread access to effective ALG - polyclonal antibodies (Ab) therapy and later with the first monoclonal Ab therapy muromonab-CD3 - , which can reduce reliance on high-dose steroids. Many improvements in medical, surgical, anesthetic, and intensive care management improved clinical results. The growth in transplanting hearts, livers, pancreases and lungs, has created the transplantation programs of the present day. CsA, which blocks the transcriptional activation of IL-2 and others cytokines in T cells, made a significant contribution to the basic science of T cell activation.

Tacrolimus (Tac) differed from other drugs in that much that its early development occurred in liver transplants, rather than in kidneys. Acting by the same mechanism as CsA, Tac binds to abundant intracellular protein to create a complex that inhibits the enzyme calcineurin. By the late 1980s, Tac was introduced for use in organ transplants. Today, it is the most common and largely used IS drug.

Mycophenolate mofetil (MMF) is an agent derived from the older drug, mycophenolic acid, which is a potent inhibitor of de novo purine synthesis in lymphocytes and highly effective in combination with CsA and Tac in preventing acute rejection in humans.

Rapamycin (or Sirolimus-Sir) had been discovered in the 1970s as an antifungal, but the potential of its IS properties for commercial development was not recognized until the late 1980s. Large-scale trials have demonstrated its potential and have led to its recent approval for use in kidney transplantation (Table 3).

Year	Immunosuppressive milestones
1950	Glucocorticoid therapy in immune diseases
1959	6-mercaptopurine and azathioprine (AZA)
1968	Polyclonal antilymphocyte globulin (ALG)
1978	First clinical use of cyclosporine (CsA)
1981	Introduction of murine monoclonal anti-CD3 to reverse rejection
1989	First clinical results with tacrolimus (Tac)
1991	First report of clinical use of mycophenolate mofetil (MMF)
1998	First report of clinical use of rapamycin (Sirolimus-Sir)

Table 3. A timeline in transplant immunosuppression.

As the third millennium begins, new humanized or chimeric protein products are becoming available (anti-Il2 receptors; anti-CD2; anti-CTL4 Ig; anti-CD3; anti-CD40 ligand; …). Gene therapy and new classes of agents such as FTY720, FK778, peptides and antisense oligonucleotides are currently being evaluated to determine their potential. The new priority is reduction in toxicity with equivalent efficacy. However, immunosuppression would be tailored by better laboratory measurements of the immunological status, ischemic reperfusion injuries, and stability (Halloran & Gourishankar, 2001)[13].

5. The history of Deceased Donor (DCD) transplantation in Belgium

5.1. The first cadaver – Heart Beating Donor (HBD) – kidney transplant in Belgium

In 1962, Professor G.P.J. Alexandre obtained a fellowship for a year of surgical research to be spent in the laboratory of the Harvard Medical School in Boston, under the direction of Professor Joseph Murray, in the Department of Surgery of the Peter Bent Brigham Hospital directed by Professor Francis D. Moore (Squifflet, 2003)[14]. His initial U.S. contact in Boston was with Professor Roy Calne who was packing to return to England, in whom he put his trust to look at the surviving dogs from his experiments. The dogs were receiving the BW - 57322 - the actual Azathioprine (AZA) - as well as other drug combinations including Azaserine and Actinomycin D. The later drug combination was considered good enough to be used in clinical practice (Fig. 10).

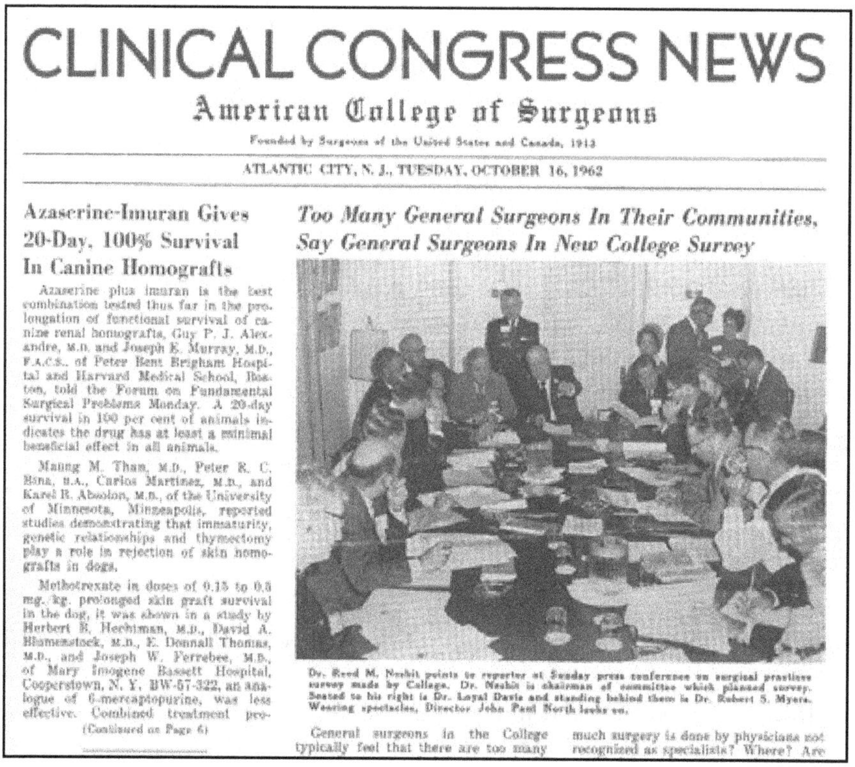
CLINICAL CONGRESS NEWS

American College of Surgeons

Founded by Surgeons of the United States and Canada, 1913

ATLANTIC CITY, N. J., TUESDAY, OCTOBER 16, 1962

Azaserine-Imuran Gives 20-Day, 100% Survival In Canine Homografts

Azaserine plus imuran is the best combination tested thus far in the prolongation of functional survival of canine renal homografts, Guy P. J. Alexandre, M.D. and Joseph E. Murray, M.D., F.A.C.S., of Peter Bent Brigham Hospital and Harvard Medical School, Boston, told the Forum on Fundamental Surgical Problems Monday. A 20-day survival in 100 per cent of animals indicates the drug has at least a minimal beneficial effect in all animals.

Maung M. Than, M.D., Peter R. C. Bina, B.A., Carlos Martinez, M.D., and Karel R. Absolon, M.D., of the University of Minnesota, Minneapolis, reported studies demonstrating that immaturity, genetic relationships and thymectomy play a role in rejection of skin homografts in dogs.

Methotrexate in doses of 0.15 to 0.5 mg./kg. prolonged skin graft survival in the dog, it was shown in a study by Herbert B. Hechtman, M.D., David A. Blumenstock, M.D., E. Donnall Thomas, M.D., and Joseph W. Ferrebee, M.D., of Mary Imogene Bassett Hospital, Cooperstown, N. Y. BW-57-322, an analogue of 6-mercaptopurine, was less effective. Combined treatment pro-

(Continued on Page 6)

Too Many General Surgeons In Their Communities, Say General Surgeons In New College Survey

Dr. Reed M. Nesbit points to reporter at Sunday press conference on surgical practices survey made by College. Dr. Nesbit is chairman of committee which planned survey. Seated to his right is Dr. Loyal Davis and standing behind them is Dr. Robert S. Myers. Wearing spectacles, Director John Paul North looks on.

General surgeons in the College typically feel that there are too many ... much surgery is done by physicians not recognized as specialists? Where? Are

Fig. 10. Proceedings of the Meeting of the American College of Surgeons, Atlantic City, October 16, 1962.

Azathioprine plus Imuran is the best combination tested; a 20-day survival in 100% of animals. Therefore, Professor G.P.J. Alexandre returned to Belgium with both drugs in his luggage. Since no chronic dialysis apparatus was available in the Department of Surgery at Saint Pierre Hospital in Louvain where Professor G.P.J. Alexandre was completing his surgical training, first candidates for renal transplantation were maintained on peritoneal dialysis, performed by medical students on a voluntary basis, in 24-hour rotation.

On June 3, 1963, a patient was brought in the Emergency Department with a head injury and a profound coma. Despite active resuscitation and vasopressive drugs administration, the patient presented all the signs of what Mollaret had previously described and named "coma dépassé" (Mollaret & Goulon)[15]. Professor Jean Morelle, who was the Chief of the Department of Surgery and also experienced in neurosurgery, took the most important decision of his career: to remove a kidney from that patient while the heart was still beating. Moreover, and by contrast to Professor Hamburger's donor management (Legendre & Kreis, 2010)[16], they stopped the mechanical ventilation, immediately after kidney procurement, waiting for the heart beat stop in the OR. No preservation fluid was used; the blood contained in the transplant was not even washed away; the graft functioned immediately without any tubular necrosis (Delayed Graft Function) and the patient's serum creatinine normalized in a few days. The patient died on day 87 from sepsis; at that time of death, three other patients had been transplanted with that effective drug IS regimen. The third patient was transplanted with a living donor kidney (patient's uncle) while the fourth, with a cadaver kidney: both had long term function, more than six years. In this way the kidney transplant program of Professor Alexandre was launched. From then on, the number of transplants performed annually has increased progressively and reached a mean stable number of 100 transplants per year in 1978 when the Department moved to Unit 22 of the Clinic Saint-Luc in Brussels and Professor Jean-Paul Squifflet joined the team. Professor Alexandre left in January 1992 while Professor Squifflet moved to Liege, CHU Sart Tilman in October 2005. From 1963 to 2005, during 42 years, 3.355 renal transplants have been performed (Table 4 and Table 5) (Squifflet J.P., 2007)[17].

Organ	First transplant	Number	
		Total	Live donor
Kidney (Total)	June 3, 1963	3.355	501
Kidney + liver	February 2, 1987	23	
Kidney + heart	February 23, 1986	8	
Pancreas (Total)	November 10, 1982	89	
Pancreas + kidney (SPK)	November 10, 1982	83 (in 82 recipients)	
Pancreas alone (PTA)	February 5, 1983	3	
Pancreas + liver	September 22, 1988	1	
Pancreas after liver	April 4, 1998	1	
Pancreas after failed Kd (SPK)	May 11, 1999	1	
(Islets after kidney)	(October 13, 2002)	(2)	

(Squifflet J.P., 2007)[17].

Table 4. Total number of Organ (Kidney and Pancreas) Transplantations at Saint Pierre Hospital in Louvain (June 3, 1963 to October 30, 1977) and Saint-Luc Hospital in Brussels (November 1, 1977 to September 30, 2005) by G.P.J. Alexandre (June 1963 to October 1991) and J.P. Squifflet (January 1978 to September 30, 2005)

Year	Application
June 3, 1963	First cadaver kidney transplant First heart beating donor First use of AZA and steroids
August 24, 1963	First living related donor renal transplant
January 20, 1965	First haemodialysis
January 20, 1966	First living unrelated donor renal transplant with thoracic duct
June 10, 1966	drainage preparation
1967	First birth of baby from mother kidney recipient
November 8,	Creation of Eurotransplant Foundation
1967	Use of home-made ALG (antilymphocytic globulins) for rejection
March 31, 1971	treatment
September 1976	First pediatric kidney transplantation
November 1977	Use of Eurocollins solution for kidney preservation
January 1978	Move from Saint Pierre Hospital in Louvain to Unit 22 Saint-Luc
	Hospital in Brussels
June 30, 1978	Induction therapy with ALG vs ATGAM
October 1982	AZA and steroids
November 10,	First ABO-incompatible living related donor transplantation
1982	Introduction of cyclosporine A (CsA)
February 5, 1983	First simultaneous kidney and pancreas transplantation in Belgium
March 1985	First pancreas transplant alone in Belgium
March 1985	Introduction of OKT3 for treating acute rejections
February 23,	Honoris Causa: Professor D.E.R. Sutherland, Professor T. Starzl,
1986	Professor J. Van Rood
June 13, 1986	First simultaneous heart and kidney transplantation
February 2, 1987	Belgian law on organ donation and transplantation (presumed
	consent)
July 15, 1987	First simultaneous liver and kidney transplantation
November 7,	Birth of (the 3rd world) baby girl after SPK transplantation
1989	Introduction of bone marrow infusion after kidney transplantation
September 23,	Introduction of deoxyspergualin in kidney transplantation

1992	First use of LoCD2a/BTI-322/MEDI-507 monoclonal Ab in a human
October 12, 1993	kidney recipient
October 18, 1993	Introduction of mycophenolate mofetil (MMF) in kidney
February 17,	transplantation
1997	Introduction of tacrolimus (Tac) in kidney transplantation
March 2, 1997	First video assisted live donor nephrectomy in Belgium
January 1998	Introduction of sirolimus (Sir) in kidney transplantation
December 1998	Start of the EURO-SPK 001 trial
January 31, 2001	Implementation of N.H.B.D. program
June 25, 2001	Introduction of FTY 720 in kidney transplantation
January 2002	Introduction of FK 778 in kidney transplantation
October 13, 2002	Start of the EURO-SPK 002 trial
	First human islet grafting

Table 5. A timeline of the kidney and pancreas transplantation Program at Saint Pierre Hospital in Louvain (June 3, 1963 to October 30, 1977) and Saint-Luc Hospital in Brussels (November 1, 1977 to September 30, 2005) by G.P.J. Alexandre (June 1963 to October 1991) and J.P. Squifflet (January 1978 to September 30, 2005).

5.2 From the brain death concept to the Belgian law on organ donation and transplantation

In November 1957, Pope Pius XII released an important statement for the Catholic Church: he defined death as the *"complete and definitive separation of the soul and the body"* and distinguished *"human life from the mere life of the organs"*. He stated also that a Christian *"has to accept the necessary treatments to preserve life and health"* but that *"usually this duty...requires only the use of ordinary means"*. The Pope declared furthermore that the treatment of a patient in deep coma without any hope of recovery may be stopped even if this provokes cardiac arrest: *"the interruption of resuscitation attempts is only indirectly the cause of cessation of life"*. For deciding when exactly the soul leaves the body, if it is when the brain is destroyed or when the heart stops beating, the Pontiff avoided to answer the question: *"the answer cannot inferred from any religious or moral principle and from that angle is not within the competence of the church"*. On the contrary, he charged the clinicians *"to give a clear and precise definition of death and the moment of death of a patient who dies in a state of unconsciousness"* (Kinnaert, 2009)[18]. It was also the period during which Mollaret and Goulon proposed the term "coma dépassé" to describe the absence and complete destruction of cerebral functions in order to stop prolonging futile resuscitation (Mollaret & Goulon, 1959)[15]. Even if the concept was admitted in the transplant community, most of the surgeons were waiting for the heart beat stop before starting the procurement (Legendre & Kreis, 2010)[16]. The further step, taken by Professor Alexandre, in disconnecting the body in the OR after the kidney procurement was eventually more difficult to accept. Indeed, even T. Starzl who had performed the first

cadaver liver transplantations in 1963 did not apply it before his participation to the Ciba symposium in London in 1966 on Ethics in Medical Progress (Squifflet 2003)[3] (Kinnaert, 2009)[18], (Ethics in Medical progress, 1966)[19]. The discussions he had with Professor Alexandre illustrate well all doubts that people had during that period.
Alexandre:"*Dr. Gierts spoke about taking organs from a dying person. I would like to make it clear that, in my opinion, there has never been and there never will be any question of taking organs from a dying person who has "non reasonable chance of getting better or resuming consciousness". The question is of taking organs from a dead person, and the point is that I do not accept the cessation of heart beats as the indication of death. We are as much concerned with the preservation of life in a dying person as with the preservation of life in a fœtus: but I think irreversible damage to the central nervous system is an indication of physiological death that permits us to take an organ from a body that is already a cadaver.*"
Starzl: "*Dr. Giertz has drawn a distinction between the Stockholm case and the practice in Belgium which seems to me to be largely quantitative. I assume that when kidneys are removed from "living cadavers" in Louvain, only one organ is removed, so that the patient is not thereby killed. How long did your patients continue to be heart-lung preparations, Dr. Alexandre? Were there any specific differences in the subsequent care of your cases and of the Stockholm patient? The Swedish patient continued to be on the respirator after the kidney was removed. If, in your practice, the respirators is turned off immediately after the kidney is removed this could very easily explain the different survival times of less than one hour in Belgium, and 48 hours in Stockholm.*"
Alexandre: "*In our nine cases we switched off the respirator immediately after the kidneys were removed. The heart beats of all the patients ceased within two or three minutes. In my opinion it is irrelevant whether a heart-lung preparation goes on for two days or even for weeks: it is still a heart-lung preparation and for us it is still a dead person.*"
Starzl: "*The notion of permitting removal of our organs while we still have a circulation is an important one. Personally I would agree to this for myself, but I could not permit this to be done to a member of my family.*"
Nevertheless, that example was followed by other teams in Belgium and in most countries. In 1968, the French Heath Authorities published the "circulaire Jeanneney" following the Ad Hoc Committee of the Harvard School of Medecine (Ad Hoc Communitie, 1968)[20]. It opened the door for the first world pancreas transplantation by Kelley and Lillehei (1966), the first heart transplantation by Christian Barnard (1967) and the first heart transplantation in France by Cabrol (1968).
In Belgium, the first lung transplantation was performed by Fritz Derom (1968), the first adult liver transplantation by P.J. Kestens (1969) and soon later (1970) in children by J.B. Otte, the first heart transplantation by G. Primo (1973) and the first pancreas transplantation by J.P. Squifflet (1982).
Finally, the Belgian Transplantation community had to wait until June 1986 to get a law on Organ Donation and Transplantation. It includes an opting out system. Indeed, the transplant surgeon cannot start any organ procurement if the donor has expressed opposition at the National Registry, or if opposition is communicated in any way to the surgeon. Until 2007, it has been a soft version of the presumed consent principle because a first degree relative could oppose the procurement. A new step was taken in 2007 by suppressing this possibility and therefore turning the presumed consent principle into a strong version. Other important elements of the Belgian Act are that death is not defined - it could be brain death or cardiac death - but must be reported by 3 physicians and violent death must be also reported to the Public prosecutor (Squifflet A.C., 2011)[21]. Like other

European countries with presumed consent laws, Belgium was, in 2007 - and is still - , one of the leading countries for Multiple Organ Donors, with 27.5 cadaver donors by million inhabitants (pmi) and 86.5 cadaver organ transplants pmi (43.0 kidneys; 22.7 livers; 8.7 lungs; 6.7 hearts; 5.3 pancreases/islets). As others, Belgium is also facing challenges such as aging donors, the use of extended criteria donors (ECD) and donors with cerebral bleeding as the main cause of death (Fig. 11) (Roels & Rahmel, 2011) [22]. That's why the Eurotransplant (ET) organization had developed its ET Senior Program (ESP) and the use of non-heart beating donors (NHBD), the so-called deceased after cardiac death donors (DCD) by opposition to the brain death donors (DBD).

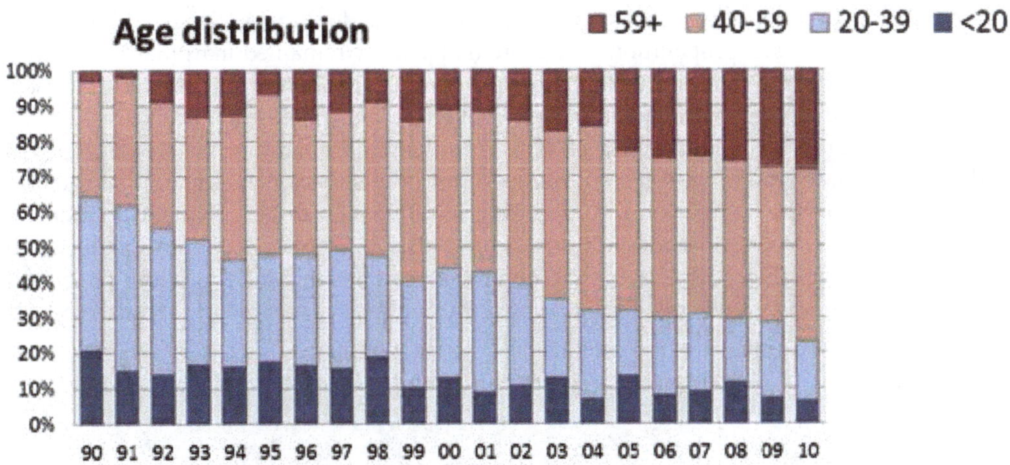

Average age 2010 effective donors: 50 yrs.
Youngest donor: 1 year - Oldest donor: 89 years.
46% women/54% men in 2010.
Fig. 11. Age distribution of (effective) donors between 1990 and 2010 in Belgium.

5.3 The first cadaver pancreas transplant in Belgium

Professor J.P. Squifflet joined Professor G.P.J. Alexandre staff in 1978. After a research fellowship in transplantation at the University of Minnesota in Professor J.S. Najarian department, under Professor D.E.R. Sutherland's supervision, he started a program in pancreatic transplantation in Brussels and performed the first Belgian simultaneous pancreas and kidney transplantation (SPK) in November 10, 1986 (Tables 4 and 5). The women recipient was also one of the first who received cyclosporine A (CsA) as the basic drug in the IS regimen. CsA was used at the dose of 14 mg/kg/day, considered today as a toxic dosage but also in combination with low doses of steroids. The second pancreas transplant was a segmental pancreas transplant alone (PTA). It was performed on a diabetic recipient with pre-end-stage renal failure, in January 1983. Unfortunately, it never functioned due to ischemic damage, pancreatitis and vascular thrombosis. It was promptly removed. By contrast, the first patient rapidly recovered from her double operation; that led to a series of 10 SPK procedures in 10 patients using a segment of pancreas anastomosed to a Roux-en-Y loop. SPK patient number 9 was transplanted in January 86 after chronic rejection of a first cadaver kidney graft. One year later, she delivered a baby girl: she was the third woman ever in the world to enjoy a successful pregnancy after pancreas transplantation. Despite her nephrologist's "disapprobation" she gave birth to a second baby boy in December 1990.

On September 22, 1989, with Professor B. de Hemptinne, J.P. Squifflet performed the first simultaneous liver and pancreas transplant on a 34-years-old man with a type 1 diabetes and a cryptogenic liver cirrhosis. One year later, the patient was back on insulin therapy with a well functioning liver graft. He asked for a second cadaveric pancreas graft that he received on April 4, 1998. Unfortunately, it stopped functioning after several months. A high level of anti-islet antibodies was demonstrated, confirming the recurrence of the type 1 diabetes auto-immune disease (Squifflet, 2007)[17].

The human islet program started in October 2002. The program benefited from the Edmonton experience but it did not succeed in reaching insulin independency with only one pancreatic organ for islet preparation. Therefore that activity remained marginal.

While moving the pancreas transplantation program to the University of Liege, a new surgical technique was implemented (De Roover et al., 2007)[23] and developed with mechanical sutures (De Roover et al., 2008)[24]. It consists in implanting the whole pancreas with a duodenal segment, with portal drainage (into the superior mesenteric vein) of the venous effluent of the pancreatic graft and exocrine diversion to the recipient duodenum. The latero-lateral duodeno-duodenostomy could be done using running sutures or mechanical staplers (Fig. 12). The advantage of that new technique is to allow pancreatic graft monitoring, and duodenal mucosa biopsy through serial endoscopy (Squifflet et al., 2008)[11].

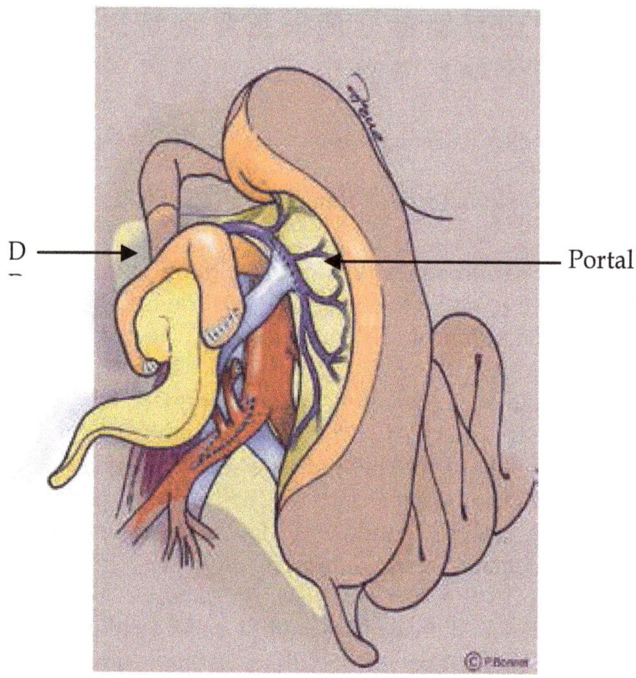

DD: latero-lateral duodeno-duodenal anastomosis.

Portal: portal venous drainage in superior mesenteric vein (De Roover et al., 2007)[23].

Fig. 12. Whole pancreas transplantation technique with enteric drainage and portal drainage.

5.4 Current challenges in Donation after Cardiac Death (DCD)

Like in Austria and Spain which have a huge activity in DBD organ procurement, in Belgium it took almost 40 years to start with DCD organ procurement (Squifflet, 2006)[25]. The main reasons are multiple.

In 1995, the first international workshop on DCD - during that period, one was speaking of Non-Heart-Beating Donors (NHBD) - took place in Maastricht (The Netherlands) where the 4 categories of DCD were defined and published with 12 statements and recommendations (Kootstra et al., 1995)[26]. That was eventually approved by the European Council.

"1. The fact that NHBD organs have to be considered for transplantation is a direct result of the shortage of donor organs in view of the fact that the waiting list continues to increase. The use of NHBD organs can be valuable way to enlarge the number of organs for transplantation.

2. Only sparse data are available on the potential number of NHBDs and the cost of the procedure. More information should be collected to evaluate the efficiency of the procedure.

3. The concept of NHBD is evolving. Therefore, it is important to show that the results are good. Inclusion of NHBD data in registries is necessary.

4. For flush out and preservation methods, one should use solutions that are state of the art. Machine perfusion for kidneys should be considered.

5. No NHBD program should be started without a written protocol approved by the local medical ethical committee.

6. For better understanding and consistency, future reports on analysis concerning procurement and transplantation of NHBD organs should refer to the "Maastricht Categories".

I	*dead on arrival*
II	*unsuccessful resuscitation*
III	*awaiting cardiac arrest*
IV	*cardiac arrest in a brain-dead donor*

7. Category II and III NHBD procedure should only be started 10 minutes after cessation of cardiac massage and artificial ventilation to ensure the "dead-donor rule".

8. Warm ischemia time in NHBDs should be counted from the moment of cardiac arrest until the start of hypothermic flush out, irrespective of the period of cardiopulmonary resuscitation.

9. Better methods for viability testing of NHBD organs should be developed.

10. As in HBD procedures, the diagnosis of death in a NHBD has to me made by (a) physician (s) independent of the procurement team.

11. Public education and openness concerning NHBD are mandatory to keep public trust and to prevent backfiring on the HBD programs.

12. Opting-out or presumed consent systems allow placement of a preservation device before contact with the family. In countries with opting-in legislation, legal approval for placement of such devices should be sought."

Between 1995 and 2003, the Belgian National Council of Physicians established rules for implementing the DCD program according to the local law. Moreover, all 7 transplant centers had to get a formal approval from their own local Ethical Committee.

Finally, it was obvious that such a DCD program could not start without having access to machine perfusion for kidney preservation and re-conditioning. With the help of ET, a large international multicentric study was set up, comparing cold storage and machine perfusion for kidney preservation. In brief, the study demonstrated that 1 year kidney graft survival was 12% higher in recipient of a machine perfused graft which presented a PO delayed graft function (DGF) compared to recipients of a cold storage preserved graft. The length of DGF was also significantly shorter as well as the time for GFR recovery (Moers et al., 2009)[13] (Jochmans et al., 2010)[27]. That study helped the Belgian Centers to implement the use of DCD without jeopardizing the DBD procurement rate (Fig. 13).

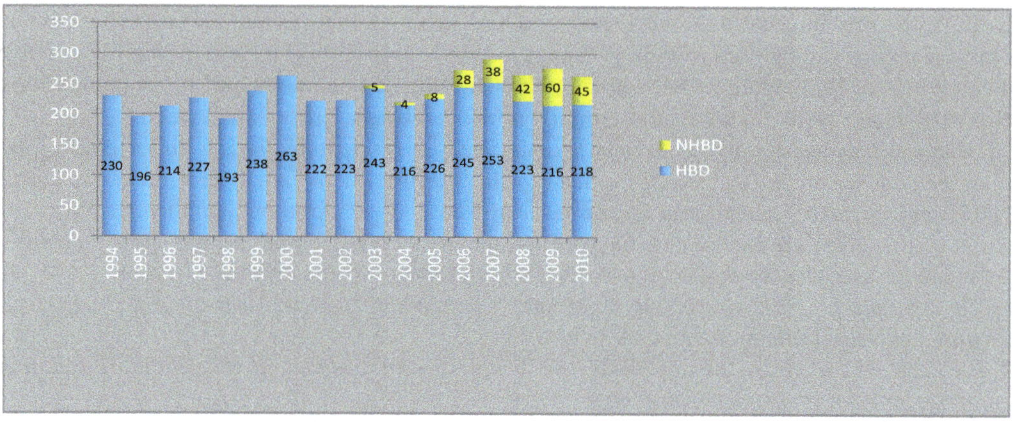

Fig. 13. Effective donor number in Belgium between 1994-2010.
In 2009: 44% University Hospitals - 56% collaborative Hospitals.

At the University of Liege (Le Dinh et al., 2011)[28], the use of DCD had as consequence to double the number of donors (Fig. 14 a), to double the number of kidney transplants (Fig. 14 b), and to 1 ½ time increase the number of liver transplants (Fig. 14 c). But it remains several issues to be solved.

5.4.1 The length of the « no touch » period

The Maastricht statement/recommendation n°7 is proposing a 10 min no-touch period after cessation of cardiac massage for Categories II and III. Indeed Category IV does not need a no-touch period as the cardiac arrest is occurring in a DBD. By contrast, 10 min might be too long if one considers that in categories II and III, the brain has already suffered from irreversible injuries. Then, the Pittsburgh School of Medicine protocol proposes a 2 min waiting time (Institute of Medicine, 1997)[29]. Today, there is a national consensus between all Belgian Centers to declare that a no-touch period of 5 minutes could be enough, but it has not been formally set up yet.

5.4.2 The comfort therapy

Even if intensivists are respecting and protecting all dying patients, they agree to avoid futile sufferances while accompanying the patient in his agonic phase. By contrast, others (Feng S., 2010)[30] think that obstacle against administration of drugs could be the logistics of individual and institutional informed consent for the donor and the potential organ recipients. For the above reason, most intensivists are administering what they call a comfort therapy, while withdrawing the unnecessary support. Therefore improved education of health care professionals and providers on the early recognition and special needs of this DCD population i.e. comfort therapy and implementation of clinical protocol should improve the yield of transplantable organs. Aggressive donor protocols will include early aggressive clinical management of DCD donors including comfort therapy. It requires the help of dedicated health care specialists.

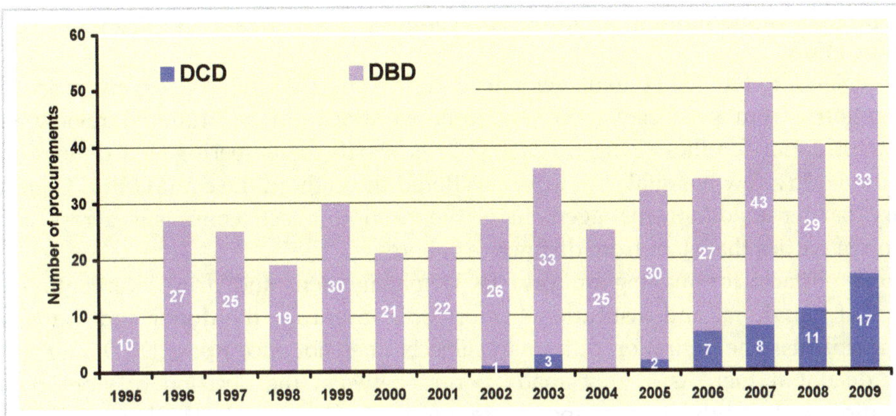

Fig. 14a

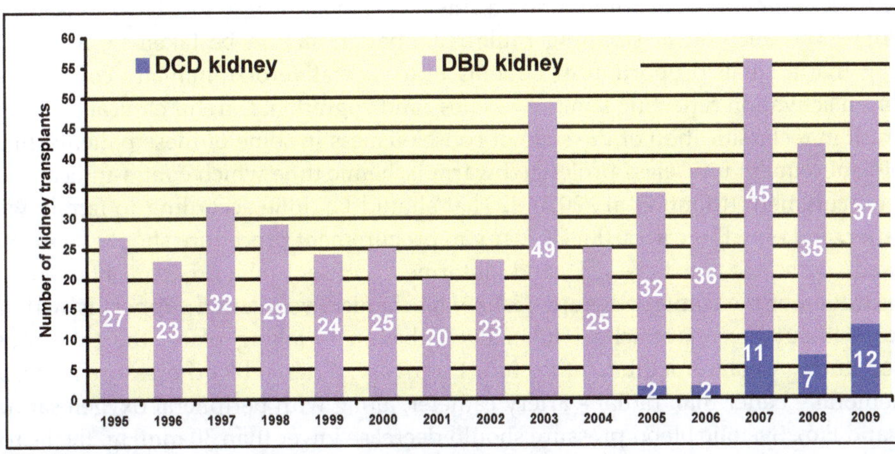

Fig. 14b

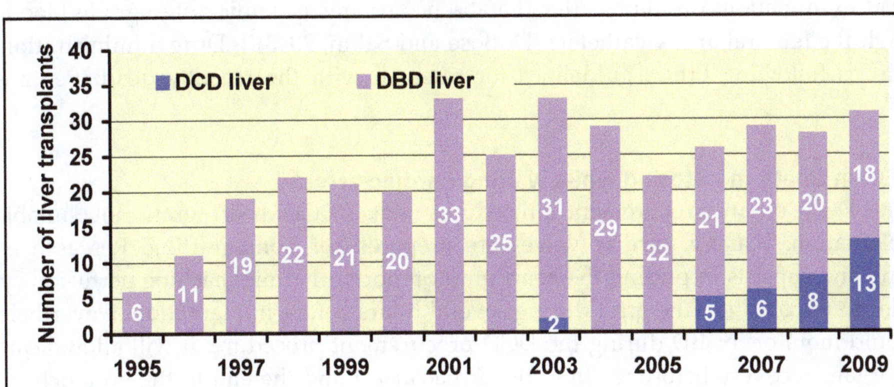

Fig. 14c

Fig. 14. Proportion of DCD/DBD donors (a), kidney (b) and liver (c) transplantations between 1995 and 2009 at the University of Liege (Hieu et al, 2011)[28].

5.4.3 The DCD management: Monitoring awaiting cardiac arrest and drug administration

Unfortunately, today DCD management varies from hospitals to organ procurement organizations, from physicians, nurses, administration and institutional review boards along with donor families (Feng S., 2010)[30]. It is worth remembering that donors are not concentrated in a few hospitals but rather scattered throughout the community. Therefore, a primary barrier to donor management is the need to reach consensus across a broad coalition of parties that stem from distinctive spheres.

A second obstacle for making uniform DCD management and drug intervention is the logistics of individual and institutional informed consent for the donor and the potential organ recipients. The definition of human subjects does not encompass DCD after they are legally dead but there is a grey shade period between the decision of stopping futile reanimation with family consent and the recognition of cardiac death, during which DCD management with drug administration takes an important place. That should require the intervention of independent well trained teams working according to ethical consensus and guidelines. The decision of stopping futile reanimation should be taken by 3 physicians, knowing that a small proportion of patients in a vegetative or minimally conscious state have brain activation reflecting some awareness and cognition. Careful clinical examination will result in reclassification of the state of consciousness in some of these patients, in order to avoid subsequent unuseless prolonged warm ischemic time which contra-indicaties DCD organ procurement (Monti et al., 2010)[31]. That should be done according to family wishes. Thereafter, and only thereafter, the DCD organ procurement procedure should be proposed, discussed with the next-of-skin, and informed consent should be obtained. After administration of the comfort therapy (5.4.2.), mechanical ventilation support is withdrawn with or without the endotracheal tube. If extubation is taking place, the tube must be replaced during organ procurement for lungs recovery. Arterial blood pressure is measured via a femoral - better than radial - artery catheter, along with peripheral oxygen saturation (Spo_2) and Fio_2. Systolic blood pressure should decrease lower than 30 mmHg, the heart rate down to zero, along without any Spo_2 waveform. The patient is pronounced dead by the physical examination 5 minutes after the absence of any systemic anterograde blood flow (through the femoral artery catheter) (DuBose and Salim, 2008)[32]. Drug administration, like heparin, is following Ethics guidelines for research with the recently dead (Pentz et al., 2005)[33].

5.4.4 Brain Death monitoring while waiting cardiac arrest

Current DCD organ procurement procedures make DCD heart graft not suitable for transplantation. Usually, cardiac valves are prepared for homografting. Research is also ongoing and consists in putting the heart graft on normothermic machine perfusion system in order to re-condition the graft during several hours before implantation. Nevertheless, if one could monitor for BD during the DCD procurement procedure, it will allow heart and other organs recovery before waiting for cardiac arrest and the end of the no-touch period, while decreasing the warm ischemic time.

The first attempt to monitor a DCD category III, controlled case for BD was done by J.M. Guerit in 2005, using the somatosensory evoked potentials (Guerit et al., 1999)[34]. By the left median nerve monitoring, he observed the disappearance of the P14 wave, while the dropping blood pressure reached the 51/27 mmHg value (Fig. 15).

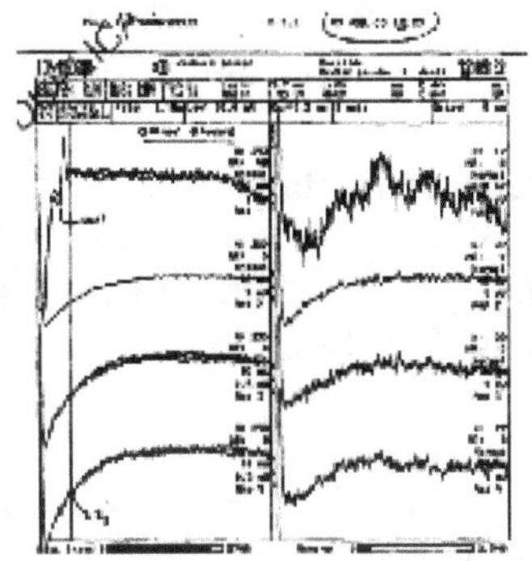

Fig. 15. The brain death (BD) monitoring during the DCD organ procurement procedure (Guerit, 2006)[36]. Disappearance of the P14 wave of somatosensory (left median nerve) evoked potentials with dropping blood pressure.

Another tool, proposed by Auyong et al. is following the bisprectal index (BIS). They presented a case series of increased BIS values during DCD procedure. If these increased BIS values could be a consequence of the catecholamic storm, which could represent a new monitoring tool of BD with the disappearance of BIS. But, limitations of BIS and electroencephelography are well known, the last one being the worst traditionally recommended tool for BD confirmation (Guerit, 2004)[35] (Guerit, 2006)[36]. Nevertheless, if these observed changes were not due to artefact, dosing of hypnotic or anaesthetic drugs might be warranted (Auyong et al., 2010)[37]. Moreover, it will open doors for recovering more DCD organs including hearts for transplantation. But it will need further manipulations to counteract the agonic phase lesions and ischemic injuries, like the intermediate use of machine perfusion for re-conditioning all grafts.

6. The living donor (LD) renal transplantation

The first attempt to LD renal transplantation took place as early as 1962 when no IS drugs were available in Belgium. Indeed, it was a first unrelated LD (LURD) kidney graft which rapidly failed (Kinnaert, 2009)[18]. Soon later, Professor Alexandre was more fortunate in performing living donor renal transplantation (LRD) using the Boston IS regimen. In 1968, he added to the IS armentorium the use of homemade antilymphocyte serum. Horses of the Belgian Police Corps and Army, disqualified for duty, were brought to the Hospital laboratories and injected with thoracic duct lymphocytes. These lymphocytes were being collected from recipients of LD kidneys who, in that period of time, were prepared, during 5 days before the operation, with drainage of the thoracic duct (TDD). After immunization, the horses were bled for extracting the antilymphocyte globulins, for injection into the recipients. Later on, Behringwerke Pharmaceuticals (Germany) took over this preparation known as the Behring horse antihuman ALG (Pressimmum ®) which was still in use until the eighties and from which thousands of patients had benefited. Initially ALG was used to treat steroid resistant acute cellular rejections. Since 1976, it had been used as induction therapy along with Aza and steroids. Moreover in LD recipients, a TDD was added to that protocol along with a per-tranplant splenectomy. In October 1982, CsA was combined to that basic IS regimen: that quadruple drug therapy was the reference treatment for more than 10 years. It allowed using low doses of each IS drug, avoiding toxic side-effects, while hoping an IS synergistic effect (Squifflet et al., 1982)[38]. During the CsA period, for LD transplantation, TDD and splenectomy were abandoned.

6.1 The pediatric renal transplantation

The real advantages of using LD kidneys over DBD during the pre CsA era became obvious with the first results obtained in the pediatric population comparing parental to cadaver donation (Fig. 16) (Squifflet et al., 1981)[39].

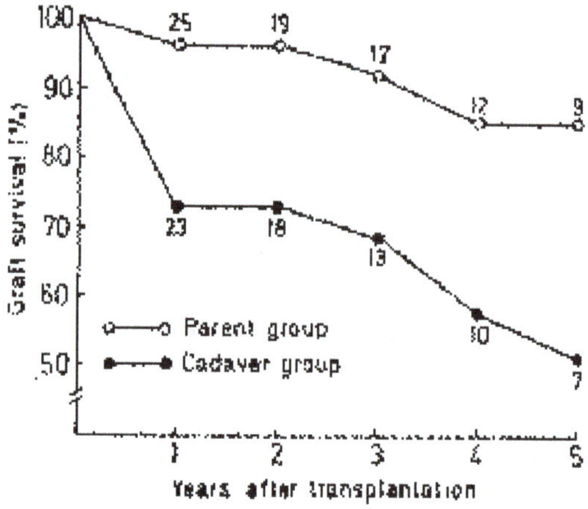

Fig. 16. **Renal Transplantation in Children.**
Graft survival in 32 parental and 35 cadaver graft in pediatric recipients during the pre CsA era (1971-1981). Numbers beside survival curses refer to the number of graft at risk. Difference between the two curses is significant ($P < 0.02$) and reaches > 30% at 5 years (Squifflet et al., 1981)[39].

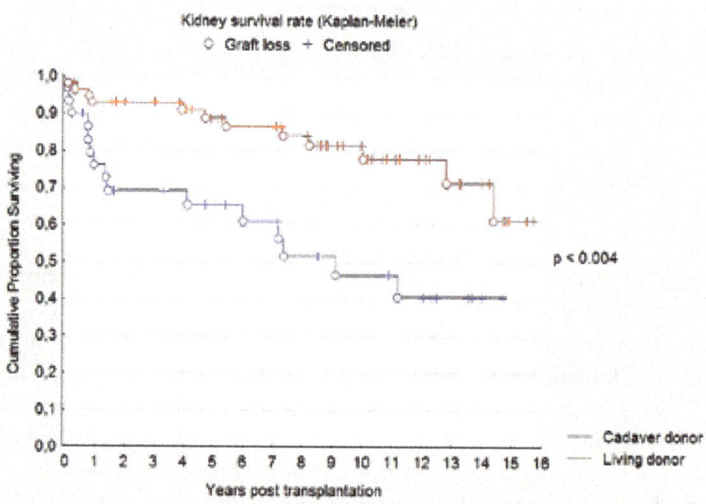

Fig. 17. **Renal Transplantation.** Kidney survival in 56 parental and 26 cadaver graft in pediatric recipients during the CsA era (1983-1994). Difference between the two curves reaches > 30% at 10 years (Malaise et al., 1995)[40].

Twenty years later during the CsA era, that was confirmed in the same pediatric population. Surprisingly, the difference in functional survival rates between the 2 subgroups remained similar but it was more than 30% at 10 years, instead of 5 years (Fig. 17). Even if one year results improved with the CsA use, the slope of the curves were parallel (Malaise et al., 1995)[40].

The children experience underlined the advantages of LD over the DBD renal transplantation. It allows donor selection according to strict medical, serological and anatomical criteria. It insures the quality of the grafts and can help for selection of potential live donors according to the HLA matching (twins, HLA identical siblings, parental...). Moreover the procedure can be programmed without any waiting on dialyse i.e. pre emptive procedure. The recipient can also be prepared by donor specific transfusions and/or pre-transplant IS therapy and/or bone marrow infusion or others. Working in 2 separate operating rooms, it can reduce ischemic injuries with a hemodynamically stable donor. Finally it increases donor self-esteem and the cadaver donor pool.

6.2 The Living Unrelated Renal Transplantation (LURD)

In looking at our LD activity (Table.5 and Fig. 18 a and b) the proportion of LD/DBD was globally 18%, but decreased slowly during the last decade, despite LD promotion.

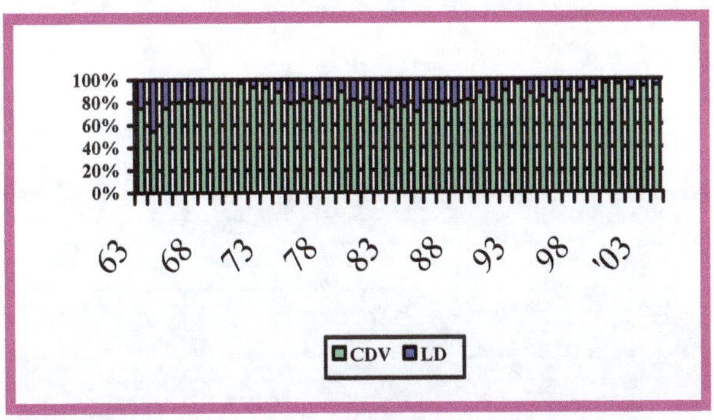

a.

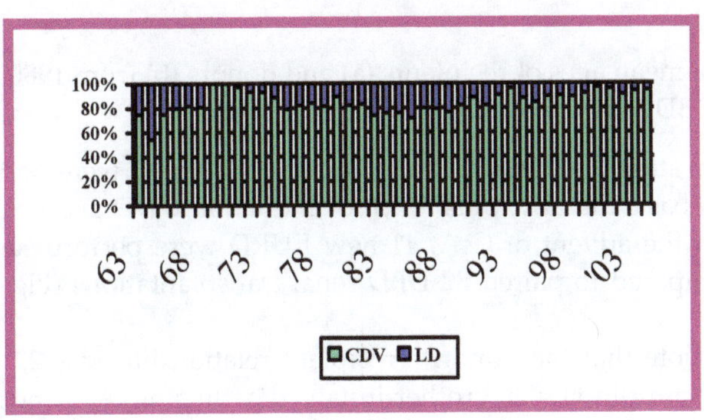

b.

a.: numbers; b.: proportion in %.

Fig. 18. LD/CDV renal transplantation (Prof. G.P.J. Alexandre and J.P. Squifflet activity) from 06/1963 to 12/2004.

The explanation of the phenomena is to be found in looking at mean ages of recipients and donors: for the recipients, it increased from 30 to 50 years and 20 to 40 years for DBD and LD respectively (Fig. 19 a); for the donors, it increased only for DBD from 25 to 40 years but remains stable for LD, around 40 years of age (Fig. 19 b). One can conclude that our selection criteria for the LD did not change over time; for the aging population of recipients, most of their LRD candidates are not fulfilling the donation criteria. Thus, LURD could be another source for renal transplantation; that source in our program, increased slowly over time (Fig. 20).

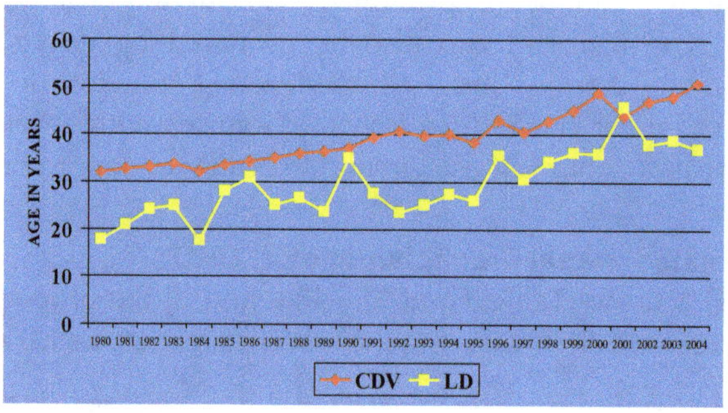

a.

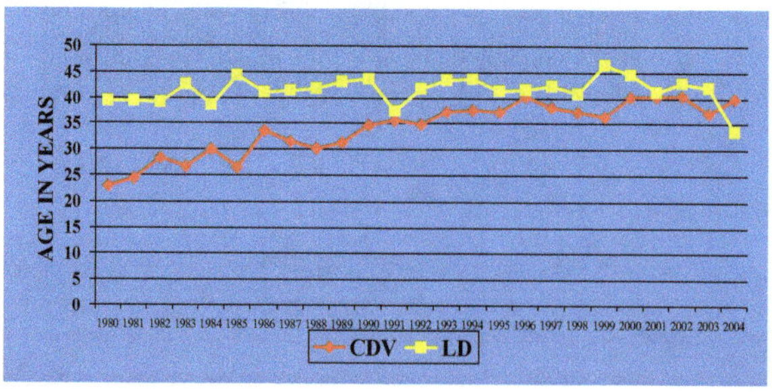

b.

Fig. 19. evolution of mean ages of recipients (a) and donors (b) from 1980 to 2004 according to donor sources: DBD red curves and LD yellow curves.

The LURD program started in 1966. During the pre CsA era, 17 were performed under AZA and Steroids as the basic therapy, plus ALG for induction, TDD and splenectomy (Squifflet et al., 1990)[41]. With the advent of CsA, 41 new LURD were performed between 1983 and 1996, and were compared to paired 82 DBD renal transplantations (Fig. 21) (Malaise et al., 1997)[42].

It is interesting to note that the donor-to-recipient relationship was 22 wife-to-husband, 9 husband-to-wife, 1 aunt-in-law, 1 brother-in-law, 1 wife's niece, 1 mother-in-law, 4 close friends and 2 family's friends. In that series, LURD renal transplantation offered similar results (Fig. 21 a and b) than DBD, despite poorer HLA-A, B and Dr matching and older donor age. The waiting time on dialysis was shorter; early better graft function was encountered in relation to the reduced total ischemia time and better preparation (conditioning) of both donors and recipients. Moreover the video-assisted donor nephrectomy technique introduced for the late cases did not increase the incentive to LD (Berney et al. 2000)[43].

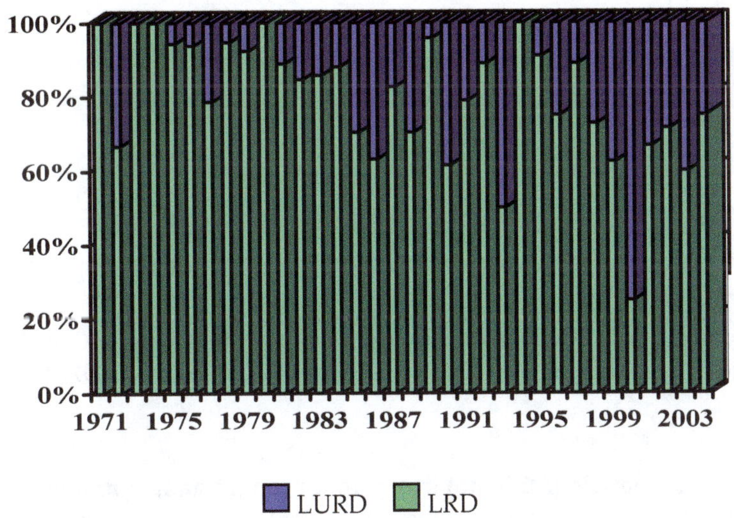

Fig. 20. Proportion LRD/LURD (Squifflet et al., 1990)[41] ; (Malaise et al., 1997)[42].

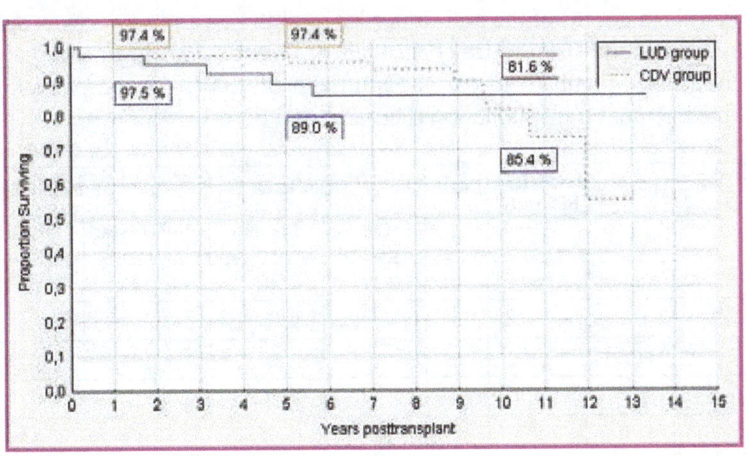

a.

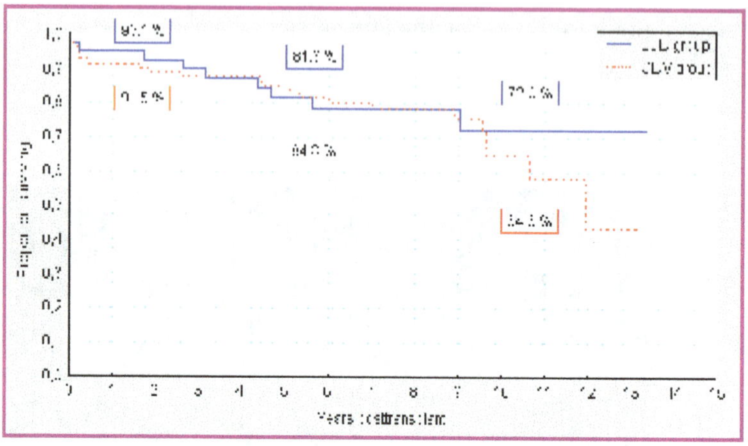

b.

Fig. 21. Comparison of LURD and DBD kidney transplantations under CsA therapy: similar actuarial patient (a.) and renal graft (b.) survival rates (Malaise et al., 1997)[42].

6.3 The ABO-incompatible (ABO-Inc) living donor renal transplantation

Early in 1981, an ABO-Inc cadaver kidney transplant was accidentally performed (blood group A1 into an O recipient). Despite a rejection crisis on the third week with a sharp increase of the anti-A iso-agglutinins, the renal function completely recovered. The patient survived more than 25 years post-transplantation with a functioning kidney graft.

Using a similar approach to that used for achieving ABO-Inc bone marrow transplantation, a series of 39 ABO-Inc live donor kidney transplants (31 related and 8 unrelated donors) was successfully performed (Table 6). The recipients received donor-specific platelet transfusions, 3 to 5 plasmapheresis to get rid of the anti-donor iso-agglutinins and underwent splenectomy at the time of transplantation (Alexandre et al., 1985)[44]. Twenty years graft survival is as high as 76% in the youngest recipients (< 15 years) (Squifflet et al., 2004)[45]. It compares favorably with ABO-compatible LD renal transplantation (Fig. 22 a. and b.).

	N :	Mean age	No RRT Before TP	Death	Graft losses		Functioning graft		
		M ± SD	%		HA Rejection	Chronic Rejection	N :	FU (year) m + sd	Creatinine (mg/dl) m + sd (Median)
Related	**31**	**20 ± 7**	**35**	**0**	**5**	**8**	**18**	**17 ± 3**	**1.9 ± 1.3 (1.5)**
Time to graft loss					11 ± 3 days	9.5 ± 4.8 yrs			
< 15 years	9	11 ± 2	55	0	0	2	7	16 ± 2	1.8 ± 0.6 (1.7)
Time to graft loss						5.5 ± 4.8 yrs			
> 15 years	22	23 ± 6	28	0	5	6	11	18 ± 3	2.0 ± 1.6 (1.4)
Time to graft loss					11 ± 3 days	11 ± 4 yrs			
Unrelated	**8**	**37 ± 9**	**12**	**2**	**4**	**3**	**1**	**20**	**1.0**

Table 6. Outcome of 39 ABO-Inc related and unrelated living donor (LD) kidney transplantations.

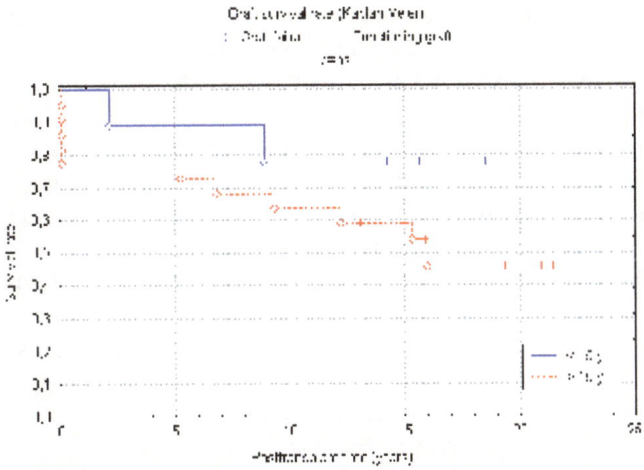

a.

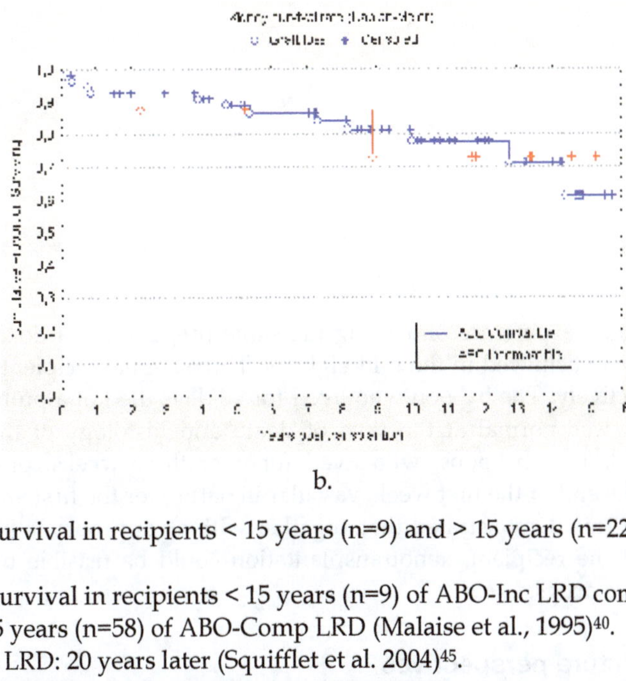

b.

a. Kidney graft survival in recipients < 15 years (n=9) and > 15 years (n=22) of ABO-Inc LRD.
b. Kidney graft survival in recipients < 15 years (n=9) of ABO-Inc LRD compared to a group of recipients < 15 years (n=58) of ABO-Comp LRD (Malaise et al., 1995)[40].
Fig. 22. ABO-Inc LRD: 20 years later (Squifflet et al. 2004)[45].

More surprising is the fact that some patients may carry very high levels of iso-agglutinins with the disappearance of all ABO blood group antigens on the endothelial cells of the transplanted kidney. Later on, Fritz Bach (Bach et al., 1997)[46] proposed the word "accommodation" to name this phenomena; probably there exists a critical period, before the third postoperative week, during which the ABO-Inc transplant is at risk for acute humoral vascular rejection. That is followed by a period of adaptation.
Today, more than 20 years later, each part of the original protocol has been further assessed or modified by different groups. Indeed, plasmapheresis was replaced by immuno adsorption columns. For deleting the last circulating iso-agglutinins, high doses of

intravenous immunoglobulins are communally used. Pre-transplant IS includes Rituximab ®, as well as at the time of transplantation, in order to avoid the splenectomy. In general, the PO IS therapy combines Tacrolimus and Mycophenolate Mofetil with r-ATG induction (Squifflet et al., 2004)[45].

Today, excellent results can be achieved: it is the demonstration that crossing the ABO barrier in LD kidneys transplantation is feasible. The same heavy protocol pertains and can also be applied for hyper immunized recipients with positive crossmatch against potential donors. Others, as well as the Belgian transplant community,

have proposed LD exchange programs (LDEP). Currently, in the Netherlands, that LDEP is very successful in helping numerous pairs of D and R from blood group O, while solving impossibilities (Fig. 23) by incorporating donations from good samaritans.

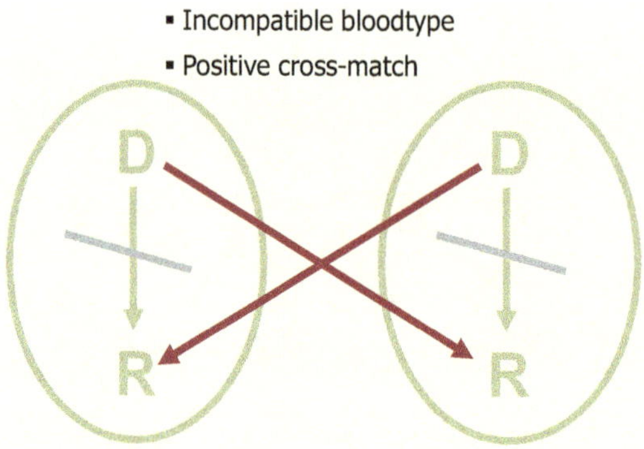

Fig. 23. Solving impossibilities with LDEP.

Based on that human experience and using the same preparation, a dozen pig-to-baboon renal xenografts were achieved in the mid-eighties. Three animal recipients survived 10, 22 and 23 days respectively. The baboon who lived for 10 days died of a pulmonary infection: the renal function was normal at the time of death and histology of the xenograft was remarkably normal. Two baboons, who lived for over three weeks, presented an acute rejection crisis at the end of the first week, vascular in nature for the first animal and cellular in the second one. This demonstrated that, together with an appropriate preparation of the donor animal and the recipient, xenotransplantation could be feasible using new potent immunosuppressive drugs.

7. Present and future perspectives

On May 28, 2002 Belgium adopted the Belgian act on Euthanasia after several months of intensive discussions (Squifflet A.C., 2011)[21]. Euthanasia is described as *'an act on purpose, performed by a third person, in order to end the life of a person who has requested for this act'*. The rules are the following:

The patient must be an adult or an emancipated minor, capable and conscious at the time of his / her request. The request is made voluntarily, is well thought out and reiterated, and is not the result of outside pressure.

The patient is in a hopeless medical condition and complains of constant and unbearable physical or mental pain which cannot be relieved.

If the person is not in the terminal phase of his illness, the 2 doctors must consult with a third doctor, either a psychiatrist or a specialist in the disease concerned.
At least one month must pass between the written request and carrying out the act.
Every euthanasia must be reported to a federal commission that regulate the practice and bring prosecutions when necessary.
Current statistics demonstrate more than 2 acts per day in Belgium and 7 per day in the Netherlands (Fig.24).

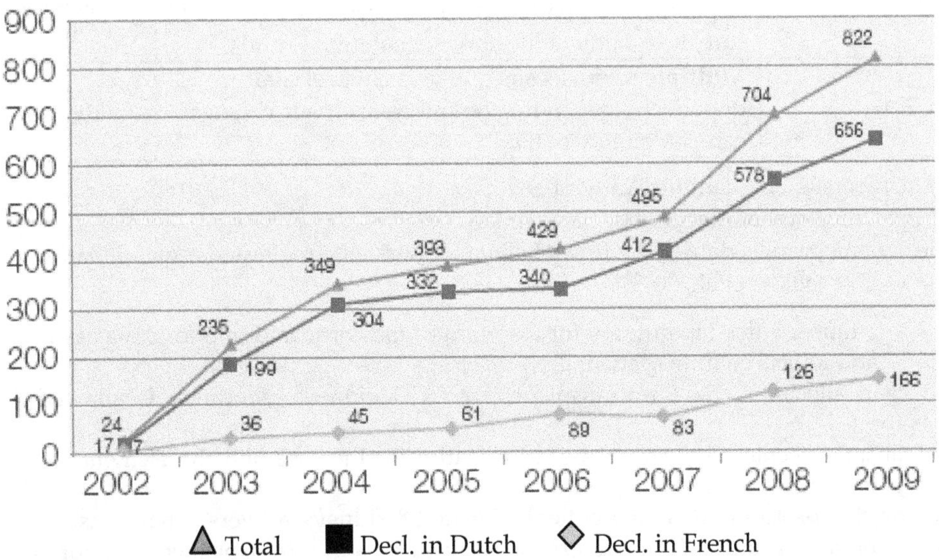

Fig. 24. Annual numbers of legal euthanasia acts in Belgium.

In January 2005, a first woman who was following the procedure of mercy killing asked for organ donation after death (Ysebaert et al., 2009)[47], (Detry et al., 2008)[48]. She was followed by 7 others persons so far. Data concerning the 4 patients are summarised in table 7 and 8 (Ysebaert et al., 2009)[47].
The organ procurement procedure which was adopted after euthanasia was as follow:

- Extensive written informed consent of donor - if possible (see patient 2) - and relatives.
- Strict separation between euthanasia request, euthanasia procedure and organ procurement.
- Euthanasia performed by 2 physicians + neurologist.
- Euthanasia in wheelchair (patients 1, 3, 4) or bed (patient 2), in a special room in the OR, in presence of the family.
- Organ retrieval after <u>clinical</u> diagnosis of cardiac death by 3 physicians.
- Procedures performed by senior staff members and nursing staff on a voluntary basis.
- Euthanasia procedure induced by overdose barbiturates, muscle relaxation and analgesia.
- Heparine given after euthanasia kit.
- The surgical procedure:
  - 3 times femoral vessels cannulation using the DBTL catheter (double balloons triple lumen) followed by a quick laparotomy for topical cooling (patients 1, 3 and 4).

Location	Age	Condition	Date of Euthanasia
1. UZA	44	**CVA** since 6 years, fixed hemliplegia, cortical blindness, special disorientation and dyspraxia.	01/2005
2. U of Lg	43	**CVA** since 4 years, locked-in syndrome, no motor recovery, central hyperthermia episodes, communication only by the eyes.	06/2006
3. UZA	47	**Multiple sclerosis** since 10 years, wheel chair dependent, depending on third parties for personal care, no quality of life, large decubitus wounds.	07/2007
4. UZA	50	**Multiple sclerosis** since 16 years, wheel chair dependent, depending on third parties for personal care, no quality of life.	10/2007

UZA: Universiteit Ziekenhuis Antwerpen
U of Lg: University of Liege, CHU Sart Tilman
Table 7. demographic data of the first 4 Belgian donors who requested organ donation after euthanasia (Ysebaert et al., 2009)[47].

  - 1 time a quick laparotomy for insertion of the aortic and inferior vena cava canule, and topical cooling (patient 2).
- Organ allocation via Eurotransplant (for DCD kidneys, allocation is allowed 4 hrs before).
- Transplant centers informed about the nature of the case and the elements of organ procurement.

Based on that protocol, the first 4 patients donated 8 kidneys, 4 livers, 3 pancreases for islet preparation and 4 lungs. All those organs were successfully transplanted without delayed graft function and need for P.O. dialysis for the kidneys (table 8).

Patient	First warm ischemic times				Outcome			
	Start – Asystoly	Asystoly – Incision	Incision – flush	Total	Kidneys	Liver	Islets	Lungs
1	12′	9′	5′	26′	2	Yes	Yes	No
2	9′	3′	5′	17′	2	Yes	No	No
3	21′	8′	5′	34′	2	Yes	Yes	2
4	6′	5′	3′	14′	2	yes	yes	2

Table 8. First warm ischemic times and outcomes of the organs procured in the first 4 Belgian donors who requested organ donation after euthanasia (Ysebaert et al., 2009)[47].

The potential number of patients asking for euthanasia who fulfilled criteria for organ donation will remain limited and was estimated to be between 5 and 10% (table 9).
That first series demonstrates that organ donation after euthanasia is feasible. It allows respecting strong patient's wish to donate that cannot be denied. The proposed procedure clearly separates euthanasia request, euthanasia procedure and organ procurement. It ensures high quality of DCD organs which might enter in a so-called Fifth Category of Maastricht, of controlled NHBD.
A step further was undertaken by a Pediatric Heart Transplantation team from Denver, Colorado (Boucek et al., 2008)[49] who procured 3 pediatric DCD hearts after a no-touch

	2003	2004	2005	2006	2007	2008	2009
Euthanasia	235	349	393	429	495	704	822
Neuromuscular disorders	22	27	16	33	48	51	58
%	9,5	7,7	4,1	7,6	9,6	7,2	7,0

Table 9. Potential number of patients fulfilling organ donation criteria among Belgian patients requesting euthanasia (Squifflet A.C., 2011)[21].

period of 3, 1.25 and 1.25 minutes. All 3 hearts were successfully transplanted into 3 children. Therefore, the Denver procedure extends the boundaries of organ donation after circulatory death, and perhaps, will require ethical discussions and revisions of the definition of death. Currently the definition of brain death requires the complete absence of all functions of the entire brain (higher-brain definition). The cardiac definition of death requires the irreversible cessation of cardiac function (impossible to reverse). Based on the Denver procedure, the last definition is not valid anymore. It means also, that in DCD organ procurement, with a neuromonitoring of brain death, and adequate analgesic drug management, cessation of cardiac beats could not be waited for, even without any no-touch period. It will also allow heart procurement, reconditioning on artificial device before implantation.

That will necessitate the revision of the dead donor rule and the endorsement of the DCD procedure by separate well trained teams.

The Belgian initiatives in the field of cadaver organ procurement have paid off in terms of number of organs available for allocation. But it remains, like in other countries, that the number of suboptimal organs is increasing for recipients of increasing age and associated morbidities. That will impair the short - and long-term graft and patient outcome.

If there is an urgent need for those centers performing living donor transplantation to turn toward cadaveric organ transplantation, there is also an urgent need for those centers which have DCD programs to turn toward living donor transplantation which offers better results.

Current situation prevails: many persons are willing to offer their organs after death in hoping to help their neighbours. Many patients with end-stage renal disease are turning to live donor kidney transplantation to improve survival and quality of life. Many healthy adults are eager and willing to accept the risk of donor nephrectomy to help their loved ones. Therefore, the responsibility is within the medical community to quantify the risks as best as possible and make the information available to those considering donation. That should be considered and will help for avoiding organ trafficking, tourism and commercialisation in the field of renal transplantation.

8. Acknoledgments

To Professor G.P.J. Alexandre, a pioneer in the field of transplantation
To Professor J. Malaise who initiated most data analysis.
Present address: University of Montreal, Quebec, Canada
Notre Dame Hospital

9. References

Küss R. & Bourget P. (1992). Une histoire illustrée de la greffe d'organes. La grande aventure du siècle. Laboratoires Sandoz, Rueil-Malmaison. ISBN: 2 - 901334 - 05 - 9 France.

Toledo-Pereyra L.H. & Toledo A.H. (2008). History of Living Donor Kidney Transplantation in : Living Donor Organ Transplantation. Gruessner R.W.G. & Benedetti E. (Eds) pp 133-138. The McGraw-Hill Companies. ISBN: 978 - 0 - 07 - 145549 - 7 USA.

Squifflet J.P. (2003). The history of organ transplantation in Belgium 1963-2003. At the honour of the Belgian pioneers in transplantation surgery. Suppl. Acta Chir Belg; 103: 5 - 62.

Squifflet J.P. (2003). From leg transplantation by St Cosmas and St Damian to the Modern Era. Suppl. Acta Chir Belg; 103: 6 - 9.

Squifflet J.P., Sutherland D.E.R., Rynasiewicz J.J., Bentley F.C., Florak G. and Najarian J.S. (1983). Technical aspects of segmental pancreatic grafting in rats. Microsurgery; 4: 61 - 66.

Murray J.E. (2011). Ronald Lee Herrick Memorial: June 15, 1931 - December 27, 2010. Am J of Transplant; 11: 419.

Groth C.G. & Longmir W.P. (2000). Historical landmarks in Clinical Transplantation. World J. Surg; 24: 755 - 843.

Squifflet J.P., Pirson Y., Gianello P., Van Cangh P., and Alexandre G.P.J. (1981). Safe Preservation of human renal cadaver transplants by Euro-Collins Solution up to 50 hours. Transplant Proc; 8: 693 - 696.

Squifflet J.P., Gruessner R.W., and Sutherland D.E.R. (2008). The history of Pancreas Transplantation: Past, Present and Future. Acta Chir Belg; 108: 367 - 378.

10. Squifflet J.P., de Hemptinne B., Gianello P., Balladur P. , Otte J.B., and Alexandre G.P.J. (1990). A new technique for en-bloc liver and pancreas harvesting. Transplant Proc; 22: 2070 - 2071.

Moers C., Smits J., Maathuis M.H., Treckmann J., Van Gelder F., Napieralski B., Van Kasterop M., Van der Heide H.J., Squifflet J.P., Van Heurn E., Kirste G., Rahmel A., Leuvenick H., Paul A., Pirenne J.and Ploeg R. (2009). Machine perfusion or cold storage in deceased donor kidney transplantation. N Engl J Med; 360: 7 - 19.

Turka L.A. (2001). Historical overview of immunobiology and transplantation research. In: Norman and Turka (Eds). Primer on transplantation. American Society of Transplantation National Office. Pages: 1 - 15. ISBN: 0 - 9660150 - 1 - 0

Halloran P.F. & Gourishankar S. (2001). Historical overview of pharmacology immunosuppression. In: Norman and Turka (Eds). Primer on transplantation. American Society of Transplantation National Office. Pages: 73 - 75. ISBN: 0 - 9660150 - 1 - 0

Squifflet J.P. (2003): The History of Transplantation at the Catholic University of Louvain-Belgium. 1963-2003. Suppl Acta Chir Belg; 103: 10 - 20.

Mollaret P. and Goulon M. (1959). Le coma dépassé (Mémoire préliminaire) Rev Neurol ; 101 : 3 - 15

Legendre C. and Kreis H. (2010). A tribute to Jean Hamburger's contribution to organ transplantation. Am J Transplant; 10: 2392 - 2395.

Squifflet J.P. (2007) Pancreas Transplantation at the University of Louvain Saint-Luc Hospital in Brussels (Belgium) and The Euro SPK trial. In: Corry R.J. and Shapiro R. (Eds). Informa Health care USA, Inc - pp 433 - 440. IBSN: 0 - 8247 - 3

Kinnaert P. (2009) Some historical Notes on the diagnosis of death. The Emergence of the Brain Death Concept. Acta Chir Belg; 109: 421 - 428.

Organ transplants: practical possibilities (1966). In: Wolstenholme GEW and O'Connor

M. (Eds). Ethics in medical progress: with special reference in transplantation. CIBA foundation Symposium. Boston, Little Brown. pp 65 - 77.

Ad Hoc Committee of the Harvard Medical Scool (1968). A definition of irreversible coma. J Amer Med Ass; 205: 85 - 8.

Squifflet A.C. (2011). Le cadre juridique belge du prélèvement et de la transplantation d'organes: choix éthiques et résultats pratiques. Ethica Clinica: in Press.

Roels L. and Rahmel A. (2011). Strategies to meet organ shortage. The European experience. Transpl Int; 24: 350 - 367.

De Roover A., Coimbra C., Detry O., Van Kemseka C., Squifflet J.P., Honore P., and Meurisse M. (2007). Pancreas graft drainage in recipient duodenum: preliminary experience. Transplantation; 84: 795 - 7.

De Roover A., Detry O., Coimbra C., Squifflet J.P., Honore P., and Meurisse M. (2008). Exocrine pancreas graft drainage in recipient duodenum through side-to-side duodeno-duodenostomy. Transpl Int; 21: 707.

Squifflet J.P. (2006). Why did it take so long to start a NHBD program in Belgium? Acta Chir Belg; 106: 485 - 488.

Kootstra G. and Loveras J., Ploeg R., Squifflet J.P., Van Der Vliet (1995): Statement on Non-Heart-Beating Donor programs. Transplant Proc; 27: 2965.

Jochmans I., Moers C., Smits J.M. et al. (2010) Renal resistance during machine perfusion is a risk factor for delayed graft function and poorer graft survival. Am J. Transplant ; 10 (suppl 4): 107.

Ledinh H., Meurisse N., Delbouille M.H., Monard J., Hans M.F., Bonvoisin C., Weekers L., Joris J., Kaba A., Damas P., Damas F., Lambermont B., Kohnen L., De Roover A., Honore P., Squifflet J.P., Meurisse M., and Detry O. (2010). Contribution of Donors after Cardiac Death to the Deceased Donor Pool: 2002 to 2009. University of Liege Experience. Transplant Proc; 42: 4369 - 4372.

Institute of Medicine (ed) (1997). Non-Heart-Beating Organ Transplantation: Medical and Ethical Issues in Procurement. In: Washington, DC; National Academy Press; 1997.

Feng S. (2010). Donor intervention and organ preservation: where is the science and what are the obstacles? Mini review. Am J Transplant; 10: 1155 - 1162.

Monti M.M., Vanhaudenhuyse A., Coleman M.R., Boly M., Pickard J.D., Tsibanda L., Owen A.M. and Laureys S. (2010). Willful modulation of brain activity in disorders of consciousness. N Engl J Med; 352: 579 - 89.

DuBose J. and Salim A. 2008; Aggressive Organ Donor Management Protocol. Journal of Intensive Care Medicine; 23: 367 - 375.

Pentz R.D., Cohen C.B., Wicclair M., De Vita M.A., Lederman Flam A., Youngner S.J., Hamric A.B., Mc Cabe M.S., Glover J.J., Kittiko W.J., Kinlaw K., Keller J., Asch A., Kavanagh J.J., and Arap W. (2005). Ethics guidelines for research with the recently dead. Nature Medicine; 11: 1145 - 1149.

Guerit J.M., Fischer C., Facco E., Tinuper P., Murri L., Ronne-Engström E., Nuwer M. (1999). Standards of clinical pratice or EEG and EPs in comatose and unresponsive states. Electroencephalogr Clin Neurophysiol; 52: 117 - 131.

Guerit J.M. (2004). The concept of brain death. In: Machado C., Shewmon D.A. (eds). Brain death and disorders of consciousness. Kluwer Academics, New-York, pp 15 - 22.

Guerit J.M. (2007). Electroencephalography: the worst traditionally recommended tool for brain death confirmation. Intensive Care Med; 33: 9 - 10.

Auyong D.B., Klein S.M., Gan T.J., Roche A.M., Olson D. and Habib A.S. (2010). Processed electroencephalogram during donation after cardiac death. Anesth Analg; 110: 1428 - 1432.

Squifflet J.P., Rynasievicz J., Sutherland D.E.R., Field J., Heil J., and Najarian J.S. (1992). Combined immunosuppressive therapy with Cyclosporin A and Azathioprine: a synergistic effect in three or four experimental models. Transplantation; 34: 315 - 318.

Squifflet J.P., Pirson Y., Van Cangh P., Otte J.B., Van Ypersele de Strihou C., and Alexandre G.P.J. (1981). Renal Transplantation in Children. A comparative study between parental and well-matched cadaveric grafts. Transplantation ; 32: 278 - 282.

Malaise J., Baldi A., Setola P., Mourad M., Pirson Y., and Squifflet J.P. (1995). Renal Transplantation in Children : a comparative study between parental and well-matched cadaver grafts. Br. J. Surg 82, suppl: 128 and Eurosurgery; 5: 261 - 264.

Squifflet J.P., Pirson Y., Poncelet A., Gianello P., and Alexandre G.P.J. (1990). Unrelated living donor kidney transplantation. Transplant Int; 3: 32 - 35.

Malaise J., Mourad M., Besse T., Jamar F., Baldi A., Setola P., De Meyer M., Pirson Y., ans Squifflet J.P. (1997). Living Unrelated Kidney Transplantation. Transplantation Proc ; 29 : 2770 - 2772.

Berney T., Malaise J., Mourad M., Morel P. and Squifflet J.P. (2000). Laparoscopic and open live donor nephrectomy: a cost/benefit study. Transplant Int ; 13: 35 - 40.

Alexandre G.P.J., Squifflet J.P., De Bruyere M., Latinne D., Moriau M., Ikabu N. (1985). Splenectomy as a prerequisite for successful human ABO-incompatible renal Transplantation. Transplant Proc ; 17: 138 - 143.

Squifflet J.P., De Meyer M., Malaise J., Latinne D., Pirson Y., and Alexandre G.P.J. (2004). Lessons learned from ABO-incompatible living donor kidney transplantation. Clinical and Experimental Transplantation; 2: 208 - 212.

Bach F.H., Ferrant C., Hechenleitner P., Mark W., Koyamada N., Miyatake T. et al. (1997). Accommodation of vascularised xenografts: host Th2 cytokine environment. Nat Med; 3: 196 - 204.

Ysebaert D., Van Beeumen G., De Greef K., Squifflet J.P., Detry O., De Roover A., Delbouille M.H., Van Donink W., Roeyen G., Chapelle T., Bosmans J.L., Van Raemdonck D., Faymonville M.E., Laurey S., Lamy M. and Cras P. (2009). Organ procurement after euthanasia: Belgian experience. Transplant proc; 41: 585 - 6.

Detry O., Laureys S., Faymonville M.E., De Roover A., Squifflet J.P., Lamy M., Meurisse M. (2008). Transpl Int; 21: 915.

Boucek M.M., Mashburn C., Dunn S.M., Frizell R., Edwards L., Pietra B., and Campbell D. (2008). Pediatric Heart Transplantation after declaration of cardiocirculatory death. N Engl J Med; 359: 669 - 675; 709 - 714.

4

The Impact of Donor Type and Quality on Renal Transplant Outcomes

Hung Do Nguyen[1], Kenneth Yong[1,2], Rebecca Croke[1] and Wai H Lim[1,2]
[1]*Sir Charles Gairdner Hospital, Department of Renal Medicine, Western Australia*
[2]*University of Western Australia, Western Australia*
Australia

1. Introduction

Renal transplantation improves survival of patients with end-stage kidney disease (ESKD) (Wolfe, McCullough et al. 2009). In most countries, including the United States and Australia, there continues to be a growing disparity between the limited availability of deceased-donor kidneys compared to potential transplant candidates. In contrast, live-donor kidney transplantation has been steadily increasing over time. It has been well established that the type (live or deceased donor kidneys) and quality (donor age and presence of donor comorbidities) of donor kidneys have a significant impact on renal allograft outcomes. In this chapter, we will focus on both live-donor and deceased donor kidney transplantation and the impact of donor factors and types on graft and patient outcomes. With the continuing shortage of deceased donor kidneys coupled with a growing number of older transplant candidates, there has been a greater acceptance of using older donor kidneys, including increased utility of expanded criteria donor (ECD) and donation after cardiac death (DCD) kidneys. We will look at the impact of using ECD and DCD kidneys on graft and patient survival, and to identify modifiable factors that may improve transplant outcomes in recipients receiving ECD and DCD kidneys. Finally, we will discuss whether the implementation of utility-based allocation strategies for deceased donor kidneys is an appropriate way forward to provide a balance between utility and equity in the distribution of deceased donor kidneys.

2. Live-donor kidney transplantation

Since its introduction over 50 years ago, live-donor kidney transplantation is associated with better graft and patient outcomes compared with deceased donor kidney transplantation. The majority of live-related kidney transplantation is from siblings and parents, although spousal donation is becoming increasingly more common. There have been many live donor factors that have been identified which could affect transplant outcomes and this will be discussed in greater details in this chapter.

2.1 Trends In live donor transplantation

Live-donor renal transplantation has increased considerably over time, with some countries like the United States and Australia reporting an increase of at least 50% over the past decade(Horvat, Shariff et al. 2009). Even in countries without a deceased donor renal transplant program such as the Middle East and Asia, live-donor renal transplantation continues to grow substantially(Ghods and Savaj 2006; Horvat, Shariff et al. 2009). It is currently estimated that live-donor renal transplantation accounts for over 40% of total renal transplant numbers worldwide. According to the Australia and New Zealand Dialysis and Transplant (ANZDATA) Registry report, the proportion of live-donor renal transplantation has increased from 31% in 1998 to 44% in 2008 (Figure 1)(Campbell, McDonald et al. 2009). Similar increases have been reported in other countries including Europe and the United States (De Meester 1998; Oosterlee and Rahmel 2008; Horvat, Shariff et al. 2009; US Organ Procurement and Transplantation Network and Scientific Registry of Transplant Recipients 2009; ERA-EDTA Registry 2010).

Within the United States, Europe and Australia, the increased rates of live-donor renal transplantation are directly attributable to growth of live-unrelated donor (LURD) kidney transplants (Oosterlee and Rahmel 2008; Campbell, McDonald et al. 2009; US Organ Procurement and Transplantation Network and Scientific Registry of Transplant Recipients 2009; ERA-EDTA Registry 2010). In Australia, the proportion of LURD has increased substantially from 31% of overall live-donor transplants in 2000 to 50% in 2008. The majority of live-related donor (LRD) kidney transplants are from parental or sibling donors, whereas spousal donation accounts for the majority of LURD transplants. Furthermore, the adoption of laparoscopic donor nephrectomy techniques coupled with low rates of short- and long-term complications of kidney donation has also contributed significantly to the expansion of live-donor transplantation (Bia, Ramos et al. 1995; Schweitzer, Wilson et al. 2000).

Finally, there is greater acceptance of older live-donors over the past decade despite donor age having been shown to affect renal transplant outcomes. In the United States, the proportion of older donors >50 years age has increased by almost 7% between 1999 and 2008, with similar proportional increase in other countries (US Organ Procurement and Transplantation Network and Scientific Registry of Transplant Recipients 2009).

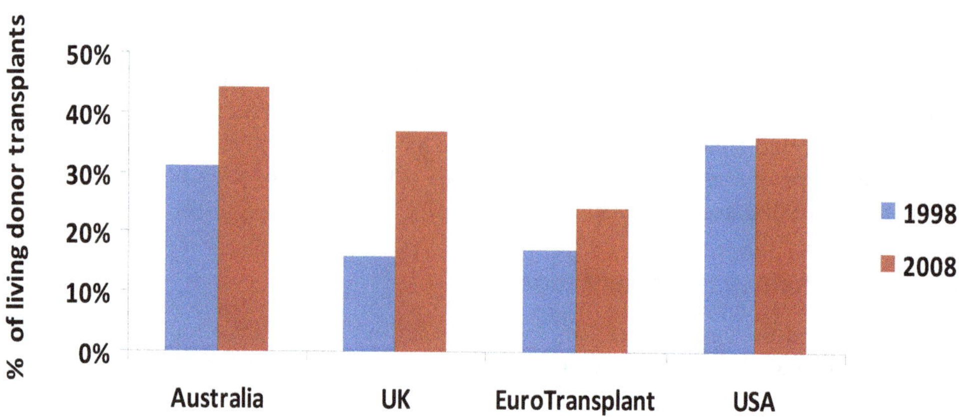

Fig. 1. Living donor transplants as proportion of total transplants.

2.2 Outcome of live compared to deceased-donor kidney transplantation

Live-donor transplantation is associated with superior graft and patient outcomes compared with deceased-donor transplantation (Table 1) (Terasaki, Cecka et al. 1995; Gjertson and Cecka 2000; Campbell, McDonald et al. 2009; US Organ Procurement and Transplantation Network and Scientific Registry of Transplant Recipients 2009). In addition, the introduction of pre-emptive live-donor renal transplantation provides ESKD patients the option of avoiding dialysis (Mange, Joffe et al. 2001; Meier-Kriesche and Kaplan 2002; Liem and Weimar 2009). Finally, it has been established by several large single centre and registry studies that the superior outcomes of live-donor transplantation occur independently of human leukocyte antigen (HLA)-matching and donor or recipient characteristics (Terasaki, Cecka et al. 1995; Gjertson and Cecka 2000; Fuggle, Allen et al. 2010).

Large registry analyses from the United States, Europe and Australia have demonstrated a significant graft and/or patient survival advantage and possibly reduction in rejection risk in pre-emptive live-donor transplants compared to non-pre-emptive live-donor transplants, possibly related to avoidance of dialysis exposure (Donelly, Oman et al. 1995; Mange, Joffe et al. 2001; Milton, Russ et al. 2008). However, one study suggested that short duration of dialysis of <90 days prior to transplant had comparable graft survival to pre-emptive transplant recipients (Milton, Russ et al. 2008). Interestingly, unlike pre-emptive live-donor transplantation, pre-emptive deceased donor transplantation does not appear to be associated with improved graft or patient survival compared to non-pre-emptive deceased donor transplantation (Kessler, Ladriere et al. 2011).

		1 year graft/ patient survival	5 year graft/ patient survival	10 year graft/ patient survival
Australia	Live	96.8%/98.7%	87.5%/94.1%	68.8%/86.7%
	Deceased	91.6%/96.4%	80.8%/89.0%	58.6%/72.6%
United States	Live	95.7%/98.3%	80.4%/90.2%	57.0%/76.5%
	Deceased	90.5%/95.2%	67.3%/80.7%	41.0%/60.6%

Table 1. Unadjusted 1, 5 and 10-year graft and patient survival rates following primary living and deceased donor transplantation in Australia & United States in 2008 (Campbell, McDonald et al. 2009; US Organ Procurement and Transplantation Network and Scientific Registry of Transplant Recipients 2009).

2.3 Effect of donor characteristics on live-donor kidney transplant outcomes

2.3.1 Donor gender

A disproportionately greater number of female donors have been observed in live-donor programs in most countries, including the United States and Australia(Kayler, Meier-Kriesche et al. 2002; Campbell, McDonald et al. 2009). In Australia, female donors accounted for 53% and 62% of overall LRD and LURD donors respectively, the latter likely to reflect the growth in spousal donation (Campbell, McDonald et al. 2009). The reason for the greater proportion of female donors remains unclear although differences in medical (higher rates of cardiovascular disease in men) and psychosocial (financial issues and differing perception towards donation between genders) factors may be contributing (Bloembergen, Port et al. 1996; Schaubel, Stewart et al. 2000; Zimmerman, Donnelly et al. 2000).

In deceased donor kidney transplants, female donors have been shown to be associated with higher rates of rejection, poorer post-transplant graft function and possibly reduced graft and patient survival (Vereerstraeten, Wissing et al. 1999; Zeier, Dohler et al. 2002). In live-donor kidney transplantation, large single centre studies have suggested that female donors are associated with a greater risk of rejection and poorer post-transplant graft function (Oien, Reisaeter et al. 2005; Oien, Reisaeter et al. 2007), but this association has not been observed in large registry analyses (Kayler, Rasmussen et al. 2003; Lim, Chang et al. 2007). The failure to account for differences in donor-recipient body mass in these studies may in part explain the conflicting results between studies. It is plausible that the inverse association between female donors and post-transplant graft function may be attributed to 'inadequate' nephron mass from smaller female donors into larger male recipients with subsequent hyperfiltration injury and decline in renal function (Brenner, Cohen et al. 1992; Brenner, Lawler et al. 1996). Supporting this explanation, *Poggio et al* demonstrated that donors with larger kidney volume (typically donors with larger body sizes and male donors), as determined by 3D helical computed tomography scanning, were associated with lower rejection risk and improved post-transplant radionuclide glomerular filtration rate (GFR) (Poggio, Hila et al. 2006). However, selective transplantation of donor and recipient pairs based on size-matching remains debatable.

2.3.2 Donor-recipient relationship

A number of large single centre studies and registry analyses including United Network of Organ Sharing (UNOS) and ANZDATA have demonstrated similar graft and patient outcomes between LRD and LURD transplants, even though LURD were more likely to be older donors and often have poorer HLA-matching (Figure 8)(Terasaki, Cecka et al. 1995; Gjertson and Cecka 2000; Humar, Durand et al. 2000; Lim, Chang et al. 2007). Early studies have indicated that husband-to-wife (Terasaki, Cecka et al. 1997; Rosenberg, Jones et al. 2004) and child-to-mother live-donor transplants were associated with an increased risk of rejection and graft failure (Cecka 1995; Mahanty, Cherikh et al. 2001), possibly related to prior exposure to donor HLA antigens during pregnancy (Miles, Schaubel et al. 2008; Fuggle, Allen et al. 2010). In a recent ANZDATA analysis of 1989 primary live-donor renal transplants between 1995 and 2004, *Lim et al* reported that the risk of graft and patient survival was similar between LRD and LURD transplants. In this study, parental donors were associated with an increased risk of acute rejection at 6 months (odds ratio [OR] 1.69, 95% confidence interval [CI] 1.13-2.53) and lower GFR at 1 and 3 years post-transplant, but this did not translate to inferior graft or patient survival (Lim, Chang et al. 2007). In contrast, husband-to-wife and child-to-mother transplants were not associated with poorer graft outcomes in this study. Analysis of the UNOS database suggested that in recipients with genetic-predisposed ESKD such as focal segmental glomerulosclerosis (FSGS), type I diabetes and polycystic kidney disease (PKD), LRD kidney transplants may be associated with poorer graft outcomes compared with LURD transplants but this association remains debatable (Futagawa, Waki et al. 2005).

2.3.3 Expanded-criteria live donors

As with deceased donors, certain live donor characteristics have been identified that may have a significant impact on renal allograft outcomes. The identification of these donor characteristics in the assessment of potential live donor-recipient pairing may help in the selection of the most appropriate live donor to achieve the best graft outcomes. A large retrospective chart review of 264 live donor-recipient pairs transplanted between 1997 and 2003 at Cleveland clinic demonstrated that older donor age ≥45 years (compared with <45 years), donor radionuclide GFR ≤110mL/min (compared with >110mL/min), donor systolic blood pressure ≥120mmHg (compared with <120mmHg) and donor cholesterol ≥200mg/dL (compared with <200mg/dL) were associated with a greater risk of acute rejection, delayed graft function (DGF), poorer post-transplant graft function and/or graft loss at 2 and 3 years post-transplantation in the adjusted model. What was interesting about this study were the additive negative effects of increasing number of donor factors on graft function. In this study, there was no association between donor uric acid, fasting glucose, gender or race and graft outcomes (Issa, Stephany et al. 2007). Other studies have demonstrated a similar strong independent relationship between live donor GFR and post-transplant graft function (Poggio, Hila et al. 2006).

The recent meta-analyses by *Iordanous Y et al* of living expanded criteria kidney donors demonstrated that older live donors were associated with poorer composite outcomes of graft and patient survival compared to younger donors (meta-analysis of 12 studies, 72% vs. 80%, unadjusted relative risk [RR] of survival 0.89, 95% CI 0.83-0.95). However, the association between donor age and survival appeared to diminished over time (1980 - RR 0.79, 95% CI 0.65-0.96 compared to 1990 - RR 0.91, 95% CI 0.85-0.99), possibly related to the use of more potent immunosuppression (Iordanous, Seymour et al. 2009). The relationship between donor hypertension or lipid level and graft outcomes in this study remains unclear. Studies examining the association between donor obesity and donor urinary abnormalities (i.e. presence of proteinuria and/or haematuria pre-donation) are lacking. When examining live donor-recipient age difference, *Ferrari P et al* demonstrated that live donor-recipient pairs with ≥30 years age difference had similar graft and patient outcomes as those with lesser donor-recipient age difference suggesting large discrepancy in donor-recipient age difference should not discourage the decision for transplantation (Ferrari, Lim et al. 2011).

It is important to acknowledge that these are retrospective studies and therefore do not clearly establish causality between live donor factors and renal graft outcomes. Nevertheless, identifying unfavorable live donor characteristics could complement the assessments of recipients in stratifying their post-transplant risk of graft dysfunction or failure.

3. ABO-incompatible and desensitization programs

The complexity of live- and deceased donor transplantation has evolved over the years such that many transplanting centres are performing ABO-incompatible transplants and desensitizing highly allo-sensitized transplant candidates to improve their transplant potential. Other innovative programs that have been established to enhance live-donor transplantation include the paired kidney exchange program (as a strategy to overcome incompatible transplants) and tumour-resected kidney transplant program whereby patients with small renal tumours are considered for kidney donation following radical nephrectomy and resection of renal tumour.

3.1 ABO-incompatible live-donor transplants

Alexandre et al first described transplantation across the blood group barrier in 1987, but there has since been a broad expansion of this program worldwide (Alexandre G 1987). With the greater availability of more potent immunosuppression coupled with the capability to measure isohemagglutinin antibodies, the outcomes of ABO-incompatible live-donor kidney transplantation are comparable to compatible live-donor kidney transplantation (Crew and Ratner 2010). However, there continues to be an early significant risk of antibody-mediated rejection (AMR). The concept of blood group incompatible transplantation involves the removal of isohemagglutinin antibodies (i.e. antibodies formed against blood group antigen A and/or B) to low levels using immunoabsorption technique (ABO antibody-specific) or plasmapheresis (not ABO antibody-specific) thereby avoiding hyperacute rejection following transplantation. Although splenectomy was once considered standard practice pre-blood group incompatible transplantation to prevent early AMR, the introduction of anti-CD20 antibody rituximab has largely eliminated the need for splenectomy achieving equivalent outcomes. However, the need for pre-transplant rituximab remains debatable (Tanabe, Ischida et al. 2009).

Tanabe et al recently reported on the outcome of 800 ABO-incompatible kidney transplants in Japan performed since 1989. The reported 5-year graft and patient survival in this cohort was 79% and 90% respectively (Tanabe K 2007). Acute AMR occurred in up to 30% of transplant recipients resulting in early graft loss in 10% of recipients with refractory AMR (Crew R 2010). Although acute AMR may be treated successfully with further immunoabsorption or plasmapheresis, recipients who develop AMR have poorer graft survival (AMR and no AMR - graft survival of 84% and 100% at 3 years and 49% and 95% at 8 years) and a greater risk of developing transplant glomerulopathy, especially in recipients with concurrent pre-transplant donor specific antibodies (DSA) (Einecke, Sis et al. 2009; Toki, Ishida et al. 2009). Acute AMR is less common after 3 months post-transplant, presumably related to the development of accommodation, a phenomenon of persistent anti-donor antibody in the absence of allograft injury (Dehoux and Gianello 2009).

3.2 ABO-incompatible deceased donor transplants

In 1991, an Organ Procurement Transplant Network (OPTN)/UNOS variance has approved a voluntary national allocation of blood group A2 and A2B deceased donor kidneys into blood group B and O transplant candidates to improve their transplant potential, although this allocation practice had already been adopted into clinical practice by the Midwest Transplant Network since 1986 (Nelson, Shield et al. 2002). As a result of this practice, 31% more blood group B transplant candidates with low anti-A IgG titres received a transplant achieving comparable graft survival as those who had received blood group B kidneys using conventional immunosuppression (10 year graft survival was 72% and 69% respectively) (Bryan, Nelson et al. 2004; Bryan, Winklhofer et al. 2005). Recent analysis of the United States Renal Data System (USRDS) database between 1995 and 2006 demonstrated that blood group O and B recipients (n=238) who had received blood group A2 kidneys had significantly shorter waiting-time compared to blood group compatible transplants (n=149,880). Graft loss and patient survival were similar in blood group A2 to B or O recipients and blood group compatible recipients (Hurst, Sajjad et al. 2010). These favourable reports suggest that this strategy should be considered in allocation programs to enhance the transplant potential of appropriate blood group B and O transplant candidates with low anti-A titres.

3.3 Desensitization of highly-sensitized patients for live-donor transplantation

There is an increasing number of transplant candidates who are allo-sensitized to HLA as a result of previous exposure to HLA antigens, typically following blood transfusions, prior transplantation and pregnancy. The presence of high levels of class I and/or II DSA (i.e. anti-HLA antibodies with reactivity against the potential donor leading to positive complement-dependent cytotoxicity [CDC] cross-match) is associated with poorer graft outcomes, including the development of acute and chronic AMR, transplant glomerulopathy and late graft loss (Eng, Bennett et al. 2008; Gloor, Winters et al. 2010; Eng, Bennett et al. 2011; Mujtaba, Goggins et al. 2011). A study by *LeFaucheur et al* demonstrated that the presence of DSA significantly reduces graft survival rates compared to recipients without DSA (1 year graft survival - 81% and 94% respectively and 8 years graft survival 47% and 78% respectively) (Lefaucheur, Suberbielle-Boissel et al. 2008) (Table 2). In addition, recent study by *Mujtaba M et al* demonstrated that the 3-year graft survival in highly-sensitized patients with lower total DSA (i.e. total mean fluorescent intensity [MFI] of <9500) was 100% compared to 76% in those with higher total DSA (i.e. total MFI >9500; $p = 0.022$) (Mujtaba, Goggins et al. 2011).

Studies reporting the utilization of desensitization technique to allow transplantation in highly-sensitized transplant candidates have focused predominantly on live-donor transplantation, which allows early planning and implementation of treatment at a suitable time. With the greater understanding of HLA antigens and anti-HLA antibodies, innovative techniques have been established to allow live-door transplantation across a 'positive CDC cross-match' barrier. Combinations of rituximab, plasmapheresis and/or intravenous immunoglobulin (IVIg) have been used successfully to desensitize highly allo-sensitized transplant candidates, therefore allowing live-donor transplantation to occur safely (Jordan, Vo et al. 2003; Gloor and Stegall 2010). The typical desensitization regimens involve either a single high dose of IVIg or combination plasmapheresis with low dose IVIg, although the latter may be more effective in achieving a negative CDC cross-match (Gloor, DeGoey et al. 2003; Stegall, Gloor et al. 2006). The addition of rituximab remains debatable and unsubstantiated and splenectomy has largely been eliminated from most desensitization protocols (Locke, Zachary et al. 2007). Current literature indicates that transplantation could safely proceed if DSA intensity is lowered sufficiently to render a negative CDC cross-match and/or an IgG titre of ≤16 by isohemagglutination. Following successful transplantation, ongoing monitoring of DSA and early recognition of AMR is crucial to avoid early graft loss. On re-exposure to donor antigens against which the recipient is sensitized, memory B lymphocytes in their spleen, bone marrow and lymph nodes undergo an amnestic reaction leading to the development of antibody-producing cells, which can produce high levels of DSA within days or weeks suggesting positive cross-match kidney transplantation requires both pre- and post-transplantation interventions to continually suppress DSA levels. Despite advances in desensitization techniques, AMR and transplant glomerulopathy occur in over 30% and 45% respectively in live donor positive cross-match kidney transplantations (Gloor J 2010).

3.4 Desensitization of highly-sensitized patients on deceased donor wait-list

Desensitization of deceased donor transplant wait-list candidates with multiple anti-HLA antibodies to enhance their transplant potential remains debatable due to the uncertain availability of deceased donor kidneys and these patients may remain on the deceased donor transplant wait-list indefinitely (Table 2). *Vo et al* reported the successful transplantation of 6 highly sensitized patients who received deceased donor kidneys following desensitization with IVIg (2g/kg on days 0 and 30) and rituximab (1g on days 7 and 22) over a 4-week period. These patients were on the deceased donor wait-list for 144±89 months (range 60-324 months), but had waited only an additional 5±6 months for a transplant. These patients achieved excellent graft and patient outcomes despite having a greater risk of acute rejection (Vo, Lukovsky et al. 2008). The same group reported an additional 45 successful deceased donor transplants in highly sensitized patients using a similar but modified desensitization approach using one instead of two doses of rituximab. In this cohort, desensitized patients waited for an additional 4.2±4.5 months before receiving a deceased donor graft. Overall graft failure and death at 2 years were 80% and 91% respectively, but almost 30% of graft loss was directly attributed to AMR (Vo, Peng et al. 2010).

	Number of patients	AMR incidence (%)	1-year DCGS (%)	2-year DCGS (%)
Lefaucheur et al (2008)	43	35	89	89
Thielke et al (2009)	51	32	93	81
Magee et al (2008)	28	39	92	89
Gloor et al (2010)	119	41	89	89
Haririan et al (2009)	41	12	90	85
Vo et al (2008)	16	30	94	Not reported
Vo et al (2010)#	76	29	87	84

Table 2. Incidence of antibody mediated rejection (AMR) and death-censored graft survival (DCGS) following positive-crossmatch kidney transplantation. #Stratified by donor type - DCGS at 1 and 2 years for live donor (LD) 90% and 90%; for deceased donor (DD) 82% and 80%.

4. Innovative live-donor programs

4.1 Paired kidney exchange

Blood group or cross-match incompatibility between a potential donor-recipient pair is often a major barrier for kidney transplantation. Paired kidney exchange (PKE), which was first described in 1986 (Rapaport F 1986), circumvents the incompatibility by allowing a live-donor to direct the donated kidney to a different but compatible recipient, with the intent that another donor will donate to the first donor's designated recipient (Delmonico 2004). Most PKE programs involves the use of computer-generated algorithms to create potential donor-recipient pairings using virtual databases containing patient characteristics along with blood group types and degree of sensitization (de Klerk, Keizer et al. 2005). There are several alternatives to the conventional 2-way or 3-way kidney paired donation types, such that an altruistic donor could create a domino paired donation (i.e. kidneys from altruistic donor set off a chain of simultaneous transplants terminating in a donation to a candidate on the deceased donor wait-list) (Gentry, Montgomery et al. 2011). Although overcoming incompatibility remains the primary focus of PKE, donor and recipients pairs may participate in the exchange in the hope of finding a better HLA-matched kidney or younger kidney amongst other reasons. Match rates for incompatible pairs can be as high as 50% (de Klerk M 2006) and as a result can increase transplant activity even in small populations by almost 10% (Ferrari P 2009). Successful PKE programs have been established in the Netherlands, South Korea, United Kingdom, United States and more recently Australia.

4.2 Tumour-resected kidney transplant program

Transplantation of donor kidneys following *ex-vivo* resection of small kidney tumours is a novel source of donor kidneys that was first described in 1995 (Penn I 1995). Although these kidneys are clearly outside the standard criteria for donor kidneys coupled with the small but potential transmission of donor-derived malignancy into recipients, the success of such program in many countries is encouraging.

The largest reported case series of utilizing donor kidneys with small renal cancers comes from Australia. In this single-centre program, 43 patients were transplanted with kidneys removed from patients with <3cm incidentally detected renal cell cancer, majority of which were patients undergoing radical nephrectomy for presumed renal cell cancer. In this program, a vigorous informed consent was undertaken and only older transplant candidates >60 years of age or those with significant comorbidities were eligible to receive these kidneys (Nicol D 2008). In this program, patient survival at 1 and 5 years of recipients of tumour-resected kidney transplants was 92% and 88% respectively, compared to 98% and 74% patient survival for patients on the deceased donor wait-list (n=153) and 99% and 97% patient survival for recipients of LURD renal transplants (n=120; log rank score 10.4, P = 0.005) (Brook, Gibbons et al. 2010). There was one tumour recurrence occurring at 9 years post-transplantation, but it was unclear whether this was donor-derived. An additional 22 similar successful cases from United States and Japan were reported with no documented tumour recurrence (Buell J 2005; Mannami, Mannami et al. 2008).

5. Deceased donor kidney transplantation

There continues to be an enormous disparity between the availability of deceased-donor kidneys and potential recipients. This problem is further exacerbated by a greater acceptance of older ESKD patients for renal replacement therapy. In Australia, acceptance of ESKD patients aged 70-74 years for renal replacement therapy has increased from 390 per million population (pmp) in 2004, to 469 pmp in 2008 (McDonald, Excell et al. 2009). Furthermore, the proportion of potential transplant candidates aged >65 years on the deceased donor wait-list has increased by 21% between 2005 and 2008 (Chadban, McDonald et al. 2006; Campbell, McDonald et al. 2009). The Scientific Registry of Transplant Patients (SRTR) has recorded a similar increase of prevalent potential recipients aged ≥70 years on the deceased donor wait-list, rising from 114 in 1990 to 2544 in 2004 (Rao, Merion et al. 2007). There has been little increase in deceased donor rates worldwide. In Australia, deceased donor rates have remained low at 11 donors pmp in 2009 (10 pmp in 2005), compared to 34 pmp in Spain, 24 pmp in United States and 17 pmp in the United Kingdom (Excell, Hee et al. 2010; Fabre, Murphy et al. 2010). However, there has been an increase in acceptance of older donor kidneys in Australia, with the number of deceased donors aged ≥55 years increasing 1.8-fold between 2001-03 to 2007-09 (Excell, Hee et al. 2010). Kidneys from older donors are associated with poorer graft outcomes including late graft loss, chronic allograft nephropathy and higher risk of cardiovascular mortality (Meier-Kriesche, Cibrik et al. 2002; Oppenheimer, Aljama et al. 2004); this is partially offset by the reduction in mortality associated with reduced wait-list time. In addition, female-to-male donation, major donor kidney weight/recipient weight inadequacy, cerebrovascular accidents (CVA) as the cause of donor death and the presence of donor comorbidities such as diabetes have an adverse impact on graft and/or patient survival (Feldman, Fazio et al. 1996; Giral, Nguyen et al. 2005; Ahmad, Cole et al. 2009; Shaheen, Shaheen et al. 2010). However, utilization of kidneys from deceased donors who had developed acute renal failure prior to organ procurement does not appear to have an unfavorable effect on graft outcome (Deroure, Kamar et al. 2010). A continuous kidney donor risk index has been developed using registry data to quantify expected graft survival for any given set of donor characteristics relative to a healthy 40-year old donor and may be useful as a decision-making tool at the time of the deceased donor kidney offer (Rao, Schaubel et al. 2009). However, the significance of such index in the different transplant eras or population groups remains unclear. In the remaining chapter, we will focus primarily on the use and outcomes of ECD and DCD donor kidneys, which have become important source of deceased donor kidneys over the last decade.

5.1 Expanded-criteria donor (ECD) kidneys (Table 3)

With the ongoing shortage of deceased donor kidneys coupled with the continued growth of potential transplant candidates, there has been an increase utilization of ECD kidneys. Compared with non-ECD kidneys, ECD kidneys are associated with poorer graft outcomes. Between 2005 and 2009 in Australia, there has been a 1.3-fold increase in the number of ECD kidneys (Excell, Hee et al. 2006; Excell, Hee et al. 2010)

In 2002, OPTN/UNOS Board of Directors established a definition of ECD kidneys, which was based on a retrospective review of 29,068 recipients from SRTR database (Port FK 2002). The term ECD kidneys was assigned based on a ≥70% greater risk of developing graft failure when compared to younger donor kidneys (aged between 10 and 39 years) and defined as any donor aged ≥60 years, or any donor aged 50-59 years, with two of the following three donor criteria: CVA death, terminal creatinine >133μmol/L, or hypertension (Metzger, Delmonico et al. 2003). Although the concept of ECD focuses primarily on advanced donor age, other risk factors such as CVA, hypertension, diabetes and high serum creatinine were also taken into account (Cosio, Qiu et al. 1996; Ojo, Leichtman et al. 2000). Multiple studies have demonstrated that recipients of ECD kidneys have better survival compared to potential recipients on the waiting-list but long-term outcomes associated with ECD grafts remains unclear (Wolfe, Ashby et al. 1999; Ojo, Hanson et al. 2001).

Further modification of the definition of ECD kidneys has been proposed in an attempt to further improve the stratification and identification of donor kidneys with increased risk of early graft dysfunction or graft loss. In 2001, *Nyberg et al* devised the Deceased Donor Score (DDS), which incorporated several donor-derived factors that have been shown to independently affect graft outcomes (Nyberg SL 2001; Nyberg SL 2003). However, this score has not been adopted widely for clinical application.

In a retrospective study of 2845 French transplant recipients aged ≥60 years, ECD kidneys were associated with poorer graft survival compared to non-ECD kidneys (Savoye, Tamarelle et al. 2007). The difference in graft survival was 6.2% at 12 months and 14.2% at 5 years (adjusted relative risk [RR] of graft failure associated with ECD kidneys compared to non-ECD kidneys was 1.98, $p<0.01$). Nonetheless, survival of ECD recipients was superior to potential recipients remaining on the waiting list (adjusted RR of potential recipients on waiting-list compared to recipients of ECD and non-ECD kidneys were 2.32 and 3.78 respectively, $p<0.0001$). Similarly, analysis of the SRTR between 1990 and 2005 demonstrated that recipients aged ≥70 years receiving ECD or non-ECD deceased donor kidneys had a 56% lower mortality risk compared to wait-listed dialysis patients aged ≥70 years (RR 0.59; 95%CI 0.53, 0.65; $p<0.0001$), and this benefit persisted in elderly patients with diabetes and hypertension (Rao, Merion et al. 2007). As the unadjusted 1-year graft and death-censored graft survival (DCGS) of elderly transplant recipients were 81% and 90% respectively; and were 67% and 85% respectively at 3years, this suggested that a considerable proportion of these recipients die with functioning grafts.

A retrospective analysis of ANZDATA of 4466 deceased donor transplants between 1991 and 2005 reported poorer outcomes in recipients of ECD kidneys, compared to non-ECD kidneys (Collins, Chang et al. 2009). Compared to non-ECD kidneys, ECD kidneys were associated with poorer graft function and a greater risk of DGF, acute rejection and death-censored graft failure (DCGF).

The observed reduction in graft survival in recipients of ECD kidneys is likely related to an increase in glomerulosclerosis with the associated reduction in functional nephron mass, which has been shown to correlate with an increased risk of DGF, graft loss and poorer graft function (Gaber, Moore et al. 1995). On average, the adjusted graft survival of ECD kidneys is 8% lower at 1 year and up to 20% lower at 3-5 years compared to non-ECD kidneys (Ojo AO 2001).

Although ECD kidneys are associated with poorer outcomes compared to non-ECD kidneys, the contribution of donor age, especially the upper acceptable age limit on graft outcomes amongst ECD grafts remains unclear. In a retrospective analysis of the UNOS/OPTN database, the impact of donor age on 9580 ECD kidneys were examined (Chavalitdhamrong, Gill et al. 2008). There was no association between donor age and acute rejection, although ECD kidneys from donors aged ≥70 years had poorer function at 12 months compared to grafts from younger ECD donors. In an adjusted model, ECD kidneys from donors aged ≥70 years were associated with an increased risk of graft failure and patient death compared to ECD kidneys from donors aged 50-69 years (hazard ratio [HR] 1.37 and 1.37 respectively, $p<0.01$). When stratified by recipient age, ECD kidneys from donors aged ≥70 years (compared to ECD 50-69 years) were associated with an increased risk of DCGF for recipients aged 41-60 years (HR 1.48, 95%CI 1.06, 2.06; $p=0.02$) but not for older recipients aged >60 years (HR 1.12, 95%CI 0.86, 1.46; $p=0.40$), suggesting that older ECD kidneys may have a smaller unfavourable impact in older recipients. In contrast, an Italian study demonstrated that 3-year graft and patient survival was similar in recipients receiving ECD kidneys from donors >75 years and <75 years (Collini, Kalmar et al. 2009). This inconsistent finding may be explained by the greater use of double kidneys (from donors >75 years) in the Italian study.

As ECD kidneys are more susceptible to peri-transplant insults, strategies to reduce cold ischemic time, improve donor kidney preservation (Burdick JF) and preventing or reducing reperfusion injury using agents such as superoxide dismutase (Land W) or platelet-

activating factor receptor antagonists (Grino JM) may be beneficial. However, these strategies have not translated to improvement in renal graft outcomes. Initial avoidance of calcineurin-inhibitors (CNI) in early post-transplant period has been suggested to reduce the risk of DGF in recipients of ECD kidneys but this approach has not been adopted widely.
Although there is a lack of consensus amongst transplant physicians and surgeons regarding the allocation of ECD kidneys, most would advocate selective utilization of these kidneys for older recipients (particularly avoiding recipients <40 years) (Merion, Ashby et al. 2005; Schold and Meier-Kriesche 2006), for recipients with extended wait-time (Carter, Chan et al. 2005; Cecka, Cohen et al. 2006) or to consider dual graft transplantation into a single recipient to avoid unnecessary discard of older donor kidneys (Waiser, Schreiber et al. 2000; Tan, Alfrey et al. 2004).

	Donor/recipient groups	Graft outcome	Patient outcome
Collins M et al 2009 ANZDATA (n=4466)		*1/5y DCGS**	*1/5y patient survival**
	Non-ECD <50y	94% / 88%	97% / 92%
	Non-ECD 50-59y	91% / 84%	97% / 90%
	ECD 50-59y	87% / 81%	97% / 89%
	ECD ≥60y	87% / 71%	96% / 87%
Collini A et al 2009 Single centre (n=192)		*1/3y graft survival*	*10y patient survival*
	ECD >75y	73% / 64%	81% / 81%
	ECD <75y	82% / 71%	92% / 90%
Savoye E et al 2009 Single centre (n=2845)		*1/5y graft survival#*	*1/5y patient survival*
	Expanded criteria 0^	93% / 83%	ECD - 97% / 67%
	Expanded criteria 1^	87% / 74%	Non-ECD - 98% / 91%
	Expanded criteria 2^	87% / 65%	
	Expanded criteria 3^	83% / 55%	
Chavalitdhamrong D et al 2008; OPTN/UNOS database (n=9580)		*3/5y graft survival**	*3/5y patient survival**
	ECD 50-69y	69% / 55%	82% / 71%
	ECD ≥70y	62% / 44%	75% / 58%

Table 3. Effect of expanded criteria donor on renal transplant outcomes. *p<0.05; #analysis in patients aged ≥60 years, ^expanded criteria risk factors including donor aged >60 years, donor hypertension, donor diabetes, donor death from cerebrovascular accident. Abbreviation: ANZDATA - Australia and New Zealand Dialysis and Transplant Registry, ECD - expanded criteria donor, OPTN - Organ Procurement Transplant Network, UNOS - United Network of Organ Sharing, y - year(s). Adapted from Lim et al (Nephrol Dial Transplant 2010).

5.2 Donation after cardiac death donor kidneys

Over the last decade, the number of brain-death donors has steadily declined, in part attributed to changes in neurosurgical practice (Jüttler, Schwab et al. 2007). However, the use of DCD donor kidneys has increased substantially. In Australia, the number of DCD donors has increased from 1 to 42 between 2000 and 2009 (Excell, Hee et al. 2010), whereas in the United Kingdom, the proportion of DCD of all deceased donors has increased by 29% between 2000 and 2009 (Transplant 2010). The prolonged warm ischaemic period that invariably accompanies DCD kidney transplants is likely to explain the greater incidence of

DGF (Locke, Segev et al. 2007). As a result, DCD kidneys are more likely to be allocated locally to minimize cold ischaemic time. Recent analysis of the UK transplant registry demonstrated that compared with brain-death donor kidney transplants, recipients of controlled DCD donor kidneys of Maastricht category 3 (defined as donors awaiting cardiac arrest following withdrawal of life-sustaining treatment in intensive care unit (Kootstra, Daemen et al. 1995)) was associated with a significantly greater risk of DGF but lower risk of acute rejection up to 3 months post-transplant (Figure 2). For primary but not repeat renal allograft recipients of DCD kidneys, overall 5-year graft survival was comparable to primary and repeat renal allograft recipients of brain-death donor kidneys in unadjusted and adjusted models. Repeat renal allograft recipients of DCD kidneys have a greater risk of primary non-function compared to primary renal allograft recipients of DCD kidneys. Increasing donor and recipient age, as well as prolonged cold ischaemic time but not the presence of DGF or HLA-matching were associated with poorer graft outcomes in primary renal allograft recipients of DCD kidneys (Summers, Johnson et al. 2010). With comparable transplant outcomes between brain-death and controlled DCD donor kidneys, DCD kidneys are considered an acceptable source of donor kidneys although particular attention in reducing cold ischaemic time and avoidance of large donor-recipient age differences and avoidance of allocating DCD kidneys to repeat renal allograft recipients may be appropriate.

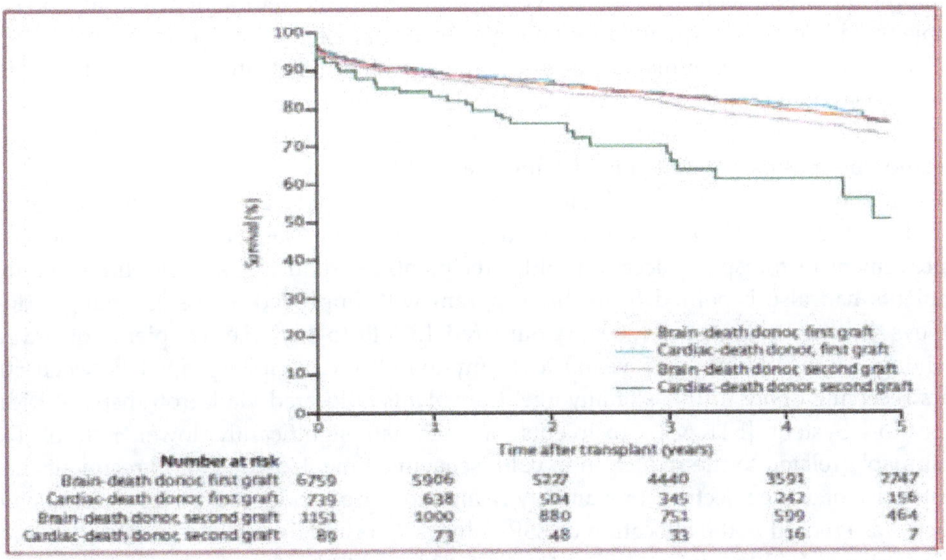

Fig. 2. Kaplan-Meier survival estimates comparing brain-death and cardiac-death donor grafts, stratified by primary and repeat grafts (adapted from Summers et al 2010).

5.3 Utility-based allocation strategies to maximise overall functioning graft years

Allocating younger donor kidneys to older potential recipients has raised concerns amongst many transplant physicians and surgeons, as many older recipients will die with functioning grafts. If these younger kidneys were re-allocated from older to younger recipients, a proportion may have continued to function for a substantial period in younger recipients. As older recipients have reduced life expectancies, adopting an allocation strategy that better matches the life expectancy of the donor kidney with that of the recipient may be more appropriate (Meier-Kriesche, Schold et al. 2005). Allocation strategies that have been examined included the concept of donor-recipient age-matching and the creation of a kidney allocation score (KAS) to improve the utility of deceased donor kidneys. These strategies will be discussed in this chapter.

5.3.1 Age-matching

Allocation of deceased donor kidneys according to donor-recipient age-matching avoids the allocation of younger donor kidneys to older recipients and older donor kidneys to younger recipients according to a single donor and recipient age cut-off value. The Eurotransplant Seniors Program (ESP) is an example of an age-matching allocation model that has been successfully implemented in the allocation of deceased donor kidneys.

5.3.1.1 Eurotransplant seniors program

The foundation of ESP, which was established in 1999, was to preferentially allocate older donor kidneys ≥65 years to ABO-compatible, unsensitized older recipients ≥65 years receiving a primary graft (Cecka, Cohen et al. 2006). The ESP was designed to match the functional potential of donor kidneys ≥65 years to the functional requirements of older recipients aged ≥65 years. Although a degree of age-matching already occurred prior to the development of ESP such that the very young donor kidneys were seldom allocated to older recipients, this may be explained by younger healthier potential recipients near the top of the list declining a suboptimal donor graft, and therefore retain their place on the waiting list until a younger donor kidney becomes available. Similar practice also occurs in countries such as the United States and Australia where age-matching is not part of the standard allocation process (Segev 2009; Lim, Chang et al. 2010).

In ESP, donor kidneys were distributed locally to reduce cold ischaemic time, in an attempt to reduce the risk of DGF. Consequently, this program has not only resulted in an improvement in transplant access in older recipients by reducing wait-list times, younger recipients had also benefited from this program with improved access to younger donor kidneys (Smits, Persijn et al. 2002). Compared to 'old-to-any' (i.e. recipients of any age receiving a donor kidney ≥65 years) and 'any-to-old' (i.e. recipients aged between 60-64 years receiving donor kidneys of any age) transplants (allocated via Eurotransplant Kidney Allocation System [ETKAS]), recipients of ESP had significantly lower risk of DGF; presumably related to the reduction in cold ischaemic time. However, ESP recipients had a greater risk of acute rejection, presumably related to a greater degree of HLA-mismatch(es), which was ignored in the allocation of ESP kidneys. One and 5-year DCGS in ESP recipients were similar to 'old-to-any' recipients (1 year - 83% and 81% respectively; 5 years - 67% for both groups) but were inferior compared to 'any-to-old' recipients (1 year 90% and 5 years 81%) (Table 4). When stratified by donor age, the 1 and 5-year graft survival in the ESP group was 75% and 47% compared to 74% and 53% for 'any-to-old' recipients with older donors aged ≥60 years ($p=0.38$) and 85% and 67% for 'any-to-old' recipients with younger donors aged <60 years ($p<0.001$) suggesting older recipients receiving older donor kidneys allocated through the ETKAS system had similar outcome as ESP recipients. Although the risk of DGF was reduced in ESP recipients, this remained an important predictor of graft outcomes indicating that DGF may have a greater adverse impact on graft outcome in older recipients receiving older donor kidneys. It is conceivable that strategies to reduce the risk of DGF in ESP recipients (e.g. attempts to further reduce cold ischaemia) may lead to an improvement in graft and patient outcomes. An important and often overlooked finding in this study is that younger recipients of older donor kidneys have poorer survival, similar to that of the 'any-to-old' recipients allocated through the ETKAS system (Table 4).

Eurotransplant Senior DR-compatible Program is a new future initiative of the ESP to preferentially allocate kidneys to recipients with 0 HLA-DR mismatches and therefore potentially reducing the risk of rejection (de Fijter 2009). The outcome of this approach will be prospectively evaluated in the coming years.

5.3.1.2 Simulated age-matching allocation of deceased donor kidneys

In Australia, utilization of older donors has steadily increased, with donors aged ≥55 years increasing from 134 to 241 between 2001-03 and 2007-09 (i.e. an increase of 16% of overall donors) (Excell, Hee et al. 2010). A recent ANZDATA registry study of 4616 renal transplant recipients has demonstrated that the adoption an age-matching allocation model would lead to substantial improvement in the number of functioning graft years and associated cost savings (Lim, Chang et al. 2010). In this study, recipients ≥55 years had more than a 2.5-fold increased risk of death with functioning graft compared to recipients <55 years (HR 2.84, 95%CI 1.97, 4.10 for 0-1 year; HR 2.78, 95%CI 2.19, 3.53 for 1-8 years and HR 4.44, 95%CI 3.10, 6.35 for >8 years; all p-values <0.01). However, the risk of early (<1 year) and late (>8 years) DCGF was similar in younger and older recipients. Compared with younger donor grafts, older donor grafts ≥60 years were associated with a significant increased risk of DCGF, death with functioning graft and poorer post-transplant graft function. The application of an age-matching allocation model to this cohort would result in an additional 262 mean functioning graft years, which equates to $11.8-21.7 million dialysis cost savings (cost per patient per year on dialysis $45,000-$83,000) (Cass, Chadban et al. 2006). Similarly, analysis of the SRTR database of 74,998 deceased donor transplants performed between 1990 and 2002 demonstrated that if older recipients aged 60-64 years received younger donor grafts aged 15-50 years, the application of age-matching allocation would have increased graft life by 27,500 years, with estimated cost savings in excess of 1 billion dollars (Meier-Kriesche, Schold et al. 2005). However, at an individual level, the absolute impact of age-matching appears less impressive. In the ANZDATA study by *Lim et al*, Younger recipients of younger donor kidneys would on average have an additional 3 functioning graft years compared to older recipients receiving younger donor kidneys (11.6 vs 8.7 mean graft years respectively) and the negative impact of older donor kidneys on functioning graft years appears to be greater for younger compared to older recipients (9.3 vs 7.1 mean graft years respectively) (Table 4).

Retrospective analysis of the OPTN database demonstrated that for every 1 year increase in donor age, the risk of graft failure (HR 1.01, p<0.001) and death with functioning graft (HR 1.004, p<0.001) was increased substantially (Moers, Kornmann et al. 2009). The negative impact of donor age on graft survival appears maximal between donors aged between 36 to 40 years (Keith, Demattos et al. 2004). In a simulated age-matching allocation system, the reallocation of older donor grafts ≥65 years from younger recipients <65 years (old-to-young) to older recipients ≥65 years (old-to-old) would result in an absolute reduction in 10-year graft survival by 8% (from 21% to 13%, p<0.001), whereas reallocation of donor kidneys <65 years from recipients ≥65 years (young-to-old) to younger recipients <65 years (young-to-young) would result in an improvement in 10-year graft survival by 7% (19% to 26%, p=0.40). Unlike the ANZDATA study, there was no net benefit of implementing an old-for-old allocation system with regards to overall functional graft years (Table 4).

5.3.2 Kidney allocation score

In 2004, a subcommittee of the UNOS/OPTN recommended that the establishment of a Kidney Allocation Score (KAS) based on Life Years From Transplant (LYFT - measures transplant utility), combined with panel reactive antibody (PRA), Donor Profile Index (DPI - measures donor quality) and dialysis time (measures transplant equity) could potentially lead to an increase in the total number of life years gained from a restricted number of available deceased donor kidneys (Wolfe, McCullough et al. 2009; OPTN 2010). LYFT is defined as the additional years of life that a potential transplant recipient could expect to gain as a consequence of the transplant as compared to not receiving a transplant. LYFT is calculated from an equation generated by statistical modeling of historical data combining

	Donor/ recipient groups	Graft outcome	Patient outcome
Frei U et al 2008 ESP/ETKAS^ (n=3539)		*5y patient DCGS**	*5y patient survival**
	D/R ≥55 (ESP)	67%	60%
	D ≥65 / R - any age	67%	71%
	D - any age / R 60-64	81%	74%
Lim W et al 2010 ANZDATA (n=4616)		*Mean graft years*	NR
	D <60 / R <55	11.6	
	D <60 / R ≥55	9.3	
	D ≥60/ R <55	8.7	
	D ≥60 / R ≥55	7.1	
Keith D et al 2004 OPTN Registry (n=50,322)		NR	*10y patient survival*
	D 30-41/ R 0-40		82%
	D 30-41 / R ≥55		45%
	D ≥55 / R 0-40		76%
	D ≥55 / R ≥55		35%
Moers C et al 2009 OPTN Registry (n=99,860)		*10y graft survival*	*DFG*
	D <65 / R <65	NR	NR
	D <65 / R ≥65	19%	56%
	D ≥65/ R <65	21%	40%
	D ≥65 / R ≥65	NR	NR
Waiser et al 2000 Single centre (n=1269)		*8y graft survival**	*DFG*
	D ≤55 / R ≤55	50%	11%
	D ≤55 / R >55	53%	27%
	D >55/ R ≤55	21%	2%
	D >55/ R >55	57%	26%

Table 4. Effect of age-matching allocation on graft and patient outcomes. *p<0.05; ^Prospective data. Abbreviation: ESP - Eurotransplant Senior Program, ETKAS - Eurotransplant Kidney Allocation System, ANZDATA - Australia and New Zealand Dialysis and Transplant Registry, OPTN - Organ Procurement Transplant Network, D - donor, R - recipient, DCGS - death-censored graft survival, DFG - death with functioning graft, y - year(s), NR - not reported. Adapted from Lim et al (Nephrol Dial Transplant 2010).

the observed biological effects of patient and donor characteristics on survival. The equation created had a C-value of 0.75, that is the equation predicted the potential transplant recipients with the longer lifetime 75% of the time, although the equation may be inaccurate for the prediction of lifetimes for potential transplant candidates with characteristics that differ from the historical group. A C-value of 0.75 is comparable to the model for end-stage liver disease (MELD) with a C-value of 0.64, commonly used by many transplanting centres to prioritize patients for liver transplantation based on expected survival (Sharma, Schaubel et al. 2008). In addition, based on DPI, the kidneys with the longest survival potential will be allocated according to the combined score of LYFT (80% of total score) and dialysis time/PRA (20% of total score), whereas kidneys with lesser potential for long-term survival will be allocated according to dialysis time and PRA, such that better donor kidneys are allocated to younger potential recipients, who will have the longest expected LYFT. Older potential recipients, who will have a lower expected LYFT and potential recipients with the longest dialysis time will be less likely to receive better donor kidneys but may have an advantage in being allocated shorter-lived kidneys more rapidly (i.e. shorter waiting-time). If deceased donor kidney allocation was based on the KAS, there would a total expected increase in LYFT of 2642 years during a single year of allocation as compared with the current allocation system in the United States.

A perception that organ allocation is occurring in an inequitable manner could potentially reduce organ donor rates. Nevertheless, the utilization of KAS may improve allocation based solely on age-matching, with other patient factors such as diabetes, which are known to adversely affect graft and patient survival, are taken into account in the calculation of LYFT (Machnicki, Pinsky et al. 2009).

5.3.3 Positives and negatives of implementing utility-based allocation models

It remains unclear whether the implementation of utility-based allocation models will achieve a better balance between utility and equity. While kidney transplantation is more cost effective than dialysis, it will take considerable time for the expected lower long-term cost to offset the high initial cost associated with transplantation. In older recipients who are more likely to die with a functioning graft, the expense of transplantation may not be acceptable, on an economic basis, especially with a high-quality donor kidney.

Although adoption of an allocation model based on LYFT is likely to increase functioning graft years, this model is difficult to implement and may even be perceived as being discriminatory to potential 'high-risk' potential recipients (e.g. indigenous and highly sensitised potential recipients) who will have a higher predicted graft loss, resulting in a lower LYFT (Young and Gaston 2000; Young and Gaston 2005). The applicability of LYFT based on historical data to more recent eras and patient cohorts, where there may be differing clinical practices and use of novel immunosuppressive agents remains uncertain. In addition, the optimal weighting of DPI, dialysis time or other factors in the calculation of KAS remains undecided. Although not directly considered in the KAS and age-matching allocation models, KAS may indirectly take into consideration social equity and possibly quality of life, assuming that younger recipients receiving younger donor kidneys will have a longer lifespan and therefore greater contribution to society compared to older recipients (Laupacis, Keown et al. 1996). In contrast, age-matching allocation is simpler but chronological age is often a poor estimate of physiological age and therefore, allocation policy based solely on age-matching could potentially disadvantage a number of healthy older potential recipients.

6. Conclusion

With the continuing shortage of deceased donor organs coupled with the increased utilization of marginal live and deceased donors including ECD and DCD donor kidneys, there have been considerable interest in examining the outcomes of these grafts. Over the last decade, there has been an expansion of innovative transplant programs, including paired exchange and tumour-resected kidney transplant programs, which has helped to overcome incompatible transplants and increase donor kidney pool respectively. In this chapter, understanding the association between live and deceased donor characteristics and transplant outcomes will assist clinicians and potential recipients in the informed process of donor selection as well as the prediction of graft outcomes following transplantation.

7. References

Ahmad, M., E. Cole, et al. (2009). "Impact of deceased donor diabetes mellitus on kidney transplant outcomes: a propensity score-matched study." Transplantation 88(2): 251-60.

Alexandre G, S. J., De Bruyère M, Latinne D, Reding R, Gianello P, Carlier M, Pirson Y (1987). "Present experiences in a series of 26 ABO-incompatible living donor renal allografts." Transplant Proceedings 19(6): 4538-4542.

Bia, M. J., E. L. Ramos, et al. (1995). "Evaluation of living renal donors. The current practice of US transplant centers." Transplantation 60(4): 322-7.

Bloembergen, W. E., F. K. Port, et al. (1996). "Gender discrepancies in living related renal transplant donors and recipients." J Am Soc Nephrol 7(8): 1139-44.

Brenner, B. M., R. A. Cohen, et al. (1992). "In renal transplantation, one size may not fit all." J Am Soc Nephrol 3(2): 162-9.

Brenner, B. M., E. V. Lawler, et al. (1996). "The hyperfiltration theory: a paradigm shift in nephrology." Kidney Int 49(6): 1774-7.

Brook, N., N. Gibbons, et al. (2010). "Outcomes of transplants from patients with small renal tumours, live unrelated donors and dialysis wait-listed patients." Transpl Int 23(5): 476-83.

Bryan, C., P. Nelson, et al. (2004). "Transplantation of A2 and A2B kidneys from deceased donors into B waiting list candidates increases their transplantation rate." Clin Transpl: 127-33.

Bryan, C., F. Winklhofer, et al. (2005). "Improving access to kidney transplantation without decreasing graft survival: long-term outcomes of blood group A2/A2B deceased donor kidneys in B recipients." Transplantation 80(1): 75-80.

Buell J, H. M., Thomas M, Munda R, Alloway R, First M, Woodle E (2005). "Donor kidneys with small renal cell cancers: can they be transplanted?" Transplant Proceedings 37(2): 581-582.

Burdick JF, R. J., McBride MA, Kauffman HM, Bennett LE (1997). "National impact of pulsatile perfusion on cadaveric kidney transplantation." Transplantation 64(12): 4.

Campbell, S., S. McDonald, et al. (2009). Transplant Waiting List. The Thirty Second Report Australia and New Zealand Dialysis and Transplant Registry. S. McDonald, L. Excell and B. Livingston. Adelaide.

Campbell, S., S. McDonald, et al. (2009). Chapter 8 : Transplantation. ANZDATA Registry 32nd Annual Report. Adelaide, South Australia, Australia and New Zealand Dialysis and Transplant Registry (ANZDATA).

Carter, J., S. Chan, et al. (2005). "Expanded criteria donor kidney allocation: marked decrease in cold ischemia and delayed graft function at a single center." Am J Transplant 5(11): 2745-53.

Cass, A., S. Chadban, et al. (2006). Economic impact of end-stage kidney disease in Australia. K. H. Australia.

Cecka, J., B. Cohen, et al. (2006). "Could more effective use of kidneys recovered from older deceased donors result in more kidney transplants for older patients?" Transplantation 81(7): 966-70.

Cecka, J. M. (1995). "Living donor transplants." Clin Transpl: 363-77.

Chadban, S., S. McDonald, et al. (2006). Transplant Waiting List. The Twenty Ninth Report: Australia and New Zealand Dialysis and Transplant Registry. S. McDonald, S. Chang and L. Excell. Adelaide.

Chavalitdhamrong, D., J. Gill, et al. (2008). "Patient and graft outcomes from deceased kidney donors age 70 years and older: an analysis of the Organ Procurement Transplant Network/United Network of Organ Sharing database." Transplantation 85(11): 1573-9.

Collini, A., P. Kalmar, et al. (2009). "Renal transplant from very old donors: how far can we go?" Transplantation 87(12): 1830-6.

Collins, M., S. Chang, et al. (2009). "Outcomes of transplantation using kidneys from donors meeting expanded criteria in Australia and New Zealand, 1991 to 2005." Transplantation 87(8): 1201-9.

Cosio, F., W. Qiu, et al. (1996). "Factors related to the donor organ are major determinants of renal allograft function and survival." Transplantation 62(11): 1571-6.

Crew, R. and L. Ratner (2010). "ABO-incompatible kidney transplantation: current practice and the decade ahead." Curr Opin Organ Transplant 15: 526-30.

Crew R, R. L. (2010). "ABO-incompatible kidney transplantation: current practice and the decade ahead." Current Opinion in Organ Transplantation 15: 526-530.

de Fijter, J. (2009). "An old virtue to improve senior programs." Transpl Int 22(3): 259-68.

de Klerk, M., K. Keizer, et al. (2005). "The Dutch national living donor kidney exchange program." Am J Transplant 5(9): 2302-5.

de Klerk M, W. M., Haase-Kromwijk B, Claas F, Weimar W (2006). "A highly efficient living donor kidney exchange program for both blood type and crossmatch incompatible donor-recipient combinations." Transplantation 82(12): 1616-1620.

De Meester, J. (1998). Kidney: Donation, Waiting Lists and Transplants. Eurotransplant International Foundation Annual Report 1998 [internet]. B. Cohen, G. Persijn and J. De Meester. Leiden (Netherlands), Eurotransplant.

Dehoux, J. and P. Gianello (2009). "Accomodation and antibodies." Transpl Immunol 21: 106-10.

Delmonico, F. (2004). "Exchanging kidneys - advances in living-donor transplantation." N Engl J Med 350(18): 1812-14.

Deroure, B., N. Kamar, et al. (2010). "Expanding the criteria of renal kidneys for transplantation: use of donors with acute renal failure." Nephrol Dial Transplant 25(6): 1980-6.

Donelly, P., P. Oman, et al. (1995). "Predialysis living donor renal transplantation: Is it still the 'gold standard' for cost, convenience and graft survival." Transplant Proc 27: 1444-6.

Einecke, G., B. Sis, et al. (2009). "Antibody-mediated microcirculation injury is the major cause of late kidney transplant failure." Am J Transplant 9(11): 2520-31.

Eng, H., G. Bennett, et al. (2011). "Donor HLA Specific Antibodies Predict Development and Define Prognosis in Transplant Glomerulopathy." Hum Immunol.

Eng, H., G. Bennett, et al. (2008). "Anti-HLA donor-specific antibodies detected in positive B-cell crossmatches by Luminex predict late graft loss." Am J Transplant 8(11): 2335-42.

ERA-EDTA Registry (2010). ERA-EDTA Annual Report 2008 [internet]. Amsterdam (Netherlands).

Excell, L., K. Hee, et al. (2006). ANZOD Registry Report 2006. Australia and New Zealand Organ Donation Registry. L. Excell, K. Hee and G. Russ. Adelaide.

Excell, L., K. Hee, et al. (2010). ANZOD Registry Report 2010. Australia and New Zealand Organ Donation Registry. L. Excell, K. Hee and G. Russ. Adelaide.

Excell, L., K. Hee, et al. (2010). ANZOD Registry Report 2010. ANZOD Registry Report. L. Excell, K. Hee and G. Russ. Adelaide, Australia and New Zealand Organ Donation Registry.

Fabre, J., P. Murphy, et al. (2010). "Presumed consent: a distraction in the quest for increasing rates of organ donation." BMJ 341: c4873.

Feldman, H., I. Fazio, et al. (1996). "Recipient body size and cadaveric renal allograft survival." J Am Soc Nephrol 7(1): 151-7.

Ferrari, P., W. Lim, et al. (2011). "Effect of donor-recipient age difference on graft function and survival in live-donor kidney transplantation." Nephrol Dial Transplant 26(2): 702-8.

Ferrari P, W. C., Christiansen F (2009). "Paired kidney donations to expand the living donor pool: the Western Australian experience." The Medical Journal of Australia 190(12): 700-703.

Frei, U., J. Noeldeke, et al. (2008). "Prospective age-matching in elderly kidney transplant recipients--a 5-year analysis of the Eurotransplant Senior Program." Am J Transplant 8(1): 50-7.

Fuggle, S. V., J. E. Allen, et al. (2010). "Factors affecting graft and patient survival after live donor kidney transplantation in the UK." Transplantation 89(6): 694-701.

Futagawa, Y., K. Waki, et al. (2005). "Living-unrelated donors yield higher graft survival rates than parental donors." Transplantation 79(9): 1169-74.

Gaber, L., L. Moore, et al. (1995). "Glomerulosclerosis as a determinant of posttransplant function of older donor renal allografts." Transplantation 60(4): 334-9.

Gentry, S., R. Montgomery, et al. (2011). "Kidney paired donation: fundamentals, limitations, and expansions." Am J Kidney Dis 57(1): 144-51.

Ghods, A. J. and S. Savaj (2006). "Iranian Model of Paid and Regulated Living-Unrelated Kidney Donation." Clinical Journal of the American Society of Nephrology 1(6): 1136-1145.

Giral, M., J. Nguyen, et al. (2005). "Impact of graft mass on the clinical outcome of kidney transplants." J Am Soc Nephrol 16(1): 261-8.

Gjertson, D. W. and J. M. Cecka (2000). "Living unrelated donor kidney transplantation." Kidney Int 58(2): 491-9.

Gloor, J., S. DeGoey, et al. (2003). "Overcoming a positive crossmatch in living-donor kidney transplantation." Am J Transplant 3(8): 1017-23.

Gloor, J. and M. Stegall (2010). "Sensitized renal transplant recipients: current protocols and future directions." Nat Rev Nephrol 6(5): 297-306.

Gloor, J., J. Winters, et al. (2010). "Baseline donor-specific antibody levels and outcomes in positive crossmatch kidney transplantation." Am J Transplant 10(3): 582-9.

Gloor J, W. L., Cornell L, Fix L, DrGoey S, Knauer R, Cosio F, Gandhi M, Kremers W, Stegall M (2010). "Baseline donor-specific antibody levels and outcomes in positive crossmatch kidney transplantation." American Journal of Transplantation 10: 582-589.

Grino JM (1994). "BN 52021: a platelet activating factor antagonist for preventing post-transplant renal failure. A double-blind, randomized study. The BN 52021 Study Group in Renal Transplantation." Annals of Internal Medicine 121(5): 12.

Horvat, L. D., S. Z. Shariff, et al. (2009). "Global trends in the rates of living kidney donation." Kidney Int 75(10): 1088-98.

Humar, A., B. Durand, et al. (2000). "Living unrelated donors in kidney transplants: better long-term results than with non-HLA-identical living related donors?" Transplantation 69(9): 1942-5.

Hurst, F., S. Sajjad, et al. (2010). "Transplantation of A2 Kidneys into B and O Recipients Leads to Reduction in Waiting Time: USRDS Experience." Transplantation 89: 1396-1402.

Iordanous, Y., N. Seymour, et al. (2009). "Recipient outcomes for expanded criteria living kidney donors: the disconnect between current evidence and practice." Am J Transplant 9(7): 1558-73.

Issa, N., B. Stephany, et al. (2007). "Donor factors influencing graft outcomes in live donor kidney transplantation." Transplantation 83(5): 593-9.

Jordan, S., A. Vo, et al. (2003). "Intravenous immune globulin treatment inhibits crossmatch positivity and allows for successful transplantation of incompatible organs in living-donor and cadaver recipients." Transplantation 76(4): 631-6.

Jüttler, E., S. Schwab, et al. (2007). "Decompressive Surgery for the Treatment of Malignant Infarction of the Middle Cerebral Artery (DESTINY): a randomized, controlled trial." Stroke 38(9): 2518-25.

Kayler, L. K., H. U. Meier-Kriesche, et al. (2002). "Gender imbalance in living donor renal transplantation." Transplantation 73(2): 248-52.

Kayler, L. K., C. S. Rasmussen, et al. (2003). "Gender imbalance and outcomes in living donor renal transplantation in the United States." Am J Transplant 3(4): 452-8.

Keith, D., A. Demattos, et al. (2004). "Effect of donor recipient age match on survival after first deceased donor renal transplantation." J Am Soc Nephrol 15(4): 1086-91.

Kessler, M., M. Ladriere, et al. (2011). "Does pre-emptive kidney transplantation with a deceased donor improve outcomes? Results from a French transplant network." Transpl Int 24(3): 266-75.

Kootstra, G., J. Daemen, et al. (1995). "Categories of non-heart-beating donors." Transplant Proc 27: 2893-94.

Land W, S. H., Schleibner S, Illner WD, Abendroth D, Rutili G, Arfors KE, Messmer K (1994). "The beneficial effect of human recombinant superoxide dismutase on acute and chronic rejection events in recipients of cadaveric renal transplants." Transplantation 57(2): 7.

Laupacis, A., P. Keown, et al. (1996). "A study of the quality of life and cost-utility of renal transplantation." Kidney Int 50(1): 235-42.

Lefaucheur, C., C. Suberbielle-Boissel, et al. (2008). "Clinical relevance of preformed HLA donor-specific antibodies in kidney transplantation." Am J Transplant 8(2): 324-31.

Liem, Y. S. and W. Weimar (2009). "Early living-donor kidney transplantation: a review of the associated survival benefit." Transplantation 87(3): 317-8.

Lim, W., S. Chang, et al. (2010). "Donor-recipient age matching improves years of graft function in deceased-donor kidney transplantation." Nephrol Dial Transplant 25(9): 3082-9.

Lim, W. H., S. H. Chang, et al. (2007). "Parental donors in live-donor kidney transplantation associated with increased rejection rates and reduced glomerular filtration rates." Transplantation 84(8): 972-80.

Locke, J., D. Segev, et al. (2007). "Outcomes of kidneys from donors after cardiac death: implications for allocation and preservation." Am J Transplant 7: 1797-807.

Locke, J., A. Zachary, et al. (2007). "The utility of splenectomy as rescue treatment for severe acute antibody mediated rejection." Am J Transplant 7(4): 842-6.

Machnicki, G., B. Pinsky, et al. (2009). "Predictive ability of pretransplant comorbidities to predict long-term graft loss and death." Am J Transplant 9(3): 494-505.

Mahanty, H. D., W. S. Cherikh, et al. (2001). "Influence of pretransplant pregnancy on survival of renal allografts from living donors." Transplantation 72(2): 228-32.

Mange, K. C., M. M. Joffe, et al. (2001). "Effect of the use or nonuse of long-term dialysis on the subsequent survival of renal transplants from living donors." N Engl J Med 344(10): 726-31.

Mannami, M., R. Mannami, et al. (2008). "Last resort for renal transplant recipients, 'restored kidneys' from living donors/patients." Am J Transplant 8(4): 811-8.

McDonald, S., L. Excell, et al. (2009). New patient commencing treatment in 2008. Australia and New Zealand Dialysis and Transplant Registry. S. McDonald, L. Excell and B. Livingston. Adelaide: 1-12.

Meier-Kriesche, H., D. Cibrik, et al. (2002). "Interaction between donor and recipient age in determining the risk of chronic renal allograft failure." J Am Geriatr Soc 50(1): 14-7.

Meier-Kriesche, H., J. Schold, et al. (2005). "Kidneys from deceased donors: maximizing the value of a scarce resource." Am J Transplant 5: 1725-30.

Meier-Kriesche, H. U. and B. Kaplan (2002). "Waiting time on dialysis as the strongest modifiable risk factor for renal transplant outcomes: a paired donor kidney analysis." Transplantation 74(10): 1377-81.

Merion, R., V. Ashby, et al. (2005). "Deceased-donor characteristics and the survival benefit of kidney transplantation." JAMA 294(21): 2726-33.

Metzger, R., F. Delmonico, et al. (2003). "Expanded criteria donors for kidney transplantation." Am J Transplant 3(Suppl 4): 114-25.

Miles, C. D., D. E. Schaubel, et al. (2008). "The role of donor-recipient relationship in long-term outcomes of living donor renal transplantation." Transplantation 85(10): 1483-8.

Milton, C., G. Russ, et al. (2008). "Pre-emptive renal transplantation from living donors in Australia: Effect on allograft and patient survival." Nephrology 13: 535-40.

Moers, C., N. Kornmann, et al. (2009). "The influence of deceased donor age and old-for-old allocation on kidney transplant outcome." Transplantation 88(4): 542-52.

Mujtaba, M., W. Goggins, et al. (2011). "The strength of donor-specific antibody is a more reliable predictor of antibody-mediated rejection than flow cytometry crossmatch analysis in desensitized kidney recipients." Clin Transplant 25(1): E96-102.

Nelson, P., C. r. Shield, et al. (2002). "Increased access to transplantation for blood group B cadaveric waiting list candidates by using A2 kidneys: time for a new national system?" Am J Transplant 2(1): 94-9.

Nicol D, P. J., Wall D, Griffin A, Campbell S, Isbel N, Hawley C, Johnson D (2008). "Kidneys from patients with small renal tumours: a novel source of kidneys for transplantation." British Journal of Urology International 102(2): 188-192.

Nyberg SL, M. A., Kremers WK, Thostenson JD, Larson TS, Prieto M, Ishitani MB, Sterioff S, Stegall MD (2003). "Improved scoring system to assess adult donors for cadaver renal transplantation." Am J Transplant 2(6): 6.

Nyberg SL, M. A., Rogers M, Harmsen WS, Velosa JA, Larson TS, Prieto M, Ishitani MB, Sterioff S, Stegall MD (2001). "Donor scoring system for cadaveric renal transplantation." Am J Transplant 1(2): 8.

Nyengaard JR, B. T. (1992). "Glomerular number and size in relation to age, kidney weight, and body surface in normal man (abstract)." The Anatomical Record 232(2): 7.

Oien, C. M., A. V. Reisaeter, et al. (2007). "Living donor kidney transplantation: the effects of donor age and gender on short- and long-term outcomes." Transplantation 83(5): 600-6.

Oien, C. M., A. V. Reisaeter, et al. (2005). "Gender imbalance among donors in living kidney transplantation: the Norwegian experience." Nephrol Dial Transplant 20(4): 783-9.

Ojo, A., J. Hanson, et al. (2001). "Survival in recipients of marginal cadaveric donor kidneys compared with other recipients and wait-listed transplant candidates." J Am Soc Nephrol 12(3): 589-97.

Ojo, A., A. Leichtman, et al. (2000). "Impact of pre-existing donor hypertension and diabetes mellitus on cadaveric renal transplant outcomes." Am J Kidney Dis 36(1): 153-9.

Ojo AO, H. (2001). "Survival in recipients of marginal cadaveric donor kidneys compared with other recipients and wait-listed transplant candidates." Journal of the American Society of Nephrology 12(3): 9.

Oosterlee, A. and A. Rahmel, Eds. (2008). Eurotransplant International Foundation Annual Report 2008 [internet]. Leiden (Netherlands), Eurotransplant.

Oppenheimer, F., P. Aljama, et al. (2004). "The impact of donor age on the results of renal transplantation." Nephrol Dial Transplant 19(Suppl 3): iii11-iii15.

OPTN. (2010). "Kidney allocation policy development." http://optn.transplant.hrsa.gov/kars.asp.

Penn I (1995). "Primary kidney tumors before and after renal transplantation." Transplantation 59(4): 480-485.

Poggio, E., S. Hila, et al. (2006). "Donor kidney volume and outcomes following live donor kidney transplantation." Am J Transplant 6(3): 616-24.

Port FK, B.-G. J., Metzger RA, Dykstra DM, Gillespie BW, Young EW, Delmonico FL, Wynn JJ, Merion RM, Wolfe RA, Held PJ (2002). "Donor characteristics associated with reduced graft survival: An approach to expanding the pool of kidney donors." Transplantation 74(9): 5.

Rao, P., R. Merion, et al. (2007). "Renal transplantation in elderly patients older than 70 years of age: results from the Scientific Registry of Transplant Recipients." Transplantation 83(8): 1069-74.

Rao, P., D. Schaubel, et al. (2009). "A comprehensive risk quantification score for deceased donor kidneys: the kidney donor risk index." Transplantation 88(2): 231-6.

Rapaport F (1986). "The case for a living emotionally related international kidney donor exchange registry." Transplant Proceedings 18(3 (Suppl. 2)): 5-9.

Rosenberg, J. C., B. Jones, et al. (2004). "Accelerated rejection following offspring-to-mother and husband-to-wife transplants." Clin Transplant 18(6): 729-33.

Savoye, E., D. Tamarelle, et al. (2007). "Survival benefits of kidney transplantation with expanded criteria deceased donors in patients aged 60 years and over." Transplantation 84(12): 1618-24.

Schaubel, D. E., D. E. Stewart, et al. (2000). "Sex inequality in kidney transplantation rates." Arch Intern Med 160(15): 2349-54.

Schold, J. and H. Meier-Kriesche (2006). "Which renal transplant candidates should accept marginal kidneys in exchange for a shorter waiting time on dialysis?" Clin J Am Soc Nephrol 1(3): 532-8.

Schweitzer, E. J., J. Wilson, et al. (2000). "Increased rates of donation with laparoscopic donor nephrectomy." Ann Surg 232(3): 392-400.

Segev, D. (2009). "Evaluating options for utility-based kidney allocation." Am J Transplant 9: 1513-8.

Shaheen, M., F. Shaheen, et al. (2010). "Impact of recipient and donor nonimmunologic factors on the outcome of deceased donor kidney transplantation." Transplant Proc 42(1): 273-6.

Sharma, P., D. Schaubel, et al. (2008). "Re-weighting the model for end-stage liver disease score components." Gastroenterology 135(5): 1575-81.

Smits, J., G. Persijn, et al. (2002). "Evaluation of the Eurotransplant Senior Program. The results of the first year." Am J Transplant 2: 664-70.

Stegall, M., J. Gloor, et al. (2006). "A comparison of plasmapheresis versus high-dose IVIG desensitization in renal allograft recipients with high levels of donor specific alloantibody." Am J Transplant 6: 346-51.

Summers, D., R. Johnson, et al. (2010). "Analysis of factors that aff ect outcome after transplantation of kidneys donated after cardiac death in the UK: a cohort study." Lancet 376: 1303-11.

Tan, J., E. Alfrey, et al. (2004). "Dual-kidney transplantation with organs from expanded criteria donors: a long-term follow-up." Transplantation 78(5): 692-6.

Tanabe K (2007). "Japanese experience of ABO-incompatible living kidney transplantation." Transplantation 84(12 Suppl): S4-7.

Tanabe, K., H. Ischida, et al. (2009). "Evaluation of two different preconditioning regimens for ABO-incompatible living kidney donor transplantation. A comparison of splenectomy vs. rituximab-treated non-splenectomy preconditioning regimens." Contrib Nephrol 162: 61-74.

Terasaki, P. I., J. M. Cecka, et al. (1997). "Spousal and other living renal donor transplants." Clin Transpl: 269-84.

Terasaki, P. I., J. M. Cecka, et al. (1995). "High survival rates of kidney transplants from spousal and living unrelated donors." N Engl J Med 333(6): 333-6.

Toki, D., H. Ishida, et al. (2009). "Acute antibody-mediated rejection in living ABO-incompatible kidney transplantation: long-term impact and risk factors." Am J Transplant 9(3): 567-77.

Transplant, N. H. S. B. a. (2010). "Transplant activityin the UK, 2008–2009." from http://www.organdonation.nhs.uk/ukt/statistics/transplant_activity_report/current_activity_reports/ukt/2008_09/transplant_activity_uk_2008-09.pdf.

US Organ Procurement and Transplantion Network and Scientific Registry of Transplant Recipients (2009). US Organ Procurement and Transplantion Network and the Scientific Registry of Transplant Recipients Annual Report 2009: Transplant Data 1999-2008, US Department of Health and Human Services.

Vereerstraeten, P., M. Wissing, et al. (1999). "Male recipients of kidneys from female donors are at increased risk of graft loss from both rejection and technical failure." Clin Transplant 13(2): 181-6.

Vo, A., M. Lukovsky, et al. (2008). "Rituximab and intravenous immune globulin for desensitization during renal transplantation." N Engl J Med 359: 242-51.

Vo, A., A. Peng, et al. (2010). "Use of intravenous immune globulin and rituximab for desensitization of highly HLA-sensitized patients awaiting kidney transplantation." Transplantation 89: 1095-102.

Waiser, J., M. Schreiber, et al. (2000). "Age-matching in renal transplantation." Nephrol Dial Transplant 2000(15).

Wolfe, R., V. Ashby, et al. (1999). "Comparison of mortality in all patients on dialysis, patients on dialysis awaiting transplantation, and recipients of a first cadaveric transplant." N Engl J Med 341(23): 1725-30.

Wolfe, R., K. McCullough, et al. (2009). "Predictability of survival models for waiting list and transplant patients: calculating LYFT." Am J Transplant 9(7): 1523-7.

Young, C. and R. Gaston (2000). "Renal transplantation in black Americans." N Engl J Med 343(21): 1545-52.

Young, C. and R. Gaston (2005). "Understanding the influence of ethnicity on renal allograft survival." Am J Transplant 5: 2603-4.

Zeier, M., B. Dohler, et al. (2002). "The effect of donor gender on graft survival." J Am Soc Nephrol 13(10): 2570-6.

Zimmerman, D., S. Donnelly, et al. (2000). "Gender disparity in living renal transplant donation." Am J Kidney Dis 36(3): 534-40.

5

Novel Renal Transplant-Related Surgical Approaches in the 21st Century

Shih-Chieh Jeff Chueh and Bashir R. Sankari
Glickman Urological and Kidney Institute, Cleveland Clinic, and Cleveland Clinic Lerner College of Medicine, OH USA

1. Introduction

The surgical procedures of implanting a kidney graft into the extraperitoneal iliac fossa has not changed much since its inception in 1950s; whereas the other renal transplant-related surgical approaches have been dramatically updated recently, especially with the commencement of urological laparoscopic surgery. The mile-stone advancement is the laparoscopic live donor nephrectomy (LDN). Conventional open LDN technique has been alleged as a hurdle for expanding live donor programs. Minimally invasive surgery approaches, like laparoscopic LDN, have been advocated to overcome this obstacle (Boulware et al., 2002). A variety of laproscopic LDN approaches will be detailed.

1.1 Pre-operative evaluation of live kidney donor

The eligibility as a living donor is subject to the regulations of the respective local Health Authorities. In the United States the United Network of Organ Sharing (UNOS) operates Organ Procurement and Transplantation Network (OPTN) under contract with the Health Resources and Services Administration (HRSA) of the U.S. Department of Health and Human Services (HHS), which was established by the United States Congress under the National Organ Transplant Act (NOTA) of 1984 and provides policies of live kidney donors to be abided by. Under UNOS/OPTN policy, relatives, loved ones, friends, and even individuals who wish to remain anonymous may serve as live donors. Donating an organ is a personal decision that should only be made after fully informed about the possible risks and benefits. Live donors should be older than 18 years old, in good overall physical and mental health and free from uncontrolled high blood pressure, diabetes, cancer, HIV/AIDS, hepatitis, and organ diseases. Pre-operative assessments exclude incompatibility between the donor and the recipient and also confirm the proper functioning of the donor's bilateral kidneys, and ensure that the risks of surgery and anesthesia are acceptable (OPTN, 2006; UNOS, 2009).

1.2 Which kidney to harvest?

Usually left kidney is preferred for live donation because the left renal vein is longer, which makes the implantation surgery easier and safer. In specific situations like: complex vascular or ureteral structures of the left kidney, significant inferiority of the right renal function relative to the left, right renal stone, etc., right kidney will be harvested for transplantation.

2. Laparoscopic live donor nephrectomy

2.1 History of laparoscopic live donor nephrectomy

Kavoussi and Clayman performed first laparoscopic nephrectomy for a cancerous kidney (Clayman et al., 1991). Ratner and Kavoussi first reported a successful laparoscopic live donor nephrectomy (LLDN, Ratner et al., 1995). Initially there were concerns about graft function and donor's safety with such procedure, and only limited centers routinely performed such procedure (Jacobs et al., 2004; Su et al., 2004). With more experience it revealed non-inferiority of the LLDN results, as compared with those of the open LDN. The benefits of the LLDN include smaller wounds, less pain, earlier resumption of oral intake, and faster recuperation and earlier return to previous life style and to work. Nowadays, LLDN has been the surgery of choice for harvesting a kidney from a live donor (Kercher et al.,2003; Troppmannet al., 2003; Tooher et al., 2004; Velidedeoglu et al., 2002).

2.2 Techniques of laparoscopic live donor nephrectomy

2.2.1 Hand-assisted laparoscopic live donor nephrectomy

2.2.1.1 Immediate preoperative preparation

The most important pre-operative conditioning of the live donor is vigorous hydration to combat the detrimental effect of pneumoperitoneum on the kidney function. Usually before the kidney is harvested 3~6 liters of fluid has been given to the donor to ensure good renal perfusion and diuresis. The operation is carried out under general anesthesia; an oro- or nasogastric tube is necessary to decompress the stomach, and a urethral catheter drains the bladder and helps monitoring urine output. Continuous or frequent blood pressure monitoring during the surgery to ensure mean arterial blood pressure about 100 mmHg, and a central line to ensure central line pressure around 10 mmHg help the kidneys well perfused. At the initiation of renal hilar dissection and right before the transection of the renal vessels, 12.5 grams of Mannitol are given to protect the kidneys and to induce diuresis.

2.2.1.2 Left hand-assisted LLDN (Chueh et al., 2002a; Hollenbeck et al., 2004)

The donor is positioned in an oblique flank position with the operating table flexed at the waist and all the pressure points are well padded. First, around the navel a 7-cm midline incision is made, or alternately a Pfannenstiel incision, if the donor's body size allows the intra-abdominal hand to reach the kidney. The incision is deepened layer by layer into the peritoneal cavity. A hand-assisted device (HAD) is set-up at this site. With one hand in the abdomen through the HAD, the insertion sites of the ports are tented up by the operator's fingers to ensure safe insertion of the trocars. The working port is located in the anterior axillary line about the level of the umbilicus, and the laparoscopic port can be at the left lower abdomen between the umbilicus and the anterior superior iliac crest (making sure to avoid injuring the inferior epigastric artery) or in the midline (epigastrium) above the HAD. The pneumoperitoneum of the abdominal cavity was then insufflated up to 10-12 mmHg, and a 30 degree laparoscope is used for the whole procedure.

The dissection begins by taking down the descending colon along the white line of Toldt to expose the kidney and ureter. Special attention must be exercised to the tissue planes between the structures: the Gerota fascia and soft tissues in front of the ureter needs to be preserved with the ureter, whereas the Gerota fascia in front of the kidney can be taken down with the colon, so the color of the kidney can be visualized during the dissection and abundant soft tissues around the ureter can be preserved to ensure good blood supply to the

ureter. Initial series showed higher rate of ureteral complications and urine leakage when no special attention to preserve the ureteral blood supply was exerted (figure 1; Bartlett, 2002).
The take-down of the descending colon extends from its distal junction with the sigmoid colon up to its splenic flexure, and it further extends cranially up to the lateral parietal attachment of the spleen; i.e.: the phrenicocolic and splenophrenic ligaments are divided. This extensive take-down facilitates the colon, spleen and the pancreatic tail to fall off the main operative field and helps to harvest a long ureter (figure 1b). The intra-abdominal hand is used freely for retracting the colon, spleen and pancreas away from the operative field, and for some blunt dissection between the kidney and the surrounding soft tissues. Pressure on the kidney or the renal vessels, either by the intra-abdominal fingers or by any instruments, is absolutely forbidden.
Further dissections aim at the tributaries of the left renal vein: namely, the gonadal, adrenal and lumbar veins. The gonadal vein is dissected along its medial side and off the underlying psoas muscle; whereas the majority of its lateral border is kept intact to preserve the blood supply to the ureter, except near its entrance into the left renal vein where it is dissected circumferentially and transected to expose a window for further dissection of the lumbar vein(s) and the left renal artery. The gonadal vein is controlled and transected again distally near the iliac vessels. The lumbar vein(s) usually drain into the posterior surface of the left renal vein. Its dissection is facilitated by elevating the gonadal vein stump or the lower margin of the renal vein. The lumbar vein is often quite short and might be multiple. The division of the lumbar vein(s) further opens up the window to dissect the renal artery. The dissection of the upper margin of the left renal vein leads to the insertion point of the left adrenal vein into the renal vein, which is usually more medial to that of the gonadal vein. The adrenal vein is controlled and divided. The adrenal gland was dissected off the upper pole of the kidney with special attention not to interfere with upper pole branch(es) of the renal artery if there is any extra-hilar early branching of the renal artery.
The left renal vein is dissected medially beyond its anterior crossing of the aorta. The renal artery is first partially dissected without any grasping or compression of the artery to avoid arterial spasm. Then the lateral, posterior and superior surfaces of the kidney were dissected off its surrounding attachments along the plane of the renal capsule, while leaving some soft tissues attached to the capsule for further traction. The adipose and soft tissues around the renal hilum and those in the triangle between the low pole of the kidney and the ureter (golden triangle, figure 1b*) are preserved to ensure adequate blood flow to the ureter.
The posterior and superior surfaces of the renal artery are then further freed when the kidney is flipped forward. The arterial dissection is carried out proximally to include its take-off from the aorta in order to facilitate retrieving longer artery.
The ureter is dissected medial to the gonadal vein to leave abundant tissues around it all the way down to its crossing at the iliac vessels, where it is transected immediately before the division of the renal pedicle to avoid torsion of the kidney (figure 1a and 1b). Only the distal ureter is clipped, and the proximal end of the ureter is left open to observe and ensure brisk urine output. The dissection of the upper pole and posterior-upper part of the kidney sometimes might be difficult because of the limited angles of the pivot function of the laparoscopic ports. Special care must be exerted not to put pressure on the renal parenchyma during this part of the dissection.
After making sure that the kidney is attached to the body only by the renal vessels the kidney is held up gently with the intra-abdominal hand, and the renal artery is first ligated at its origin from the aorta. Then the renal vein is controlled at the point of its crossing to the

aorta or even more medially if the dissection allows. This sequence of vessel ligations prevents congestive stasis of blood in the kidney. The control of the renal pedicles have been performed with either a standard laparoscopic vascular stapler (usually 3 rows of staplers on both sides of a dividing knife), Endo TA™ 30 stapler (only a triple staggered row of titanium staples, Covidien), polymer locking clips (Hem-o-lok, Weck, Teleflex), or laparoscopic metal clips (for artery only). The Endo TA stapler and the polymer locking clips provide the advantage of preserving maximal graft vascular length, which makes the implantation vascular anastomosis easier; whereas the use of conventional laparoscopic vascular stapler sacrifices 4 mm of the graft vascular length because 3 rows of staggered staplers at the end of the vessels need to be excised before anastomosis.

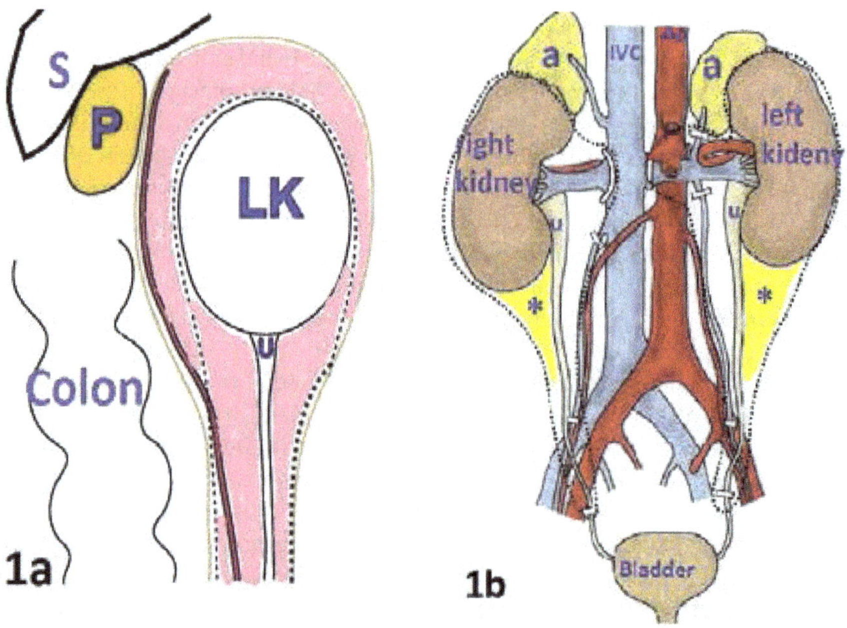

Fig. 1. Schematic planes of dissection during various nephrectomies. 1a. sagittal view. LK= left kidney, P= pancreatic tail, S= spleen, u= left ureter, painted pink area= perirenal soft tissues inside Gerota's fasia, dotted line= dissection plane during LDN, red line= anterior dissection plane during radical nephrectomy. 1b. coronal view. a= adrenal gland, Ao= aorta, IVC= inferior vena cava, u= ureter, *= Golden triangle, tubular structures painted in red= arteries, tubular structures painted in blue= veins, rectangle areas over vessels or ureter= sites of ligating vessels or ureter, dotted lines= planes of dissection during LDN.

Even though there have been several papers reporting successful applications of Hem-o-lok clips in controlling the pedicles during LLDN (Chueh et al., 2004; Ponsky et al., 2008), however, LLDN had been indicated by the manufacturer of the Hem-o-lok clip as a contraindication for the use of the polymer locking clips in 2006, and FDA announced a product recall, too (FDA, 2006), because Hem-o-lok clips may become dislodged following ligation of the renal artery after laparoscopic donor nephrectomy; and cases of delayed bleeding leading to severe morbidities or even mortality of the donor after using the Hem-o-lok clips. This issue has been further pointed out when UNOS first sent a notice to its members and FDA regarding the Hem-o-lok clip in 2008. More recently, UNOS and

American Society of Transplant Surgeon (ASTS) again sent a letter to their members to emphasize the importance of this issue, and urge the centers those perform live donor nephrectomy not use this clip for LLDN. Possible technical explanations for the complication might be related to that some harvesting surgeon just applied one Hem-o-lok clip over the artery in order to retrieve longer artery, and the Hem-o-lok clip slipped off an arterial stump that was left too short, or due to that the polymer clip(s) were weakened because of some thermal energy damage during the operation, and they fell apart in a couple days later. Hence, Endo TA™ 30 stapler is our current preference because of its ability of ensuring arterial seal and of harvesting longer vessels. Cold scissors cut of the renal pedicle vessels lateral (distal) to the stapler lines of the TA stapler completely frees the kidney, and the kidney is immediately retrieved out of the abdomen via the HAD wound to the back table for ex vivo perfusion and bench preparation in ice slush.

Once the kidney is delivered to the back table, the harvesting surgeon re-establishes the HAD and the pneumoperitoneum for meticulous hemostasis. Laparoscopic suction and irrigation are freely used to locate the bleeders. Attention is first focused on the transected ends of pedicles, and then the adrenal bed, lumbar vein stump, and lymphatic openings. The pneumoperitoneum is progressively decreased to 5 mmHg to ensure all minor bleeders are detected and securely controlled. Usually a drainage tube is not necessary.

The procedural sequences of LLDN are different from those of other types of laparoscopic nephrectomies because the renal pedicles are usually first ligated in the later circumstances, but in the former the pedicle vessels are initially dissected from the surrounding tissues, yet not ligated until the whole kidney is ready to be retrieved. This is to ensure a shortest warm ischemic time (WIT) of the harvested kidney for a better graft function after implantation.

A pinkish kidney with tense tone of the renal cortex and a well distended renal vein during the dissection indicate good perfusion of the kidney (and usually translated into immediate graft functioning after transplantation). But if the color is dusky or pale, or the tone of the kidney is floppy, or the renal vein is collapsed during the dissection, it indicates that the kidney is not adequately perfused and thus requires immediate attention and corrections of the donor's conditions by the surgeon and the anesthetic team must be executed. Maneuvers that might help include: more vigorous hydration, elevating the blood pressure and vasodilation of the renal artery with pharmaceutical agents, decrease the pressure of the pneumoperitoneum (5~8 mmHg), correction of any kinking or spasm of the renal artery, etc.

2.2.1.3 Right hand-assisted LLDN (Buell et al., 2004; Chueh et al., 2002a)

Only the procedural differences from the above-mentioned left hand-assisted LLDN are described below. The donor is placed similarly but with the right side up. The first camera port at the umbilicus is safely placed. After CO_2 insufflation to create pneumoperitoneum, a 7-cm subcostal oblique line corresponding to the level of right renal pedicle is marked on the skin. Three working ports, 2 at the ends of the marked line and 1 at the anterior axillary line between iliac bone and lower costal margin, are inserted. The ascending colon and the 2nd portion of the duodenum are taken down to expose the kidney and the inferior vena cava (IVC). After division of the right gonadal vein near its insertion into the IVC, and preliminary dissection of the renal pedicle and right ureter, the incision between the two working ports is connected to set-up the HAD and the surgeon's hand is inserted. The dissection of the right renal artery is done mainly when the kidney is flipped medially to expose its posterior surface. After all the dissections are completed, the ureter is transected. Then the hand is removed from the HAD, and the pneumoperitoneum is desufflated, while leaving the base wound retractor of the HAD still in place. This creates a window large enough for division of the vessels with traditional Satinsky vascular clamp to yield a full-length right renal vein with a partial IVC cuff. After the kidney is retrieved to the back table, the defect in the IVC is closed with 4-0 Prolene continuous sutures in 2 layers for meticulous hemostasis. Then the Satinsky vascular clamp is released. Some right renal donors might have longer renal vein, which can be measured from the Computed Tomography angiographic images preoperatively during the donor evaluation. In that case the HAD wound for the hand and for extracting the kidney can be moved down to a periumbilical, right Gibson, or Pfannenstiel incision. And the right kidney, after totally freed from the surrounding tissues, is pulled up laterally during the application of the Endo TA stapler, which is then pushed as medially as possible at the junction of right renal vein and the IVC to harvest a renal vein at its maximal length.

2.2.2 Pure laparoscopic live donor nephrectomy

The basic concept, planes of dissection, and the majority of the "pure laparoscopic" approach are very similar to those of the hand-assisted approach. The followings will only depict the differences:

2.2.2.1 Pure left LLDN

A working instrument, which usually enters into the operative field through a left subcostal port, substitutes all the functions of the intra-abdominal hand in the HAD approach. Without the HAD, the laparoscopic port can be at the umbilicus or left upper abdomen, depending on the body habitus of the donor. The port for the right-hand instrument is located at the same position. Another 15 mm port is created along the Pfannenstiel incision, which is later extended to 5-6 cm, with muscle split in the midline for the final extraction of the harvested kidney. An extra-large retrieving bag- EndoCatch II (Covidien, Mansfield, MA, USA) is employed through that port for helping traction during the dissection and for retrieving the kidney. Once all the dissections have been done and the ureter has been transected, the EndoCatch II is partially activated to "bag" the kidney and the ureter into the EndoCatch II bag while the edge of the bag and the string are still attached to its metallic ring; in this way, the renal pedicles can be tented up tight by elevating the Endocatch II ring (kidney) in the air. This tremendously facilitates the ligation of the renal pedicles and ensures long vessel length of the graft.

2.2.2.2 Pure right LLDN (Boorjian et al., 2004; Johnson et al., 2001)

Procedures are similar to those of pure left LLDN. The main differences are: 1. The ascending colon and the 2nd portion of duodenum, instead of the descending colon, pancreatic tail and the spleen, are taken down. 2. The right gonadal vein usually drains into the inferior vena cava (IVC), but it might also drain into the right renal vein directly. 3. There might be some small, thin-walled, innominate veins, which have higher chance to cause bleeding, draining into the right renal vein. 4. The wall of the right renal vein is thin, in comparison to that of the left renal vein, which is more prone to tear or bleeding during the procedures. 5. The length of the right renal vein is usually only 1-2 cm in length, which is much shorter than that of the left renal vein. 6. During the dissection of the upper pole of the right kidney, retraction of liver is usually necessary for better exposure. Once the kidney is completely dissected with only the renal vessels attached to the body, the kidney is bagged into the EndoCatch bag, and lifted high to tent up the renal pedicles. The right renal artery is stapled behind the IVC, and the renal vein is stapled at the IVC where it drains into, both with the Endo TA stapler, and then both vessels are transected immediately lateral (distal) to the staplers.

2.2.3 Retroperitoneoscopic live donor nephrectomy

Several teams (Bachmann et al., 2008; Sundqvist et al., 2004; Tanabe et al., 2005; Kohei et al., 2010) published successful series of retroperitoneoscopic LDN. Tanabe's revised technique usually employs a 3-port dissection technique combined with a Pfannenstiel 5-cm retrieving wound to accomplish the surgery.

The donor is in a lateral flank position, but the table is not bent. It requires a flexible laparoscope inserted through a mid-axillary port between the lower costal margin and the iliac crest, and a very experienced and skillful assistant as the telescope holder to collaborate with the operator. The surgeon develops the retroperitoneal working space, and dissects the kidney off the surrounding tissues with a pure retroperitoneoscopic dissection technique under a low 5-10 mmHg pressure of pneumo-retroperitoneum. After the kidney is totally freed (except the vascular pedicles), that Pfannestiel wound is deepened to the extraperitoneal space to connect to the previously dissected retroperitoneal space, then a Lapdisc (Hakko Medical, Tokyo, Japan) is setup at that incision and an Endocatch II retrieving device is inserted through the Lapdisc to harvest the kidney. Laparoscopic EndoGIA Stapler (Covidien, Mansfield, MA, USA) is used to control the renal artery and renal vein, or even larger gonadal vein or lumbar vein during the dissection.

The benefits of such an approach are early and direct dissection of the renal artery, no violation of the intraperitoneal organs, bowels, etc., and theoretically might lead to less post-operative ileus or bowel injury. The risks and challenges are that the retroperitoneal working space is much smaller and it is more technically demanding to operate in such circumstance without exerting unnecessary pressure on the kidney.

Summarizing their experiences with a total of more than 600 live donors operated via such approach shows that the chance of open conversion was low, and the complication rates were 4.9~ 7.7 %. Mean warm ischemia time was 2.2- 4.8 minutes. And the recipients' allograft function recovered smoothly. Thus, in experienced hands retroperitoneoscopic LDN seems provide similar outcome as compared with those of laparoscopic LDN.

2.3 Comments and summary of laparoscopic LDN

Evidences showed that the post-operative pain and quality of life of the donors, either operated by the hand assisted approach or the pure laparoscopic approach are similar, and both are significantly better that those of the traditional open approach (Velidedeoglu et al., 2002; Kercher et al., 2003; Troppmann et al., 2003; Mjøen et al., 2010; Leventhal et al., 2010). Laparoscopic LDN has evolved to be the surgery of choice for live kidney donors. Yet the bottom line issues are still the donor's safety and the functional integrity of the kidney graft. The donor surgeons should work in the way that they are most confident with and have very low threshold of converting to an approach with bigger incision to ensure the ultimate basic principles. For beginners it might be easier and safer to start with the hand-assisted approach, but this approach is ergonomically not friendly; and also poses some difficulty in fine handling and traction of the tissues by the left hand (fingers). Even though with the most experienced LLDN surgeon, there should always be a set of open exploration instruments immediately available in the operation suite during the LDN surgery; and the threshold of converting to a safer procedure should always be low.

3. Laparoendoscopic Single Site (LESS) live donor nephrectomy

Through the last 2 decades of developing minimally invasive surgery, urological laparoscopic surgery has gained more acceptance as a standard of care in various intra-abdominal procedures. Novel endeavors to advance this field are aimed at further mitigating morbidity and improving cosmetic outcomes. This trend has led to the development of multi-channel single-access ports, articulating instruments, and surgical techniques that could allow the laparoscopic procedures to be performed through a single small skin incision (laparoendoscopic single-site [LESS] surgery). The majority of such reports often hide the incision within the umbilicus, and transperitoneal route is typically employed. There have been reports of LESS live donor nephrectomy (LDN) in some elite transplant centers (Gill et al., 2008; Gimenez etal., 2010., Andonian et al., 2010a). We recently also successfully completed 4 cases of LESS LDN with speedy convalescence of the donors, and smooth recovery of the recipients' graft function.

3.1 Technique of LESS LDN

3.1.1 Belly-Button LESS LDN (Chueh and Sankari, submitted, 2011)

We will depict our technique of LESS LDN performed through a small incision at the belly-button. The donor is placed in a 60 degree flank position as in the pure laparoscopic LDN. A first layer transparent adhesive drape is applied over the whole abdomen after it has been prepped and draped. A 4.5 ~5-cm vertical midline incision is made around the umbilicus, and the wound is deepened layer by layer until the peritoneum cavity is entered. A GelPort® hand-assisted device (HAD) is setup at this wound. A second layer transparent adhesive drape is then applied over the abdomen, which also covers the whole GelPort and obliterates intra-operative gas leakage from the central pre-made entry/exit hole of the gel-cap. Thus the GelPort is used as the access platform for the following LESS LDN.

A 12-mm port is inserted through the gel-cap portion of the GelPort at its periphery part, but not right at the margin of its rigid ring. Pneumoperitoneal insufflation is started and a 30-degree 5 or 10-mm laparoscope is used to examine the peritoneal cavity. Another 2 laparoscopic ports, one 5-mm and one 12-mm in size, are inserted through the gel-cap portion of the GelPort under direct vision; again at the periphery of the gel-cap, forming a triangular relationship with the first port, and each port stays away from the others as far as possible. Then with a grasper in the non-dominant hand, and a cutting device in the dominant hand, the colon is taken down to expose the kidney. Most of the time two straight instruments can be used at the same time, or a grasper with a flexible angled tip and a straight cutting instrument might work better at some situations.

Then the other following procedures are very similar to those of the pure laparoscopic LDN described above. In case of difficulty dissections (e.g.: distended colon obscuring clear visualization of the renal hilum, or some bleeding requiring efficient suction to localize the bleeder), a third 5-mm working port can be inserted through the Gel-cap at a point away from the other ports for a 3rd instrument to provide effective traction or suction. The dilemma of adding the 3rd or more instruments is that although it might provide better operative field, the sword-fighting limited angles of the crowded instruments through the LESS incision might also make smooth progression of the procedures difficult. Hence the decision of how many ports necessary should be evaluated individually.

When the kidney is only attached to the body by the renal pedicles, and the ureter has been transected at its crossing of the iliac vessels, an extra-large EndoCatch II (Covidien) is

separately inserted through the gel-cap either directly or through a 15-mm port for retrieving the kidney. The EndoCatch II is opened to "bag" the kidney and its proximal ureter into the retrieval bag while the edge of the bag and the string are still attached to its metallic ring. Thus, the renal pedicles can be tightly tented up by elevating the Endocatch II ring in the air. This significantly opens up the space of the renal vessels with their body attachments (aorta and IVC) and facilitates the ligation of the renal pedicles and ensures long vessel length of the graft. The ligation of the renal artery and the renal vein is performed by applying the laparascopic Endo TA stapler (Covidien), and then the vessels are transected distal to the staple lines with scissors. If there are 2 or more renal arteries, they can be controlled separately by Endo TA staplers, or the smaller artery can ligated with Hem-o-lok or metal clips (at least 2 to 3 clips are necessary). The smaller artery is ligated first to shorten the warm ischemic time of the major portion of the kidney.
At this point, the kidney is totally freed, and the string of the EndoCatch is pulled to detach the retrieval bag from the metallic ring to keep the kidney in the bag, the 2nd layer of the transparent adhesive drape is cut around the external ring of the GelPort, and the gel-cap is released from its base fascial retractor to harvest the kidney easily without squeezing it.
Then the GelPort device is quickly assembled again, and the pneumoperitoneum is re-insufflated for meticulous hemostasis. The pressure of pneumoperitoneum is decreased to 5 mmHg to detect even mild venous or lymphatic oozing. Usually no drain tube is necessary. The GelPort devise is removed, and the wound is closed in a standard fashion.

3.1.2 Pfannenstiel LESS Live Donor Nephrectomy (Andonian et al., 2010a)

This technique is pioneered by Kavoussi et al. Their main benefit is to hide the skin incision line low in the supra-pubic area, instead of via the belly-button. Through a 5-cm Pfannenstiel incision, three 5-mm ports are placed in a triangular manner (2 at the midline [5 cm apart], and 1 at the ipsilateral rectus mucle 5 cm from the inferior port in the midline). A 5 mm flexible-tip laparoscope (EndoEye, Olympus, Japan), along with other long bariatric laparoscopic instruments, is used to perform laparoscopic donor nephrectomy in the fashion similar to the pure laparoscopic LDN. Before ligating the renal hilum, the superior midline trocar is exchanged for a 12-mm trocar to allow for an Endo-GIA stapler. After the kidney is placed in the entrapment sac, the anterior rectus fascia between the 2 midline ports is incised and the kidney is removed. After closure of the fascial defects, the Pfannenstiel incision is closed in a subcuticular manner.
Its initial outcomes are successfully in 6 patients without standard laparoscopic or open conversion; and no additional needlescopic instruments used. The median operative time, median warm ischemia time (5 minutes), and median hospital stay are similar to those of the case-matched standard laparoscopic (SL) approach. Although VAS (visual analog pain scale) scores were lower in the LESS versus SL group at each of post-operative day (POD) #2 (1.5 vs. 4) and discharge (0 vs. 2), this did not reach statistical significance (Andonian et al., 2010b).

3.2 Comments and summary of LESS LDN

The benefit of using the GelPort® as the access platform for the LESS LDN in our series is its feasibility of conversion to a standard multiple-port laparoscopic LDN or even a hand-assisted LDN in case any difficult dissections or significant bleeding occur during the procedure of LESS LDN. This offers an immediate 'exit strategy', because considerable and difficult-to-control bleedings might suddenly happen anytime during the procedure, and endangers the safety of the donor or the function of the graft. No matter what approach of

LDN is performed, cannot the bottom-line principles of ensuring the safety of the live donor and good quality of the kidney harvested be over-emphasized. Only when these 2 basic important principles can be strictly upheld, can we pursue the smaller incision and smoother recovery of the live donors. Thus, during the procedure of LESS LDN the threshold of conversion to a conventional laparoscopic LDN (either pure-laparoscopic or hand-assisted approach) should be kept low to protect the donor and the kidney. In case of a significant bleeding that cannot be adequately secured or a situation that endangers function of the kidney (e.g.: prolonged warm ischemic time), instead of continuing struggles with the LESS approach it is recommended to compress or grasp the bleeder with a grasper, and then add one or more ports outside the LESS platform, or even insert a hand into the operating field to control the situation. Use of a GelPort™ as the LESS platform during LDN gives the flexibility of different degrees of speedy conversions.

Even though there have been multiple reports demonstrating the feasibility of LESS LDN, one important basic question not well-answered so far is how many benefits or disadvantages to the live donors this technique provides in comparison to the conventional laparoscopic LDN. The answer to this question can only be achieved by an adequately powered multi-center prospective randomized comparison using tools designed to detect subtle differences in morbidity and to assess cosmetic satisfaction. The other issue is regarding the cost of the surgery. A recent report by Lunsford et al concludes that Single-site laparoscopic living donor nephrectomy offers comparable perioperative outcomes to conventional laparoscopic living donor nephrectomy at a higher cost. (Lunsford et al., 2011) More reports with detailed economic analyses are required to answer this question.

4. Other renal transplant-related laparoscopic procedures

Besides laparoscopic donor nephrectomy there are other laparoscopic or novel procedures feasible among ESRD patients with a transplant kidney (Fornara et al., 1997). These procedures aim at either problems related to the transplanted kidneys (e.g.: lymphocele, tumor in transplant kidney); or problems related to the native kidneys (e.g.: polycystic kidneys, renal cell carcinomas). Their respective details are described as follows:

4.1 Laparoscopic marsupialization of lymphoceles

Lymphocele development after renal transplantation is a well-recognized possible complication that occurs with the incidence of 0.6-26%. Lymphoceles may originate either from the lymphatic system of the recipient or the transplanted kidney. Before the laparoscopic era, the standard treatment of symptomatic lymphoceles is first puncture aspiration to differentiate between urinoma/lymphocele and to test for bacterial infection; then percutaneous drainage, with or without the injection of sclerosing solution; and finally, open marsupialization if initial approaches fail. With the advent of laparoscopic surgery, laparoscopic approaches to remove an ellipse of peritoneal wall along with the adjacent lymphocele wall, to lyse all internal lymphocele loculations, and even tuck in a piece of omentum by laparoscopic suture allow for the free flow of lymph into the peritoneal cavity and remove the pressure effect of the lymphocele on the transplant kidney, graft ureter, and even venous drainage can be achieved (Parra et al., 1992; Khauli et al., 1992).

There are many caveats in performing such procedure. Several cases of graft ureter transaction have been reported. Thus, pre-operative stenting the graft ureter should be performed whenever possible. (Abou-Elela et al., 2006; Shokeir et al., 1994). Multiple septa and loculations of the lymphoceles might lead to early recurrence or failure of the surgery. Tricks to deal with this circumstance includes transcutaneous staining of the lymphocele lining with methylene blue, and use of intraoperative ultrasonography (Schilling et al., 1995; Matin & Gill, 2001). Other tips for anatomically difficult lymphoceles lateral or inferior to the transplant kidney, which without a common wall between the lymphocele and peritoneal cavities has been reported by placing a cable of 2 internalized peritoneal dialysis catheters between the lymphoceles and the peritoneal cavity for maintaining permanent lymphoperitoneal drainage (Matin & Gill, 2000). Other potential problems associated with laparoscopic marsupialization of lymphoceles consist of injury to other organs (6%), and open conversion (6%) (Atray et al., 2004; Gruessner et al.,1995).

4.2 Laparoscopic nephrectomy for renal cell carcinoma or polycystic kidneys in native kidneys

Laparoscopic nephrectomy has been shown effective in removing diseased kidneys with tumors, even tumors larger than 7-cm in diameter. (Berger et al., 2008; Steinberg et al., 2004) Long-term oncologic outcomes (overall, cancer-specific, and recurrence-free survivals) of laparoscopic radical nephrectomy, either with pure laparoscopic or HAD technique, or with trans-peritoneal or trans-retroperitoneal approach, for renal cell carcinoma (RCC) are comparable to those of its open counterpart, with the obvious benefits of less pain, less blood loss and earlier recuperation (Colombo et al., 2008; Chung et al., 2007; Venkatesh et al., 2007; Desai et al., 2005; Nambirajan et al., 2004).

Patients with ESRD are known to have higher surgical risks (higher American Society of Anesthiologists score, higher comorbidity index, higher incidence of previous abdominal surgery, and higher incidence of hypertension), and yet they also have higher incidence of renal tumors and which does not decrease even after renal transplantation because of maintenance immunosuppression (Chueh SC et al., 2011a; Melchior et al., 2011; Navarro et al., 2008; Tollefson et al., 2010). Laparoscopic radical nephrectomy among this special patient group, even though more challenging and might be associated with slightly longer admission and higher perioperative risks, is well recognized as feasible and safe (Bird et al., 2010). Recently, there was even report of successful LESS radical nephrectomy among these patient groups (Greco et al., 2010; Chueh et al., 2011b).

Technically, laparoscopic radical nephrectomy is similar to that of the previously mentioned LDN, with their main differences depicted are as follows: 1). The sequence/ timing of pedicle ligation: during LDN in order to shorten the warm ischemic time the renal artery and renal vein are ligated right before retrieving the kidney; whereas during radical nephrectomy in order to decrease the chance of tumor cell seeding along the vessels, renal artery and vein are controlled as early as possible and before further mobilization of the whole kidney. 2). The plane of dissection (figure 1a): during LDN peri-renal fat and soft tissues are not necessary and Gerota's fascia is opened to reveal the color and tone of the kidney during the dissection; whereas during radical nephrectomy dissection is made along outside the Gerota's fascia to encompass all the soft tissues around the kidney to ensure enbloc resection. Adrenal gland is spared during LDN but it is excised during radical nephrectomy if the tumor is in the upper pole or no clear plane between the tumor and adrenal gland discerned on the images (Siemer et al., 2004). Abundant soft tissues around the ureter are mandatory during LDN; whereas ureter can be stripped during radical nephrectomy unless urothelial carcinoma is suspected preoperatively. 3). Method of specimen extraction: Some urologists morcellate the kidneys for cancerous renal specimen of radical nephrectomy to achieve key-hole wounds, whereas at least a 5-cm incision needs to be made to harvest the LDN kidney. 4). Laparoscopic setting: during LDN the pressure of the pneumoperitoneum is kept as low as possible (usually around 10-12 mmHg or less) to avoid interfering the renal perfusion and subsequent graft function; whereas during radical nephrectomy a pneumoperitoneum of 15 mmHg is usually employed.

Polycystic kidney disease (PCKD) might lead to ESRD, and renal transplant is a well-known therapy for those patients. Indications for native nephrectomies among those PCKD patients include severe fullness and early satiety, abdominal pain, recurrent urinary tract infections, recurrent hematuria, poorly controlled hypertension, need space for future transplant; and suspicion of malignancy in the enlarged kidneys. Laparoscopic nephrectomy for PCKD kidneys has been shown as a viable alternative of its open counter-part. Either transperitoneal or retroperitoneoscopic approach is feasible. Retroperitoneoscopic approach provides quicker and direct access to the renal hilum, but requires separate port wounds on each side of the body. And many papers reported the use of HAD facilitate the dissection and excision of the diseased PCKD kidneys. When compared to open surgery, the laparoscopic approach results in significantly shorter hospital stay, decreased morbidity and quicker recovery (Rehman et al., 2001; Gill et al., 2001). The use of Vacuum Curettage System (Berkeley VC-10, ACMI, Southborough, MA) to morcellate and aspirate the kidney was reported to provide a significant decrease in the overall size and allow easy extraction through the midline incision (Whitten et al., 2006).

As to when is the best timing to do the surgery, and whether simultaneous bilateral or staged surgery is safer for the patients are still in dispute. Some articles reported 60% complication rate if performed simultaneously, and thus recommend staged operation. Another report mentioned renal transplantation and ipsilateral native PCKD nephrectomy carry no significant additional morbidity compared to that of renal transplantation alone (Ismail et al., 2005; Lucas et al., 2010).

4.3 Laparoscopic nephroureterectomy and bladder cuff eecision for localized urothelial carcinomas in native upper urinary tract

Standard treatment for localized urothelial carcinoma (UC) of the upper urinary tract (UUT) is nephroureterectomy with resection of the ipsilateral distal ureter and bladder cuff. Since Clayman et al. reported in 1991 the initial case of laparoscopic nephroureterectomy (LNU), there have been reports demonstrating that LNU decreases pain and accelerates convalescence of patients (Jarrett et al., 2001). It can be done either with pure laparoscopic approach or with the help of a hand-assisted device (McNeill et al., 2000; Gill et al., 2000; Shalhav et al., 2000; Chen et al., 2001).

Operative technique of a hand-assisted nephroureterectomy (HALNU; Chen et al., 2001): The patient is placed in a 60° oblique position with no change in posture during the entire procedure. The operating table can be rotated from side to side to facilitate exposure during different parts of the surgery. Via a 7-cm lower abdominal Gibson incision, distal ureterectomy with bladder cuff resection was done according to the classic open maneuver. If this is on the side of the transplant kidney cautions need to be exerted to prevent interfering with the transplant ureter. The bladder is closed so that it is watertight with 2-0 absorbable sutures. The end of the distal ureter was double ligated, wrapped with a 4 x 4 gauze, tied up, and left in the retroperitoneum. Then a hand-assisted device (HAD) is set up at this incision, and pneumoperitoneum is insufflated. Two laparoscopic ports are inserted, under the guidance of the intraperitoneal hand and telescope. A 30° telescope is used.

Nephroureterectomy is then performed similarly to those described. The surgeon and the assistant, both facing the patient's abdomen, stand side by side. For a left HALNU, if the surgeon is ambidextrous, he/she inserts his/her right hand intraperitoneally, and operates the laparoscopic instrument with his/her left hand. If he/she is right-handed, the operator's left hand is placed intraperitoneally. For a right HALNU, the surgeon inserts his/her left hand into the HAD. After the colon is taken down, the renal vessels are first identified, dissects, then ligated and transected. An adrenalectomy is performed only when the tumor involved the upper pole parenchyma of the kidney in image studies. Then the kidney and the entire length of the ureter with the surrounding tissues are excised and removed en-bloc from the lower abdomen incision made for the HAD.

4.4 Simultaneous laparoscopic bilateral nephroureterectomy (nephrectomy) without changing body position

The incidence of UC is higher in patients with ESRD, especially in some Asian countries and countries with Balkan Nephropathy and the carcinomas are often multifocal (Liao et al., 2004). When there is UC in either one or both sides of the upper urinary tract in ESRD patients, the treatment of choice usually is simultaneous bilateral nephroureterectomy. Traditionally, open simultaneous bilateral nephroureterectomy is usually done via a long midline incision extending from the xyphoid to the symphysis pubis. To perform unilateral LNU smoothly, the patient has to be positioned at 60° oblique to a full lateral flank position for better exposure and easier dissection because the surrounding organs are displaced downward by gravity (Jarrett et al., 2001; McNeill et al., 2000; Gill et al., 2000; Shalhav et al., 2000). For laparoscopic bilateral nephroureterectomy (LBNU) to be completed in one session with the above-mentioned approach, one needs to do additional position changes to perform the nephroureterectomy on the contralateral side. This is cumbersome and prolongs operation time, and patients need to be re-sterilized and re-draped. The following is an easy and convenient maneuver to facilitate and speed up the operation.

Operative technique (Chueh et al., 2002): Two 6-inch-wide inflatable cuffs (an air tourniquet device originally used for damping blood flow during orthopedic surgery on extremities), one on each side of the back, are placed underneath the patient. The patient is placed in a supine position with his/her chest, shoulders, and thighs loosely secured by straps to the operation table, so that there is some room for the air cuff to lift the patient upwards when it is inflated. And thus the patient would not slide off the table when the table is maximally rotated to its side. Possible pressure-bearing areas (when the table is rotated and the cuff is inflated) like both sides of the thighs, hips, axillae, and shoulders and other bony prominences were well padded with soft gel pads (Action Product, Hagertown, MD, USA) to avoid neuromuscular injuries.

To begin the operation, a 7 cm infra-umbilical midline incision is made for the HAD, and a telescopic port is created immediately supra-umbilically to hide this scar. The operator and the assistant stand on the contra-lateral side of the kidney to be operated first. Then the air cuff on the ipsilateral side of the target kidney is inflated (up to 400 mmHg), and the operation table is rotated completely to the contra-lateral side (facing the operator). This brought the patients into a ~60° oblique position which make dissection of the ipsilateral kidney, ureter, and especially the renal pedicles much easier because the surrounding organs will slide down due to gravity after they are taken down from their original attachments. A 12-mm port was inserted in the ipsilateral abdomen at the midclavicular line slightly higher than the level of the umbilicus. If there is difficulty during dissection, another 5-mm port (optional) can be inserted at the sub-xyphoid midline. For hand-assisted laparoscopic nephroureterectomy (HALNU) on the left side, the surgeon inserts his/her left hand into the HAD, stands caudal to the assistant, and operates the laparoscopic instruments with his/her right hand.

For a right HALNU, if the surgeon is ambidextrous, he/she inserts his/her right hand intraperitoneally, stands caudal to the assistant and operates the laparoscopic instrument with his/her left hand. If he/she is right-handed, the assistant stands caudal to him/her, and the surgeon's left hand is placed intraperitoneally (the main 12-mm working port is moved to the right upper quadrant in this circumstance). The middle to lower ureter is first dissected and ligated (without cutting) with clips distal to the tumor to avoid squeezing tumor cells into the bladder during dissection. Then the hand-assisted laparoscopic nephrectomy is performed similarly to those described. The adrenal gland is not excised unless preoperative studies strongly suggested invasion of the tumor into the upper-pole parenchyma of the kidney. After transecting the renal pedicles and freeing the kidney and upper ureter, the specimen could be placed down to the ipsilateral pelvic cavity for later en bloc removal at the final stage of the surgery.

After completing the first side, the 12-mm working port wound on that side is closed in an air-tight manner, and the table is tilted completely to the other side. The air cuff on the first side is deflated, and insufflation of the cuff underneath the other side of the patient proceeds. The surgical team moves to the other side of the table (the side on which the kidney has been excised), inserts a new 12-mm port, and the nephroureterectomy on the second side is performed similarly. In patients with a functional renal graft, a 5-Fr. ureteral catheter was inserted into the graft ureter cystoscopically before the entire laparoscopic procedure to assist identification and protection of the graft kidney and ureter during later dissection.

After the above-mentioned procedures are done, in order to ensure complete resection of the distal ureter and bladder cuff, the operative table is brought back to a neutral position and both air cuffs are deflated. Traditional bladder cuff resection and bladder closure on both sides are performed in an open fashion through the lower midline wound originally made for the HAD. When a transplant kidney is present, dissection of the native lower ureter stays just medial to the lateral border of the native ureter on that specific side. If difficult dissection is encountered (e.g.: a heavy patient with a deep pelvic cavity and/or a patient with a stage T2-T3 lower ureteral tumor), the wound can be extended further towards the symphysis pubis to provide a clearer operative field, and two complete sets of nephroureterectomy specimens are subsequently brought out of the wound.

An intermediate term (median 35 months) follow-up of a total of 40 patients who were identified to have pathologically confirmed urothelial carcinoma of upper urinary tract, either operated by HALBNU (n=25) or by its open counterpart (OBNU, n=15) revealed that the HALBNU group was associated with less blood loss, earlier bowel recovery, less narcotic use, shorter hospital stay, and earlier convalescence. The operative time and complication rate were comparable between the two groups. There was no open conversion in the HALBNU group. The overall, cancer-specific, and bladder-recurrence-free survival were all equivalent between the HALBNU and OBNU group (Tai et al., 2009).

5. Partial nephrectomy for transplanted kidneys

Development of tumors in renal allograft represents a challenging opportunity to both urologists and transplant surgeons. We report our experience with a recent case and present our innovative approach to this problem.

5.1 Case presentation (Sankari and Chueh, submitted, 2011)

The patient has a simultaneous tumor in the native right kidney and a tumor in the transplanted kidney located in the right lower quadrant. The native right kidney was removed with a transperitoneal laparoscopic approach through an incision over the right lower quadrant. Then transplanted kidney was dissected intraperitoneally via the same incision. This allowed us to reflect the colon and avoid any intraperitoneal injury. The iliac artery above and below the kidney was encircled with vessel loops in case we needed to temporarily occlude the blood inflow. The tumor was located over the lateral mid aspect of the kidney and was intrarenal. Following dissection and exposure of the kidney, the tumor could not be palpated or visually identified. Intraoperative ultrasound was used to locate the tumor and markers was made 1 cm above and below the tumor margin. We believe a zero warm ischemia time is more favorable for kidney function outcome, particularly in solitary kidneys. Resection then proceeded quickly with circumferential resection of the tumor all the way down to the underlying renal sinus. Suturing of the deeper collecting system tissue was performed with 3:0 chromic running suture. Floseal hemastatic agent was used to control the exposed small renal vessels. And cupsular sutures with 2:0 chromic interrupted sutures were done. Blood loss was 300 ml. Resection time was 25 minutes without any warm ischemia time. Kidney function remained unchanged post operatively.

5.2 Comments on partial nephrectomy for transplanted kidneys

Kidney transplant recipients are at increased risk for malignancies (Chueh SC et al., 2011a; Navarro et al., 2008; Tollefson et al., 2010). Development of cancer depends on the duration and type of immunosuppression or association with viral infection. Renal cell carcinoma (RCC) in renal transplant recipients is the most common urologic cancer in both native kidneys and transplanted kidneys (Melchior, et al., 2011). The development of tumors in the renal allograft represents a very challenging task for the urologist and transplant surgeon to treat these malignancies, especially when the allograft kidney is still functioning. The overall incidence of de novo malignancies after renal transplant is 4-5 times higher than that of the general population (Penn I, 1998). Malignancy can arise from unnoticed transmission of tumor cells or metastasis within the graft, or they can originate from the recipient.

Transplanted and native kidneys should be screened for tumors by yearly ultrasound after transplant (Kalble T, et al., 2005). Thus tumors can be diagnosed at an early stage. If a tumor is detected in a functionless native kidney, radical nephrectomy is the treatment of choice. RCC within the renal allograft itself is a less frequent event and accounts for approximately 10% of the cases (Kalble T, et al., 2005; Melchior, et al., 2011; Penn I, 1998). Once RCC in the transplanted kidney is diagnosed, it is crucial to determine the genetic origin of the tumor by means of DNA analysis. Thus the potential transmission of tumor cells to other recipients from the same donor can be assessed (Boix, et al., 2009).

There is no consensus on treatment of RCC in the transplanted kidney. Available treatment options include ablative techniques, nephron sparing surgery and allograft nephrectomy. Nephron sparing surgery in the allograft can be a challenging procedure even for experienced urological surgeons (Chambade, et al., 2008). We applied the same surgical principles for partial nephrectomy in the non-transplant patient.

Modification of the immunosuppressive regimen for renal transplant recipients in whom the tumor developed is a matter of debate. But most centers would recommend adjustment of the medications. The mammalian target of Rapamycin (mTOR) inhibitor which is used to prevent acute rejection after renal transplant does not increase the risk of malignancy

(Campistol, 2009). This is in contrast to calcineurin inhibitors (CNI; tacrolimus and cyclosporine) and antimetabolites (mycophenolic acid and azathioprine). Consideration should be given to switch transplant recipients with RCC to mTOR inhibitor (sirolimus or everolimus) and discontinue CNIs and antimetabolites. Prednisone has no effect on tumor progress and can be continued to provide prophylaxis against renal allograft rejection. mTOR inhibitor is a growth factor inhibitor and will affect wound healing and its use should be delayed till after surgical wounds have healed.

In most cases partial nephrectomy requires temporary occlusion of the renal artery to allow for tumor resection and renal reconstruction in a relatively bloodless field (Uzzo and Novick, 2001). This is supplemented with surface cooling if warm ischemia time is expected to exceed more than 30 minutes. The risk of vascular injury though uncommon remains a potential risk of vascular occlusion (Thompson,et al., 2007). Renal artery occlusion can be avoided during open surgery in selected peripheral renal masses based on the rapidity with which hemostasis and renorraphy is possible. Vascular clamping has the potential to lead to renal ischemia and reperfusion injury which are associated with adverse outcome. Vascular clamping during open partial nephrectomy in patients with solitary kidney was associated with greater risk of renal failure and temporary dialysis than partial nephrectomy without ischemia (Wszolek et al., 2010). Duration of ischemia is found to be the strongest modifiable risk factor for decrease renal function after partial nephrectomy (Lane, et al., 2011).

Libertino described his technique for partial nephrectomy without vascular occlusion essentially achieving a 0-ischemia time (Smith, et al., 2010). The renal vessels are dissected all the way to the level of the intrarenal branches. Both renal arteries and renal veins are secured with vessel loops but not occluded. Hemostasis of the resected parenchyma is achieved with electrocautary for small vessels and suture ligation for large vessel. Pediatric clamps are used to occlude the larger vessels prior to ligation with a figure of eight 4:0 vicryl sutures. Opening in the collecting system is closed with absorbable sutures, and a JJ stent is inserted antegradely as needed. Renal parenchyma is then approximated with absorbable sutures. Throughout the procedure an assistant provides exposure with a Frazier suction tip and a Penfield neurosurgical spatula. The percentage change in estimated GFR was higher in the clamped group; yet, the transfusion rate was higher for the unclamped group.

Partial nephrectomy in transplanted kidney represents a unique opportunity to apply techniques developed in partial nephrectomies for solitary kidneys. Modification of the operation is necessary. Anatomically, the transplanted kidney is encased in a bed of scar tissues. Dissection of the renal hilum is tedious and risks injury to the renal vasculature. The dissection of the kidney is aided by performing the operation intraperitoneally. This will allow avoiding inadvertent injury to the intraabdominal organs. Proximal and distal control of the iliac artery above and below the level of the renal artery anastomosis will allow for temporary occlusion in the event of excessive bleeding. We recommend performing the operation without vascular occlusion if possible to avoid any ischemic injury to the transplant kidney.

6. Conclusions

Implantation of a kidney graft into the extraperotineal iliac fossa has not changed much surgically since its inception from 1950s; whereas the other renal transplant-related surgical approaches have dramatically been updated for the past ten more years, especially with the commencement of urological laparoscopic surgery.

The most important mile-stone advancement is the laparoscopic live donor nephrectomy. Since its original report in 1995, in spite of the initial concerns regarding the quality of the graft function and the safety issue for the live donor, laparoscopic live donor nephrectomy has been recently well recognized academically and practically as the surgery of choice for harvesting live donor kidney; which in fact was driven both by the donors' preference and by the surgeons' competence in performing this surgery. It can be performed either via a pure laparoscopic approach, in which a wound is extended at the end of the procedure to harvest the kidney; or it can also be performed via a hand-assisted approach, in which the graft is harvested from the hand-assisted incision.

More recently a newer variant of the laparoscopic surgery—laparoendoscopic single site (LESS) surgery has been evolved to the field of live donor nephrectomy in certain elite transplant centers. This technique creates a smaller and single incision to accomplish the procedure under the same surgical principles with a much steeper learning curve, and some special equipments are necessary to facilitate such operation. The ultimate value of LESS live donor nephrectomy still warrants further proof with prospective randomized data even though it is surgically feasible.

Besides the donor nephrectomy, laparoscopic surgery has also been applied to a variety of procedures related to the renal transplant recipients. Recurrent lymphoceles resistant to repeated aspiration and drainage can be managed with laparoscopic marsupilization (internal drainage into the peritoneal cavity). Incidence of renal cell carcinomas (RCC) in the native kidneys has been shown higher in the transplant recipients than that of the general population. If the RCC is still localized at diagnosis, it can be treated with laparoscopic radical nephrectomy. In certain areas around the world the incidence of urothelial carcinoma in the native upper urinary tract (ureters, renal pelvis and calyses) has also been reported much higher in the transplant recipients. With proper equipment laparoscopic bilateral nephroureterectomy with bladder cuff resection can be performed in one session through several small incisions without changing the patient's position.

Very rarely, tumor in the transplant kidneys might be found during follow-up. If the graft is still functioning, and the tumor is localized, partial nephrectomy of the transplant kidney can be used to excise the tumor while preserve the graft function.

The surgical procedures of each mentioned above have been detailed in this chapter.

7. References

Abou-Elela, A.; Reyad, I.; Torky, M.; Meshref, A. & Morsi, A. (2006) Laparoscopic marsupialization of postrenal transplantation lymphoceles. *J Endourol*. Vol. 20, No. 11, pp. 904-909.

Andonian, S.; Herati, AS.; Atalla, MA.; Rais-Bahrami, S.; Richstone, L. & Kavoussi, LR. (2010a) Laparoendoscopic single-site pfannenstiel donor nephrectomy. *Urology*. Vol. 75, No. 1, pp. 9-12.

Andonian, S.; Rais-Bahrami, S.; Atalla, MA.; Herati, AS.; Richstone, L. & Kavoussi, LR. (2010b) Laparoendoscopic single-site Pfannenstiel versus standard laparoscopic donor nephrectomy. *J Endourol*. Vol. 24, No. 3, pp. 429-432.

Atray, NK.; Moore, F.; Zaman, F.; Caldito, G.; Abreo, K.; Maley, W.& Zibari, GB. (2004) Post-transplant lymphocele: a single centre experience. *Clin Transplant*. Vol. 18, Suppl. 12, pp. 46-49.

Bachmann, A.; Wyler, S.; Wolff, T.; Gürke, L.; Steiger, J.; Kettelhack, C.; Gasser, TC. & Ruszat, R. (2008) Complications of retroperitoneoscopic living donor nephrectomy: single center experience after 164 cases. *World J Urol.* Vol. 26, No. 6, pp. 549-554.

Bartlett, ST. (2002) Laparoscopic donor nephrectomy after seven years. *Am J Transplant.* Vol. 2, No. 10, pp. 896-897.

Berger, AD.; Kanofsky, JA.; O'Malley, RL.; Hyams, ES.; Chang, C.; Taneja, SS. & Stifelman, MD. (2008) Transperitoneal laparoscopic radical nephrectomy for large (more than 7 cm) renal masses. *Urology.* Vol.71, No. 3, pp. 421-424.

Bird, VG.; Shields, JM.; Aziz, M.; De Los Santos, R.; Ayyathurai, R. & Ciancio, G. (2010) Transperitoneal laparoscopic radical nephrectomy for patients with dialysis-dependent end-stage renal disease: an analysis and comparison of perioperative outcome. *Urology.* Vol. 75, No. 6, pp. 1335-1342.

Boix, R.; Sanz, C.; Mora, M.; Quer, A.; Beyer, K.; Musulen, E.; González, C., Bayona, S.; Saladié, JM. & Ariza, A. (2009) Primary renal cell carcinoma in a transplanted kidney: genetic evidence of recipient origin. *Transplantation* Vol. 87, No. 7, pp. 1057-1061.

Boorjian, S.; Munver, R.; Sosa, RE. & Del Pizzo, JJ. (2004) Right laparoscopic live donor nephrectomy: a single institution experience. *Transplantation.* Vol. 77, No. 3, pp. 437-440.

Boulware, LE.; Ratner, LE.; Sosa, JA.; Tu, AH.; Nagula, S.; Simpkins, CE.; Durant, RW. & Powe, NR. (2002) The general public's concerns about clinical risk in live kidney donation. *Am J Transplant.* Vol. 2, No. 2, pp. 186-193.

Buell, JF.; Abreu, SC.; Hanaway, MJ.; Ng, CS.; Kaouk, JH.; Clippard, M.; Zaki, S.; Goldfarb, DA.; Woodle, ES. & Gill, IS. (2004) Right donor nephrectomy: a comparison of hand-assisted transperitoneal and retroperitoneal laparoscopic approaches. *Transplantation.* Vol. 77, No. 4, pp. 521-525.

Campistol, JM. (2009) Minimizing the risk of posttransplant malignancy. *Transplantation.* Vol. 87, Suppl. 8, S19-22.

Chen, J.; Chueh, SC.; Hsu, WT.; Lai, MK. & Chen, SC. (2001) Modified approach of hand-assisted laparoscopic nephroureterectomy for transitional cell carcinoma of the upper urinary tract. *Urology.* Vol. 58, No. 6, pp. 930-934.

Chueh, S.; Sankari, B.; Chung, SD. & Jones, JS. (2011a) Retroperitoneoscopic laparoendoscopic single site nephrectomy. *Br J Urol Intl* [Epub, in press]

Chueh, SC.; Chen, J.; Hsu, WT.; Hsieh, MH. & Lai, MK. (2002b) Hand assisted laparoscopic bilateral nephroureterectomy in 1 session without repositioning patients is facilitated by alternating inflation cuffs. *J Urol.* Vol. 167, No.1, pp.44-47.

Chueh, SC.; Flechner, S.; Goldfarb, D.; Sankari, B. & Campbell, S. (2011b) Re: Tollefson et al.: Surgical treatment of renal cell carcinoma in the immunocompromised transplant patient (Urology 2010;75:1373-1377). *Urology.* Vol. 77, No. 1, pp. 254-255.

Chueh, SC.; Lai, MK.; Lee, PH. & Chen, J. (2002a) Technical considerations in hand-assisted laparoscopic live donor nephrectomy: initial Taiwan experience from National Taiwan University Hospital. *J Formos Med Assoc.* Vol. 101, No. 1, pp. 76-79.

Chueh, SC.; Wang, SM. & Lai, MK. (2004) Use of Hem-o-lok clips effectively lengthens renal vein during laparoscopic live donor nephrectomy *Transplant Proc.* Vol. 36, No. 9, pp. 2623-2624.

Chung, SD.; Huang, KH.; Lai, MK.; Huang, CY.; Pu, YS.; Yu, HJ. & Chueh, SC. (2007) Long-term follow-up of hand-assisted laparoscopic radical nephrectomy for organ-confined renal cell carcinoma. *Urology.* Vol. 69, No. 4, pp. 652-655.

Clayman, RV.; Kavoussi, LR.; Soper, NJ.; Dierks, SM.; Merety, KS.; Darcy, MD.; Long, SR.; Roemer, FD.; Pingleton, ED. & Thomson PG. (1991) Laparoscopic nephrectomy. *N Engl J Med.* Vol. 324, No. 19, pp. 1370-1371.

Colombo, JR. Jr.; Haber, GP.; Jelovsek, JE.; Lane, B.; Novick, AC. & Gill, IS. (2008) Seven years after laparoscopic radical nephrectomy: oncologic and renal functional outcomes. *Urology.* Vol. 71, No. 6, pp. 1149-1154.

Desai, MM.; Strzempkowski, B.; Matin, SF.; Steinberg, AP.; Ng, C.; Meraney, AM.; Kaouk; JH. & Gill, IS. (2005) Prospective randomized comparison of transperitoneal versus retroperitoneal laparoscopic radical nephrectomy. *J Urol.* Vol. 173, No. 1, pp.38-41.

FDA, 2006 http://www.fda.gov/Safety/Recalls/EnforcementReports/2006/ucm120409.htm

Fornara, P.; Doehn, C.; Fricke, L.; Hoyer, J. & Jocham, D. (1997) Laparoscopy in renal transplant patients. *Urology.* Vol. 49, No. 4, pp. 521-527.

Gill, IS.; Canes, D.; Aron, M.; Haber, GP.; Goldfarb, DA.; Flechner, S.; Desai, MR., Kaouk, JH. & Desai, MM. Single port transumbilical (E-NOTES) donor nephrectomy. *J Urol.* Vol. 180, No. 2, pp. 637-641.

Gill, IS.; Kaouk, JH.; Hobart MG.; Sung, GT.; Schweizer, DK. & Braun, WE. (2001) Laparoscopic bilateral synchronous nephrectomy for autosomal dominant polycystic kidney disease: the initial experience. *J Urol.* Vol. 165, No. 4, pp. 1093-1098.

Gill, IS.; Sung, GT., Hobart, MG.; Savage, SJ.; Meraney, AM.; Schweizer, DK.; Klein, EA. & Novick, AC. (2000) Laparoscopic radical nephroureterectomy for upper tract transitional cell carcinoma: the Cleveland Clinic experience. *J Urol.* Vol. 164, No. 5, pp. 1513-1522.

Gimenez, E.; Leeser, DB.; Wysock, JS.; Charlton, M.; Kapur, S.; Del Pizzo, JJ. (2010) Laparoendoscopic single site live donor nephrectomy: initial experience. *J Urol.* Vol. 184, No. 5, pp. 2049-2053.

Greco, F.; Wagner, S.; Hoda, MR.; Weigand, K.; Inferrera, A. & Fornara, P. (2010) Single-Portal Access Laparoscopic Radical Nephrectomy for Renal Cell Carcinoma in Transplant Patients: The First Experience. *Eur Urol.* 2010 Oct 15. [Epub]

Gruessner, RW.; Fasola, C.; Benedetti, E.; Foshager, MC.; Gruessner, AC.; Matas, AJ.; Najarian, JS. & Goodale, RL. (1995) Laparoscopic drainage of lymphoceles after kidney transplantation: indications and limitations. *Surgery.* ;Vol. 117, No. 3, pp. 288-295.

Hollenbeck, BK.; Seifman, BD. & Wolf, JS. Jr. (2004) Clinical skills acquisition for hand-assisted laparoscopic donor nephrectomy. *J Urol.* Vol. 171, No. 1, pp. 35-39.

Ismai;, HR.; Flechner, SM.; Kaouk, JH.; Derweesh, IH.; Gill, IS.; Modlin, C.; Goldfarb, D. & Novick, AC. (2005) Simultaneous vs. sequential laparoscopic bilateral native nephrectomy and renal transplantation. *Transplantation.* Vol. 80, No. 8, pp. 1124-1127.

Jacobs, SC.; Cho, E.; Foster, C.; Liao, P. & Bartlett, ST. (2004) Laparoscopic donor nephrectomy: the University of Maryland 6-year experience. *J Urol.* Vol. 171, No. 1, pp. 47-51.

Jarrett, TW.; Chan, DY.; Cadeddu, JA. & Kavoussi, LR. (2001) Laparoscopic nephroureterectomy for the treatment of transitional cell carcinoma of the upper urinary tract. *Urology.* Vol. 57, No. 3, pp. 448-453.

Johnson, MW.; Andreoni, K.; McCoy, L.; Scott, L.; Rodegast, B.; Friedman, E.; Thomas, S.; Salm, J.; Gerber, DA. & Fair JH. (2001) Technique of right laparoscopic donor nephrectomy: a single center experience. *Am J Transplant.* Vol. 1, No. 3, pp. 293-295.

Kälble, T; Lucan, M.; Nicita, G.; Sells, R.; Burgos Revilla, FJ.; Wiesel, M. & European Association of Urology. (2005) EAU guidelines on renal transplantation. *Eur Urol.* Vol. 47, No. 2, pp. 156-166.

Kerche, KW.; Heniford, BT.; Matthews, BD.; Smith, TI.; Lincourt, AE.; Hayes, DH.; Eskind, LB.; Irby, PB. & Teigland, CM. (2003) Laparoscopic versus open nephrectomy in 210 consecutive patients: outcomes, cost, and changes in practice patterns. *Surg Endosc.* Vol. 17, No. 12, pp. 1889-1895.

Khauli, RB.; Mosenthal, AC. & Caushaj, PF. (1992) Treatment of lymphocele and lymphatic fistula following renal transplantation by laparoscopic peritoneal window. *J Urol.* Vol. 147, No. 5, pp. 1353-1355.

Kohei, N.; Kazuya, O.; Hirai, T.; Miyauchi, Y.; Iida, S.; Shirakawa, H.; Shimizu, T.; Ishida, H. & Tanabe, K. (2010) Retroperitoneoscopic living donor nephrectomy: experience of 425 cases at a single center. *J Endourol.* Vol. 24, No. 11, pp. 1783-1787.

Lane, BR.; Russo, P.; Uzzo, RG.; Hernandez, AV.; Boorjian, SA.; Thompson, RH.; Fergany, AF.; Love, TE. & Campbell, SC. (2011) Comparision of cold and warm ischemia during partial nephrectomy in 660 solitary kidneys reveals predominant role of nonmodifiable factors in determining ultimate renal function. *J Urol.* Vol. 185, No. 2, pp. 421-427.

Leventhal, JR.; Kocak, B.; Salvalaggio, PR.; Koffron, AJ.; Baker, TB.; Kaufman, DB.; Fryer, JP.; Abecassis, MM. & Stuart, FP. (2004) Laparoscopic donor nephrectomy 1997 to 2003: lessons learned with 500 cases at a single institution. *Surgery.* Vol. 136, No. 4, pp. 881-890.

Leventhal, JR.; Paunescu, S.; Baker, TB.; Caciedo, JC.; Kocak, B.; Gallon, L.; Friedewald, J.; Luo, X.; Kaufman, DB.; Fryer, JP. & Abecassis, MM. (2010) A decade of minimally invasive donation: experience with more than 1200 laparoscopic donor nephrectomies at a single institution. *Clin Transplant.* Vol. 24, No. 2, pp. 169-174.

Liao, CH.; Chueh, SC.; Lai, MK. & Chen, J. (2004) Transitional cell carcinoma in renal transplant recipients. *Transplant Proc.* Vol. 36, No. 7, pp. 2152-2153.

Lucas, SM.; Mofunanya, TC.; Goggins, WC. & Sundaram, CP. (2010) Staged nephrectomy versus bilateral laparoscopic nephrectomy in patients with autosomal dominant polycystic kidney disease. *J Urol.* Vol. 184, No. 5, pp. 2054-2059.

Lunsford, KE.; Harris, MT.; Nicoll, KN.; Collins, BH.; Sudan, DL.; Kuo, PC. & Vikraman, D. (2011) Single-Site Laparoscopic Living Donor Nephrectomy Offers Comparable Perioperative Outcomes to Conventional Laparoscopic Living Donor Nephrectomy at a Higher Cost. *Transplantation.* Vol. 91, No. 2, pp. e16-17.

Matin, SF. & Gill, IS. (2000) Laparoscopic marsupialization of the difficult lymphocele using internalized peritoneal dialysis catheter. *J Urol.* Vol. 163, No. 5, pp. 1498-1500.

Matin, SF. & Gill, IS. (2001) Laparoscopic ultrasonography. *J Endourol.* Vol. 15, No. 1, pp. 87-92.

McNeill, SA.; Chrisofos, M. & Tolley, DA. (2000) The long-term outcome after laparoscopic nephroureterectomy: a comparison with open nephroureterectomy. *Br J Urol Intl.* Vol. 86, No. 6, pp. 619-623.

Melchior, S.; Franzaring, L.; Shardan, A.; Schwenke, C.; Plümpe, A.; Schnell, R. & Dreikorn, K. (2011) Urological de novo malignancy after kidney transplantation: a case for the urologist. *J Urol.* Vol. 185, No. 2, pp. 428-432.

Mjøen, G.; Holdaas, H.; Pfeffer, P.; Line, PD. & Øyen, O. (2010) Minimally invasive living donor nephrectomy - introduction of hand-assistance. *Transpl Int.* Vol. 23, No. 10, pp. 1008-1014.

Nambirajan, T.; Jeschke, S.; Al-Zahrani, H.; Vrabec, G.; Leeb, K. & Janetschek, G. (2004) Prospective, randomized controlled study: transperitoneal laparoscopic versus retroperitoneoscopic radical nephrectomy. *Urology.* Vol. 64, No. 5, pp. 919-924.

Navarro, MD.; Lopez-Andreu, M.; Rodriguez-Benot, A.; Agüera, ML.; Del Castillo, D. & Aljama, P. (2008) Cancer incidence and survival in kidney transplant patients. *Transplant Proc.* Vol. 40, No. 9, 2936-2940.

OPTN, (2006) http://optn.transplant.hrsa.gov/ContentDocuments/Guidance_ProgramSpecificLivingKidneyDonorMedEvalProtocols.pdf

Parra, RO.; Jones, JP. & Hagood, PG. (1992) Laparoscopic intraperitoneal marsupialization: report on a new treatment for lymphoceles. *Surg Laparosc Endosc.* Vol. 2, No. 4, pp. 306-311.

Penn, I. (1998) Occurrence of cancers in immunosuppressed organ transplant recipients. *Clin Transpl.* 147-158.

Ponsky, L.; Cherullo, E.; Moinzadeh, A.; Desai, M.; Kaouk, J.; Haber, GP.; Chen, D.; Ng, C.; Fuchs, G.; Singh, D.; Finelli, A.; Frank, I. & Matin, S. (2008) The Hem-o-lok clip is safe for laparoscopic nephrectomy: a multi-institutional review. *Urology.* Vol. 71, No. 4, pp. 593-596.

Ratner, LE.; Ciseck, LJ.; Moore, RG.; Cigarroa, FG.; Kaufman, HS. & Kavoussi, LR. (1995) Laparoscopic live donor nephrectomy. *Transplantation.* Vol. 60, No. 9, pp. 1047-1049.

Rehman, J.; Landman, J.; Andreoni, C.; McDougall, EM. & Clayman, RV. (2001) Laparoscopic bilateral hand assisted nephrectomy for autosomal dominant polycystic kidney disease: initial experience. *J Urol.* Vol. 166, No. 1, pp. 42-47.

Schilling, M.; Abendroth, D. & Kunz, R. (1995) Treatment of lymphocele in renal transplant recipients by laparoscopic fenestration after transcutaneous staining. *Br J Surg.* Vol. 82, No. 2, pp. 246-248.

Shalhav, AL.; Dunn, MD.; Portis, AJ.; Elbahnasy, AM; McDougall, EM. & Clayman, RV. (2000) Laparoscopic nephroureterectomy for upper tract transitional cell cancer: the Washington University experience. *J Urol.* Vol. 163, No. 4, pp. 1100-1104.

Shokeir, AA.; Eraky, I.; el-Kappany, H. & Ghoneim, MA. (1994) Accidental division of the transplanted ureter during laparoscopic drainage of lymphocele. *J Urol.* Vol. 151, No. 6, pp. 1623-1625.

Siemer, S.; Lehmann, J.; Kamradt, J.; Loch, T.; Remberger, K.; Humke, U.; Ziegler, M. & Stockle, M. (2004) Adrenal metastases in 1635 patients with renal cell carcinoma: outcome and indication for adrenalectomy. *J Urol.* Vol. 171, (6 Pt 1), pp. 2155-2159, discussion 2159.

Smith, GL.; Kenney, PA.; Lee, Y. & Libertino, JA. (2010) Non-clamped partial nephrectomy: techniques and surgical outcomes. *Br J Urol. Intl.* online publication Oct 29, 2010. doi:10.1111/j.1464-410X.2010.09798.x[Epub ahead of print]

Steinberg, AP.; Finelli, A.; Desai, MM.; Abreu, SC.; Ramani, AP.; Spaliviero, M; Rybicki, L.; Kaouk, J.; Novick, AC. & Gill, IS. (2004) Laparoscopic radical nephrectomy for large (greater than 7 cm, t2) renal tumors. *J Urol.* Vol. 172, (6 Pt 1), pp. 2172-2176.

Su, LM.; Ratner, LE, Montgomery, RA.; Jarrett, TW.; Trock, BJ.; Sinkov, V.; Bluebond-Langner, R. & Kavoussi, LR. (2004) Laparoscopic live donor nephrectomy: trends in donor and recipient morbidity following 381 consecutive cases. *Ann Surg*. Vol. 240, No. 2, pp. 358-363.

Sundqvist, P.; Feuk, U.; Haggman, M.; Persson, AE.; Stridsberg, M. & Wadstrom, J. (2004) Hand-assisted retroperitoneoscopic live donor nephrectomy in comparison to open and laparoscopic procedures: a prospective study on donor morbidity and kidney function. *Transplantation*. Vol. 78, No. 1, pp. 147-153.

Tai, HC.; Lai, MK.; Chung, SD.; Huang, KH.; Chueh, SC. & Yu, HJ. (2009) Intermediate-term oncological outcomes of hand-assisted laparoscopic versus open bilateral nephroureterectomy for dialysis and kidney transplant patients with upper urinary tract urothelial carcinoma. *J Endourol*. Vol. 23, No. 7, pp.1139-1144.

Tanabe, K.; Miyamoto, N.; Tokumoto, T.; Yamamoto, H.; Ishida, H.; Kondo, T.; Okuda, H.; Shinmmura, H.; Shirakawa, H.; Shimizu, T.; Ishikawa, N. & Toma, H. (2005) Retroperitoneoscopic live donor nephrectomy: extended experience in a single center. *Am J Transplant*. Vol. 5, (4 Pt 1), pp. 739-745.

Thompson, RH.; Frank, I.; Lohse, CM.; Saad, IR.; Fergany, A.; Zincke, H.; Leibovich, BC.; Blute, ML. & Novick, AC. (2007) The impact of ischemia time during open nephron sparing surgery on solitary kidneys: a multi-institutional study. *J Urol*. Vol. 177, No. 2, 471-476.

Tollefson, MK.; Krambeck, AE.; Leibovich, BC.; Blute, ML. & Chow, GK. (2010) Surgical treatment of renal cell carcinoma in the immunocompromised transplant patient *Urology* Vol. 75, No. 6, pp. 1373-1377.

Tooher, RL.; Rao, MM.; Scott, DF.; Wall, DR.; Francis, DM; Bridgewater, FH. & Maddern, GJ. (2004) A systematic review of laparoscopic live-donor nephrectomy. *Transplantation*. Vol. 78, No. 3, pp. 404-414.

Troppmann, C.; Ormond, DB. & Perez, RV. (2003) Laparoscopic (vs open) live donor nephrectomy: a UNOS database analysis of early graft function and survival. *Am J Transplant*. Vol. 3, No. 10, pp. 1295-1301.

UNOS, 2009, http://www.unos.org/docs/Living_Donation.pdf

Uzzo, R. & Novick, AC. (2001) Nephron-sparing surgery for renal tumors. Indications, techniques and outcomes. *J Urol*. Vol. 166, No. 1, pp. 6-18.

Velidedeoglu, E.; Williams, N.; Brayman, KL.; Desai, NM.; Campos, L.; Palanjian, M.; Wocjik, M.; Bloom, R.; Grossman, RA.; Mange, K.; Barker, CF.; Naji, A. & Markmann, JF. (2002) Comparison of open, laparoscopic, and hand-assisted approaches to live-donor nephrectomy. *Transplantation*. Vol. 74, No. 2, pp. 169-72.

Venkatesh, R.; Belani, JS.; Chen, C.; Sundaram, CP.; Bhayani, SB.; Figenshau, RS. & Landman, J. (2007) Prospective randomized comparison of laparoscopic and hand-assisted laparoscopic radical nephrectomy. *Urology*. Vol. 70, No. 5, pp. 873-877.

Whitten, MG.; Van der Werf, W. & Belnap, L. (2006) A novel approach to bilateral hand-assisted laparoscopic nephrectomy for autosomal dominant polycystic kidney disease. *Surg Endosc*. Vol. 20, No. 4, pp. 679-684.

Wszolek, MF.; Kenney, PA.; Lee, Y. & Libertino, JA. (2010) Comparison of hilar clamping and non-hilar clamping partial nephrectomy for tumours involving a solitary kidney. *Br. J Urol. Intl.* 2010 Nov 11. doi: 10.1111/j.1464-410X.2010.09713.x. [Epub ahead of print]

6

Minimally Invasive Renal Transplantation

Ole Øyen
Oslo University Hospital Rikshospitalet Clinic for Specialised Medicine and Surgery, Norway

1. Introduction

During the last 20 years minimally invasive surgery (MIS) has replaced many open, conventional operations and is now important in almost every facet of abdominal surgery (Harrell & Beniford, 2005). Benefits regarding postoperative pain, convalescence, return to normal activities, and cosmetic results have been proven for a wide range of MIS procedures.

Within the field of transplantation, laparoscopic fenestration of lymphoceles in kidney recipients was first described in 1991 (McCullough et al.). Furthermore, laparoscopic living donor nephrectomy (L-LDN) has gained widespread acceptance, since the first procedure was performed in Baltimore, USA in 1995 (Ratner et al., 1995).

Reduction of tissue trauma seems particularly appropriate in the immunosuppressed population, with significantly delayed wound healing and a high "background" complication rate. Due to the immunosuppressive theraphy, the incidences of lymphoceles, wound dehiscence and incisional hernia are distinctly higher in kidney-Tx (KTx) - recipients. On this background it is rather surprising that MIS techniques for the renal transplant procedure itself, first have been reported during recent years. Possible explanations for these seemingly conservative attitudes, may include the urge for safe handling of the kidney through sufficient access, for total control during revascularization; and the present unfeasibility of automating the vascular anastomoses.

In 2002, however, a french case report on robotic-assisted (da Vinci system) kidney transplantation, from a deceased donor, was presented (Hoznek et al., 2002). Thereafter, no further cases/series of robotic-assisted KTx seem to have been published.

In 2006 a minimally invasive KTx (MIKT) technique was described in Transplantation and Transplantation Proceedings (Øyen et al., 2006); using a minimal skin incision (7-9 cm) and still giving optimal access to the anastomotic area of the iliac vessels - mostly without using scopic aid. Twentyone consecutive MIKT procedures, performed by a single surgeon was compared to a control group subjected to conventional KTx. Since then, a South Korean group has published two reports (Seong-Pyo et al., 2007; Park et al., 2008) on a video-assisted MIKT technique.

Another MIKT report was contributed by a spanish group (Rosales et al., 2010); a case report describing a laparoscopic KTx technique, without robotic assistance.

Furthermore, in 2010 a minimally invasive technique for renal auto-transplantation was reported (Øyen et al., 2010); by combining 'hand- assisted laparoscopic nephrectomy'' and

'MIKT, using the same incision (7–8 cm) for hand-assistance, kidney harvesting, and transplantation.
The MIKT procedure have so far not gained widespread acceptance and still seem to be at a "pioneer stage". However, considering the rapid evolution of MIS during the last two decades, there is little reason to believe that KTx and Auto-KTx in future will be excluded from this development.

2. The minimally invasive surgical revolution

During the last 20 years minimally invasive techniques have revolutionised surgery in general, and in particular have laparoscopic procedures replaced most conventional operations, including advanced surgery on liver, pancreas and intestines. Benefits regarding postoperative pain, convalescence, return to normal activities, and cosmetic results have been proven for a wide range of MIS procedures. The development has been facilitated by improvements in optical and hemostatic equipment (High definition imaging, Ultracision, LigaSure), miniaturization, and the introduction of robotic technology (da Vinci robot system).
The revolutionary MIS development was started by a French gynecologist, with experience from simple laparoscopic procedures like sterilisation, and he actually invented laparascopic cholecystectomy (Dubois et al., 1991). This invention, started in 1987, has indeed turned out to be the greatest revolution in surgical technique during the last 2000 years. In fact, our conventional instruments for open, conventional surgery (scalpel, scissors, forceps etc) have no further subtleties than those found in archeological findings from Pompei (to be seen in the Archeological Museum of Napoli). The great achievements in surgery during the last part of the 19th century and first part of the 20th century was actually due to developments in anesthesia and bacteriology/septicemiae - not in surgical technique.
During the last two decades of rapid MIS evolution, an almost linear correlation between incisional/tissue trauma and postoperative morbidity has been demonstrated.
Within the field of transplantation, laparoscopic fenestration of post-KTx lymphoceles was first described in 1991 (McCullough et. al.). This MIS technique has in recent years taken over as the standard treatment option for lymphoceles, replacing the traditional deroofing by laparotomy. Furthermore, laparoscopic living donor nephrectomy (L-LDN) has gained widespread acceptance, since the first procedure was performed in Baltimore, USA in 1995 (Ratner et al.). Many centres have adopted hand-assisted L-LDN techniques, because this is perceived to be faster, easier and safer than with the strictly laparoscopic technique (Wolf JSJ et al., 1998). By any method, a 6-9 cm incision is required for decent kidney extraction. With hand-assistance/handport the incision must usually be extended to 8-12 cm.

3. Robotic surgery: The da Vinci robot in renal transplantation; a case report from France (2002)

3.1 Method: The da Vinci surgical system

The *da Vinci* surgical system (Intuitive Surgical, Inc., Mountain View, California), based on robotic technology and introduced during the first years of this millennium, enabled surgeons to perform delicate and complex MIS operations, without extensive laparoscopic experience - affording excellent vision, precision, dexterity and control. The key components of the *da Vinci* surgical system included: an ergonomically designed console where the surgeon was seated while operating, , four interactive robotic arms, a high-definition 3D vision system, and proprietary so called *EndoWrist®* instruments. The.*da Vinci* system was powered by state-of-the-art robotic technology that allowed the surgeon's hand movements to be scaled, filtered and translated into precise movements of the *EndoWrist* instruments working inside the patient's body.

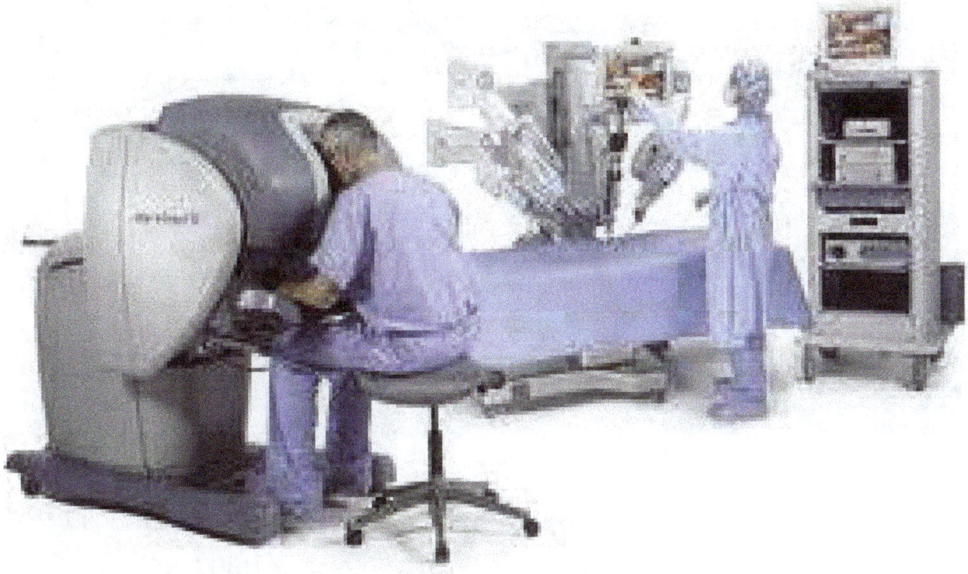

Fig. 1 The da Vinci robotic system.

During the last decade , the da Vinci system has particularly made progress within the field of laparoscopic urology, including radical prostatectomy, simple nephrectomy (not living donor nephrectomy) and pelvic lymph node dissection.

A great prospective feature of robotic surgery is the ability to dissociate the surgeon from the operative field. Specialised operations may be executed at remote hospitals, by a centralized surgeon.

3.2 Case report on 'da Vinci' KTx

The paper from 2002 (Hoznec et. al.) described a right cadaveric kidney transplanted into a 26-year-old male recipient, who had been on hemodialysis for 11 years. Surgery was done with the help of the da Vinci robot, by a "locally remote" surgeon, who completely performed vascular dissection and anastomoses, as well as ureterovesical anastomosis. The role of the assistant by the side of the patient was limited to access creation, exposure, hemostasis and maintaining traction on the running sutures performed by the robot. Operative time was 178 minutes. Robotic assistance made the vascular anastomoses feasible by stereoscopic magnification and ultraprecise visuality and manuvering. Renal perfusion was reported to be excellent with immediate diuresis. Nevertheless, postoperative acute tubular necrosis was first resolved one week post-Tx.

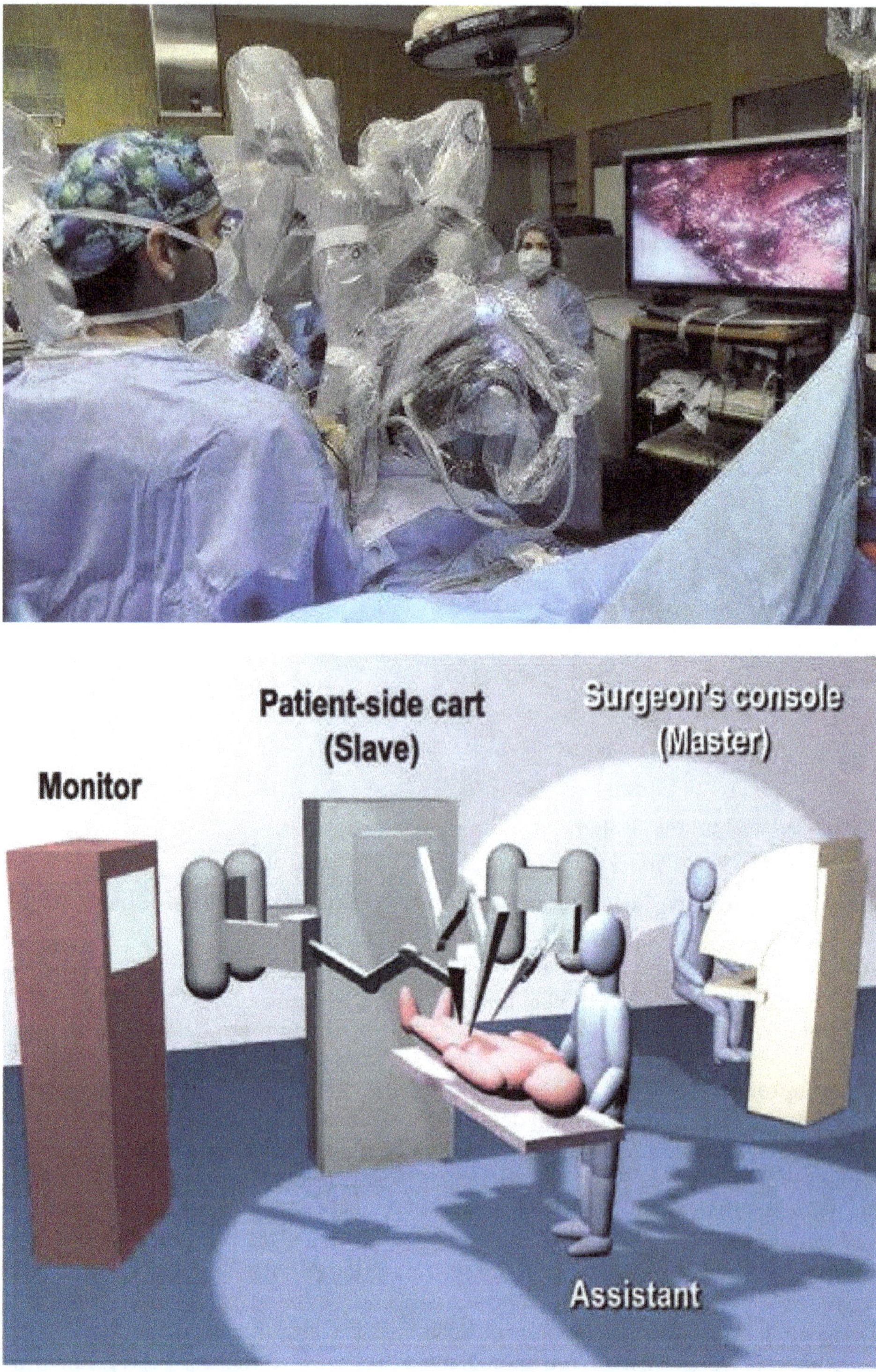

Fig. 2. The da Vinci robot system: Positioning of patient and surgeon. (Hoznek et al., 2002).

According to the authors, the case demonstrated that robotic assisted kidney transplantation was feasible. However, at that time, technical and cost hindrances was suspected to retard routine use of robots in future.

3.3 Further course/evolution of the 'da Vinci surgical system' in KTx

During recent years, the main application of the 'da Vinci robotic system' has been radical prostatectomy. In most other fields of laparoscopy, refined suturing has not been necessary, because ot the evolutionary development in stapling/clipsing devices, Ultracision and LigaSure. This is the main reason why the 'da Vinci system' has not taken over in other laparoscopic fields.

By close literature searches, the French group (nor any other group) does not seem to have reported any further 'da Vinci KTx' cases during the last decade. For the sake of completeness; the 'da Vinci KTx' case was mentioned in a review article about 'Robotic renal surgery' by the same authors (Hoznek et. al., 2004).

In the 'da Vinci KTx' paper, the size of the incision used for kidney introduction, is not indicated. The fact that a 6-9 cm incision is nevertheless required for decent implantation, and 3 hours 'da Vinci KTx' operating time, may explain why this method for KTx was not found worthy to pursue. In addition to the 6-9 cm implantation incision, the 'da Vinci' method is dependent on 2-3 laparoscopic ports (10-12 mm each), which are not necessary in the MIKT setting.

In a recent publication (Khanna & Horgan, 2011) a laboratory training and evaluation technique for robot assisted ex vivo KTx was demonstrated.

4. Minimally invasive KTx (MIKT); mostly without scopic aid – The Oslo experience (2006)

In 2005, a MEDLINE search for recent publications (years 2000-2005) containing both 'Kidney transplantation' and 'MIS' yielded 227 hits. However, a careful look at these references revealed that the great majority was about L-LDN, a few presented various MIS procedures in transplanted patients, but none of them were concerned with the transplantation procedure itself. The french da Vinci robot KTx report was not detected by our searches, because 'MIS'/'Laparoscopy' had not been included as key words..

The lack of MIKT publications in the literature was a bit surprising, for several reasons. Firstly, because MIS procedures had been described for all kinds of abdominal surgery, including sophisticated procedures, such as liver and pancreas resections. Secondly, because the potential advantages of reducing incisions/tissue trauma are probably of greater benefit in immunosuppressed patients, with significantly impaired wound healing. Possible explanations might include the urge for safe handling of the kidney through sufficient access, for total control during revascularization; and the present unfeasibility of automating the vascular anastomoses.

4.1 Developing MIKT: Method/technique

During the first years of the 21th century a MIKT technique was developed in Oslo, restricting to an appendectomy-like, approximately 8 cm long incision and with division only of the conjoined tendon (Øyen et al., 2006).

A careful and meticulous "back table" preparation of the kidney prior to transplantation was essential for MIKT, because of limited access to the parenchyma/hilus after revascularization. All redundant fatty tissue outside the "hilus-plane" was removed, to get undisturbed access for "complete" hemostatic control. All minor blood vessels, including capsular vessels, were secured by ligation or diathermy. Furthermore, the lymphatic vessels, mostly located alongside the artery, were ligated. The short right renal vein was extended by reconstruction using part of the caval tube caudally.

In the recipient, a 7-9 cm transverse incision was placed 3-5 cm above the inguinal ligament, with the medial end 2-3 cm from the midline. Only the 'conjoined tendon' and hardly any muscular tissue was divided. The iliac vessels were dissected free extraperitoneally, in a minimalistic fashion. A self-retracting system (Omnitract®) was introduced, giving medial, vascular exposure while allowing space for the kidney lateral/cranial to the skin incision. The meticulously prepared kidney was then placed in a small/fitting, lateral, retroperitoneal pouch, which has been precooled by ice sludge. All three anastomoses were performed with the kidney in this final "in situ" position. The renal vein was anastomosed to the external iliac vein ('end-to-side'). Therafter, the renal artery was anastomosed to the external iliac artery ('end-to-side'), or in most living donor cases (no aortic cuff) to the internal iliac artery ('end-to-end'). The MIKT access made it necessary to suture the back wall of the vascular anastomoses from the inside. Clamping of the vessels was done in a simplified, one-stage manner, using a Key-Lambert® clamp.

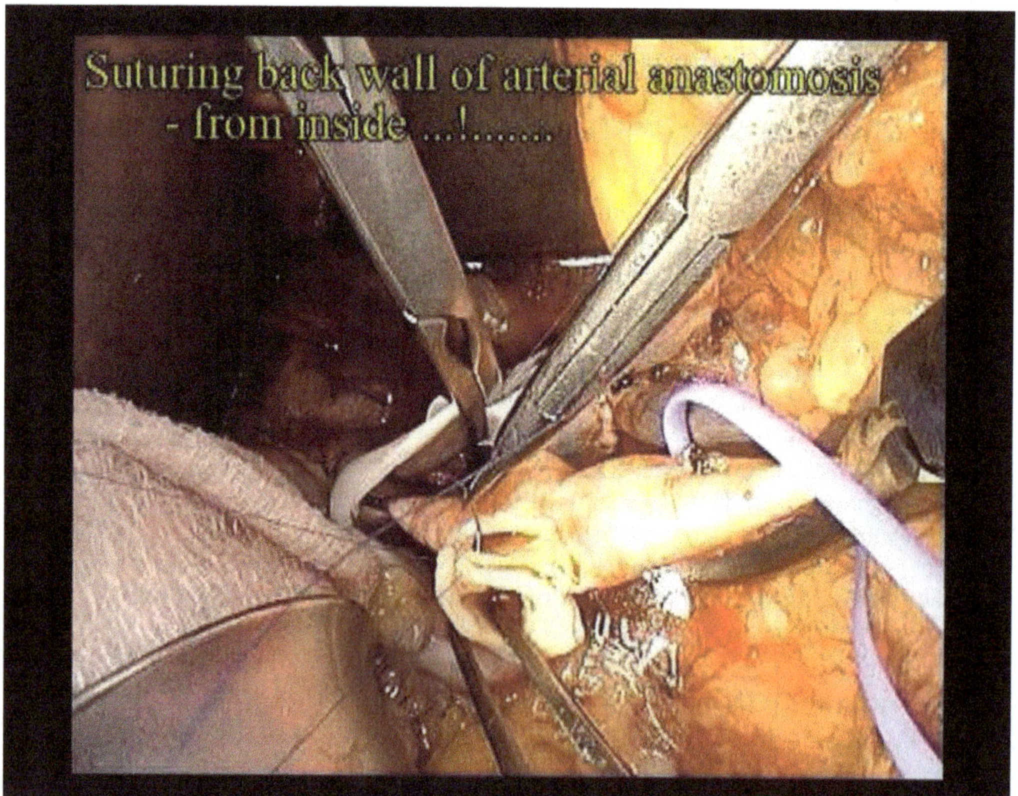

Fig. 3. Suturing the renal artery end-to-side to the external iliac artery (Clamp on renal vein).

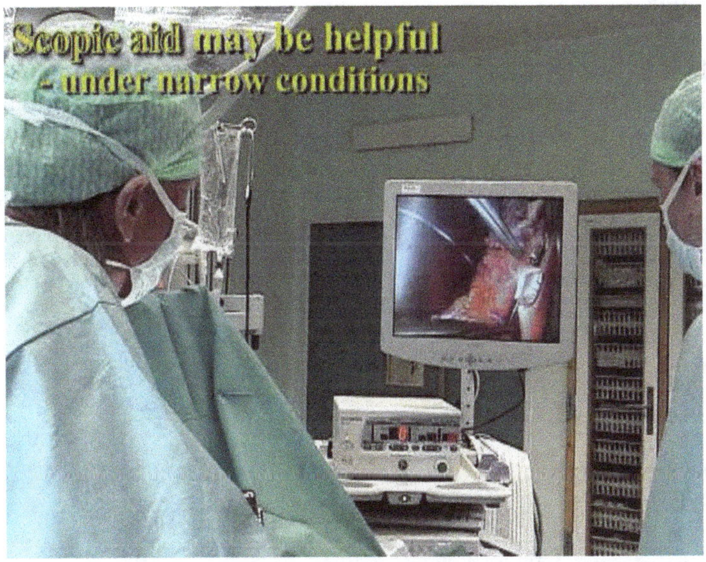

Fig. 4. MIKT scopic aid during the arterial end-to-side anastomosis.

In most cases the kidney was not moved from the neatly fitting retroperitoneal pouch after revascularization. Reimplantation of the ureter was performed by extravesical technique a.m. Lich-Gregoir, with minimal bladder dissection. Scopic aid was only found necessary in a few cases under very deep, narrow circumstances. The scope was then simply introduced through the same incision, alongside the instruments, giving a "close up" of the anstomotic area. A simplistic approach, with minimal dissection/tissue trauma was attempted at all stages.

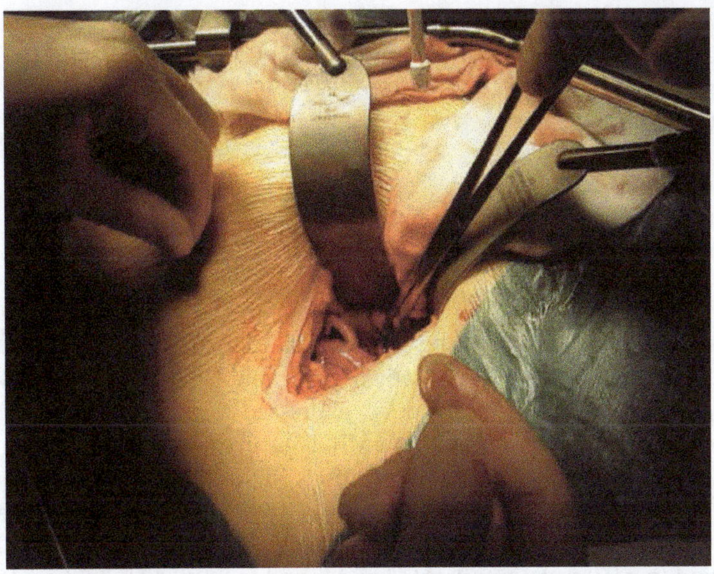

Fig. 5. After revascularisation: The perfused renal artery and vein are seen, while the kidney lies lateral to the skin incision.

4.2 MIKT: Results

A series of patients, transplanted by strict MIKT technique was then compared with matched controls subjected to conventional surgery. From December 2004 to July 2005, 21 kidney recipients were subjected to the new, minimally invasive technique. The MIKT patients constituted a consecutive series of transplantations performed by a single surgeon. A control group, subjected to conventional KTx (n=21) had been concurrently selected to match the MIKT group regarding age, sex, donor source, and primary-/retransplant status. No MIKT procedures were interrupted or converted to COKT. The results have been summarized in Table 1.

RESULTS *[mean (range)]*	MIKT n=21	Conventional Tx **n=21**	**Student t-test p-value**
Skin incision length (cm)	8,1* (7 - 9)	20,5 (17-23)	p<0,01
Operative time (min)	118* (95-140)	187 (130-270)	p<0,01
Analgesic requirementsPostop. days 0 + 1+ 2 (Morphine Equiv.; mg)	35 (3-86)	56 (20-173)	n.s. (p=0,053)
Hospitalization (days in hospital postop.)	8,2* (6-13)	12,4 (7-29)	p=0,02
Delayed graft function	10 % (2)	14 % (3)	
Measured GFR 10-12 weeks post-Tx (Cr-EDTA- Clearance; mean [range]; ml/min/1,73 m^2)	57,4 (35 – 81)	51,2 (26 – 72)	n.s. (p=0,053)
Peroperative incidents	No major	No major	
Surgical complications/reinterventions			
- Lymphocele: Reop.	2 (10 %)	3 (14 %)	
- Wound dehiscence: Reop.	0	1 (5 %)	
- Urinary obstruction: Reop.	0	1 (5 %)	
- Perirenal hemorrhage: Reop.	1 (5 %)	1 (5 %)	
- Bladder hemorrhage	0	2 (10 %)	
- Total	*3 (14 %)*	*8 (38 %)*	

Table 1. MIKT results. (extracted from Øyen et al., 2006)

Naturally, the MIKT skin incision was very much shorter. There were significant differences in favour of MIKT regarding operative time and postoperative stay in hospital. Furthermore, the analgesic requirements, expressed as morphine equivalents during postoperative days 0+1+2 were less in the MIKT group, however at non-significant levels. There were less complications and reinterventions in the MIKT recipients, totally 3 (14 %) - versus 8 (38 %) in the open KTx group. Because of the high complication rate in the control group, the total complication/reintervention rate of open KTx outside the study during the inclusion period (n = 97) were investigated and found to be 30-40 % (data not shown).

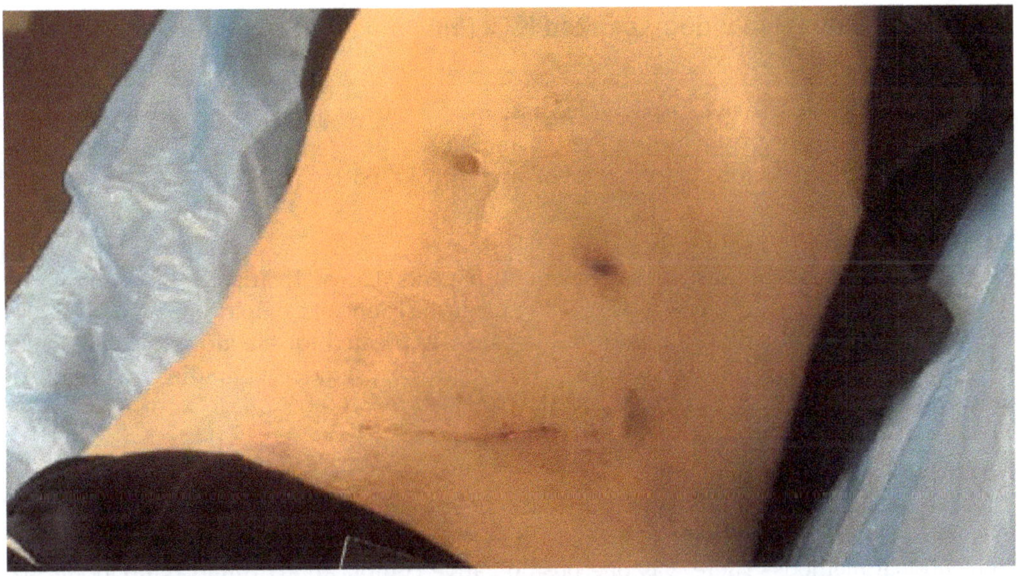

Fig. 6. Exterior result after left-sided MIKT in a slim patient, through a 7,5 cm incision.

4.3 MIKT: Discussion

Compared with L-LDN employing a 6-9 cm skin incision for kidney harvesting, the MIKT incision was only faintly larger (7-9 cm), and besides the L-LDN was dependent on 2-3 additional laparoscopic ports (5-12 mm each).

The first MIKT results were good, compared with the open, conventional KTx group and indicated that the procedure might be executed fast (because of its simplicity) and safe. By reducing incision, extent of dissection and thereby tissue trauma, the wound complications would be suspected to be reduced accordingly. Potentially it may also reduce hospitalization, and thereby the risk for nosocomial infections.

A major point about the MIKT approach (also when disregarding the results), was that reduction of tissue trauma appeared particularly appropriate in these patients, with significantly delayed wound healing and a high "background" complication rate. Due to the immunosuppressive theraphy, the incidences of wound dehiscence and incisional hernia were distinctly higher in Tx recipients, in particular after the introduction of Sirolimus/Everolimus. For simple reasons, a significant reduction of the abdominal wall incision would be anticipated to reduce these wound-related problems. Potentially, the MIKT procedure might also counteract the huge lymphocele/lymph leakage problem, by minimizing the dissection cavity and leaving less space available for fluid expansion.

Except from the single MIKT surgeon's extensive Tx experience , the distinctly shorter MIKT operating time might be explained by the simplified/minimalistic handling of the vessels, the extravesical reimplantation technique, and fast closure of a small incision.

Our data did suggest the same beneficial effects on postoperative pain/analgesia and recovery, that had been documented for a wide range of MIS procedures.

During recent years, Tx surgeons in Oslo have in part adopted the MIKT technique, by significantly reducing the size of the incision, even though not conforming strictly to MIKT. A significant reduction in overall KTx complication rates has been observed during 2008-2011, which may be partly attributed to reduced incision size and thereby tissue trauma.

5. Minimally invasive video-assisted KTx (MIVAKT) - The South Chorean experience (2007)

In 2007 a minimally invasive, partly video-assisted KTx technique (MIVAKT) was described by a South Chorean group (Seong-Pyo et al., 2007, Park et al., 2008) - obviously quite independent of the previous 'da Vinci robot' and MIKT reports.

5.1 MIVAKT: Method/Technique

The MIVAKT pocedure was carried out in 20 patients. Clinical variables were compared with the conventional KTx method. A 7-8 cm skin incision was employed. By means of a scopic balloon instrument a retroperitoneal space was created for the kidney. The vascular anastomoses and ureteroneocystostomy were performed under both direct vision and video-assisted aid.

5.2 MIVAKT: Results/Conclusion

The average length of the wound incision was 7-8 cm, placed below the belt line. The average operating time were 186 min. Less analgesics was given compared with conventional methods. There was one postoperative complication, a mild lymphocele. All patients showed normalized serum creatinine levels within 4 days post-Tx and normal findings on postoperative ultrasound and renal scintigraphy.

MIVAKT was shown to be technically feasible and might offer benefits in terms of better cosmetic outcomes, less pain, and quicker recuperation, compared with conventional KTx.

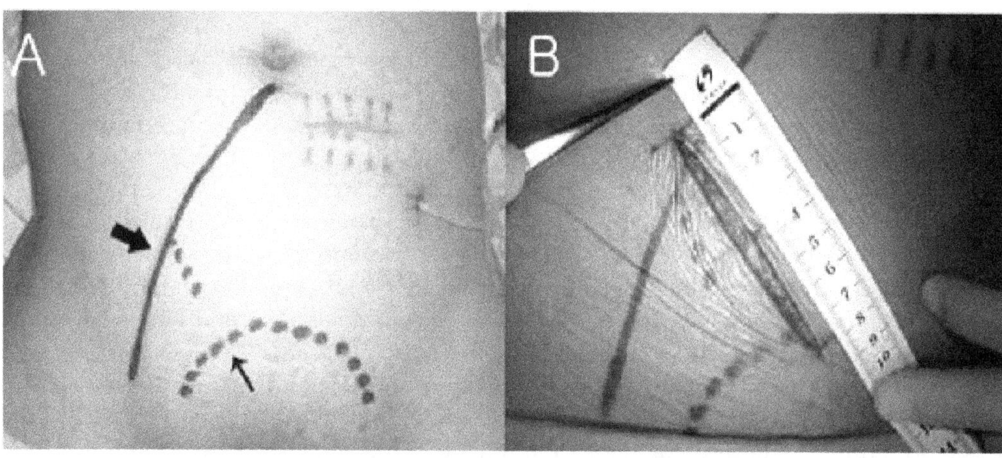

Fig. 7. (A) The location and course of the external iliac vessels (thick arrow) and the contour of the urinary bladder (thin arrow), marked preoperatively using ultrasound. (B) The 7–8 cm oblique incision. (Seong-Pyo et al., 2007)

5.3 MIVAKT: Discussion

We consider the transverse (horizontal) MIKT incision to offer better access to the iliac vessels, than the oblique MIVAKT incision. Furthermore, it is not at all necessary to use a laparoscopic balloon dissector to create the retroperitoneal space. A kidney-fitting retroperitoneal pouch is easily and safely made by hand/retractors through a minimal incision.

The video-assisted MIVAKT approach is interesting. Though, in the MIVAKT series, it seems like the vascular anastomoses for the most part were carried out under direct vision. In the MIVAKT discussion it is stated that "The grafted kidney was hung over the skin incision during the vascular anastomosis because the procedure is nearly impossible after the placing of the grafted kidney in the retroperitoneal space." This is not at all 'impossible'; but exactly what the MIKT technique is all about. Both the venous and arterial MIKT anastomoses were performed with the kidney in its final retroperitoneal position, suturing the back walls from the inside.

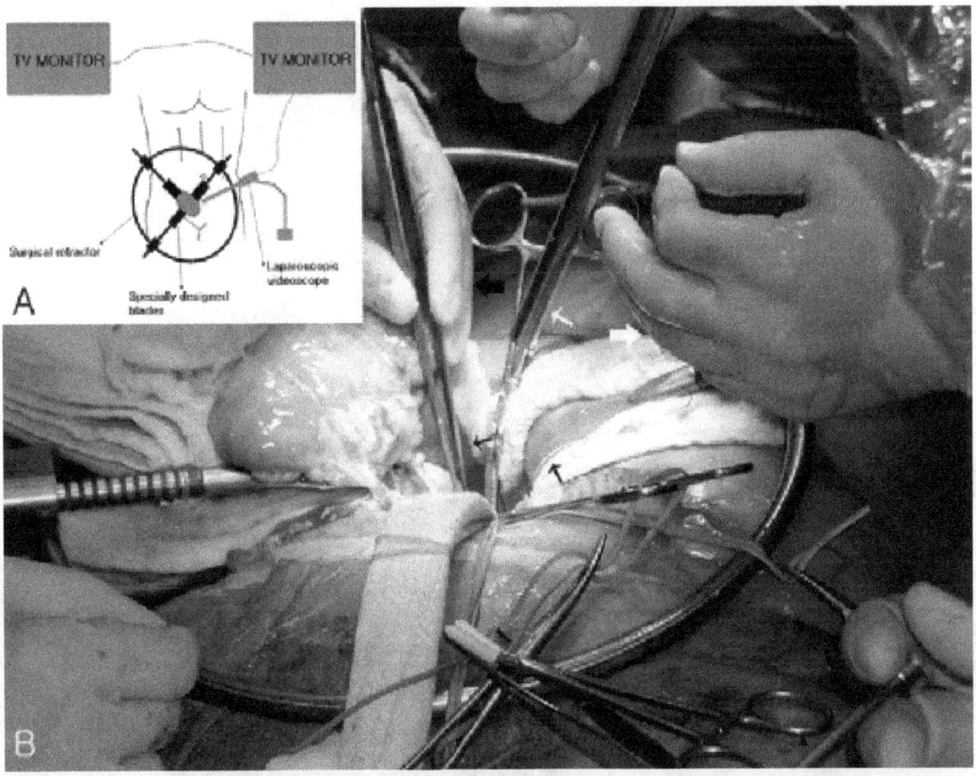

Fig. 8. (A) The circular retraction system and video-assisted TV monitoring. (B) The kidney was placed just above the skin incision during the vascular anastomoses. The laparoscope (thin white arrow) was found useful for visualisation and illumination. (Seong-Pyo et al., 2007)

6. Laparoscopic KTx – A case report from Barcelona (2010)

In 2010 a spanish group presented a case report on KTx by means of regular laparoscopic access, using 4 trocars and a Pfannenstiel incision (Rosales et al.).

6.1 Laparoscopic KTx: Method/Technique

With the recipient in the left lateral decubitus position, a hand-port was placed into a 7 cm Pfannenstiel incision. One trocar was put through the hand-port, while three more trocars were introduced in the right hemiabdomen.

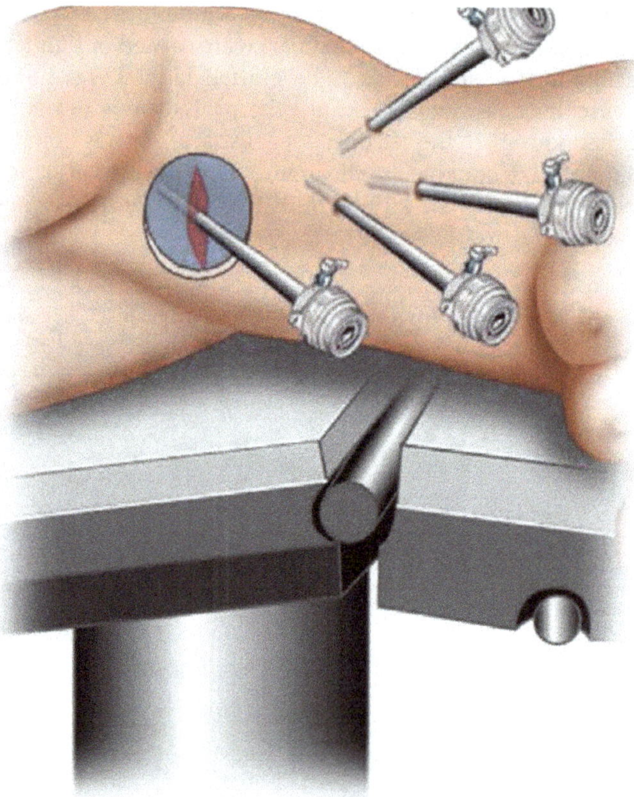

Fig. 9. Trocar positioning. Pfannenstiel incision. (Rosales et al., 2010)

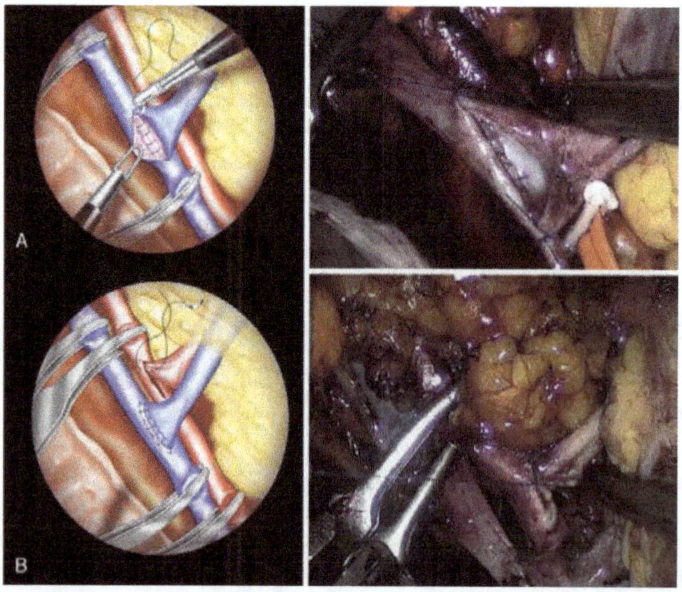

Fig. 10. Laparoscopic venous and arterial end-to-side anastomoses (Rosales et al., 2010).

By making a retroperitoneal, pelvic window ,the right external iliac vessels were dissected free. The kidney was introduced through the hand-port, and end-to-side anastomoses were performed by bulldog clamping through the hand-port and continous suture.
The ureterovesical anastomose was done by a modified Taguchi technique. Finally, the kidney graft was placed extraperitoneally by continuous suture of the peritoneal window.

6.2 Laparoscopic KTx: Results

Surgical time was 240 min, with 300 cm^3 bleeding. Cold ischemia time was 182 min. The postoperative course was uneventful and functionally satisfactory. Serum creatinine decreased progressively, to 73 µmol/l on the day of discharge. Stay in hospital was 14 days.

6.3 Laparoscopic KTx: Discussion

A laparoscopic KTx operating time of 4 hours seems too much, when MIKT can be executed in 2 hours, and with a total incision size that is probably smaller, when taking into account the 3 additional laparoscopic ports. The transverse (7-9) cm MIKT incision in the iliac fossa offers excellent direct access to the anastomotic area of the external iliac vessels. And regarding safety towards vacular incidents, the laparoscopic approach must be considered inferior.
Altogether, it seems unnecessary to perform the vascular anastomoses by laparoscopic technique - when these can be performed openly by an incision that is nevertheless needed for decent introduction/transplantation of the kidney.

7. Minimally invasive renal auto-transplantation (MI-Auto-KTx) (2010)

By combining "hand- assisted laparoscopic nephrectomy" and MIKT – using the same incision (7–9 cm) for hand-assistance, kidney harvesting, and transplantation – we have during 2009-2011 conducted "Minimally invasive renal auto-transplantation" (MI-Auto-KTx) in 6 patients. The first two MI-Auto-KTx cases have allready been documented and published (Øyen et al., 2010).

7.1 MI-Auto-KTx: Method

Laparoscopic hand-assisted nephrectomy: The handport incision (7-8 cm) was made medially in the right iliac fossa; displaced laterally compared with the usual Pfannenstiel L-LDN incision.
Extracorporeal 'back bench' preparartion: In the first case (female 38 years; renal artery aneurysm) it was possible to maintain a single arterial stem, after resection of the 16 mm aneurysm. In the second case (female 55 years; ureter lesion) three renal arteries had to be reconstructed.
MIKT: We utilized the handport incision, targeted on the iliac vessels, without extension. The meticulously prepared kidney was placed in a small/fitting, retroperitoneal pouch; and anastomosed to the iliac vessels. Reimplantation of the ureter was performed by extravesical technique.

7.2 MI-Auto-KTx: Results

Total operative times were 335 min and 434 min, respectively. In both cases the postoperative course was uneventful, and the patients were transferred to the local hospital

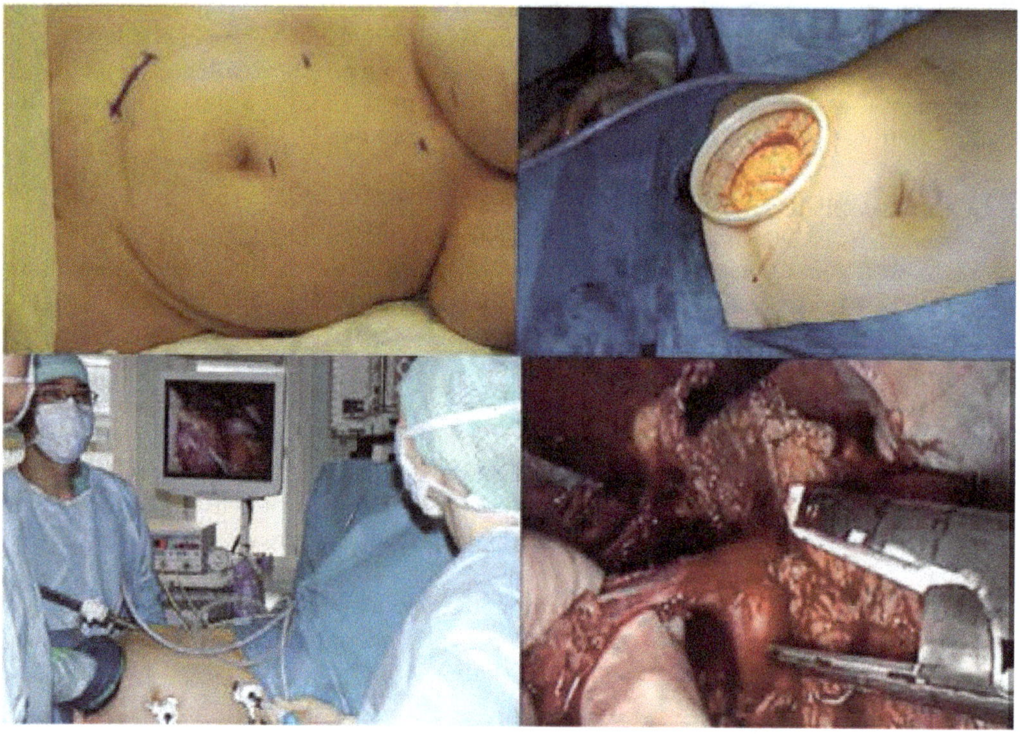

Fig. 11. MI-Auto-KTx: Laparoscopic, right-sided, hand-assisted nephrectomy; by a 7-8 cm medial "transplant incison", using GelPort and 3 trocars. The right renal vein is stapled and divided flush with the caval vein. (Øyen et al., 2010)

at day 4/day 5. When examined 3 mts postoperatively, both auto-transplants were shown to have excellent function by renal scintigraphy.

7.3 MI-Auto-KTx: Discussion

Our first two MI-Auto-KTx cases have demonstrated that a traditionally major surgical procedure, with extensive incisions/tissue trauma, can be made minimally invasive, by a similar incision as that used for L-LDN. Taking into regard the highly traumatic conventional incisions, we expect the generally proven minimally invasive benefits to be considerable.

8. Considerations about the future

The minimally invasive KTx procedures have so far not gained widespread acceptance and still seem to be at a "pioneer stage". However, considering the rapid evolution of MIS during the last two decades, there is little reason to believe that KTx and Auto-KTx in future will be excluded from this development.

Since a ≥ 6 cm incision will anyway be needed for decent introduction of the kidney (except for the possibilty of introduction through natural orifices) , we think the MIKT procedure is the most suited for further developments in this field.

9. References

Dubois F, Icard P, Berthelot G & Levard H (1991). Coelioscopic cholecystectomy: preliminary report of 36 cases. *Ann Surg*, 211: 60-2.

Harrell AG, & Beniford BT. (2005). Minimally invasive abdominal surgery: lux et veritas past, present, and future. *Am J Surg*, Vol 190, No 2, pp 239-43.

Hoznek A, Zaki SK, Samadi DB, Salomon L, Lobontiu A, Lang P & Abbou CC (2002). Robotic assisted kidney transplantation: an initial experience.. *J Urol,* Vol 167, pp 1604–06.

Hoznek A, Hubert,J, Antiphon, Gettman MT, Hemal AK & Abbou CC (2004). Robotic renal surgery. *Urol Clin N Am*, Vol 31, pp 731-76.

Khanna A & Horgan S (2011). A laboratory training and evaluation technique for robot assisted ex vivo kidney transplantation. *Int J Med Robot*. Vol 7, No 1, pp 118-122.

McCullough CS, Soper NJ, Clayman RV, So SSK, Lendrisak MD, & Hanto DW (1991). Laparoscopic drainage of a post-transplant lymphocele. *Transplantation*, Vol 51, No 3, pp 725-27.

Øyen O, Scholz T, Hartmann A & Pfeffer P (2006). Minimally invasive kidney transplantation: The first experience.. *Transpl Proc* , Vol 38, pp 2798-2802.

Øyen O, Scholz T, Hartmann A & Pfeffer P (2006). Minimal invasive kidney transplantation - The first experience. *Transplantation*, Vol 82, Suppl 2, pp 930-31.

Øyen O, Lien B, Line P-D, & Pfeffer P (2010). Minimally invasive renal auto-transplantation: The first report (2010). *J Surg Res*, Vol 164, pp e181-84.

Park SC, Kim SD, Kim JI, & Moon IS (2008). Minimal skin incision in living kidney transplantation. *Transpl Proc*, Vol 40, pp 2347-48.

Ratner LE, Ciseck LJ, & Moore RG.(1995) Laparoscopic live donor nephrectomy. *Transplantation;*, Vol 60, No 9, pp 1047-49.

Rosales A, Salvador JT, Urdaneta G, Patino D, Montllo M, Esquena S, Caffaratti J, Ponce de Leon J, Guirado L & Villavicencio H (2010). Laparoscopic kidney transplantation. *Eur Urol*, Vol 5 7, pp 164-67.

Seong-Pyo M, Jeong-Whan C, Kuyong-Jong K, Gui-Ae J, Min-Woo C, Young-Joon A & Seong-Whan K (2007). Minimally invasive video-assisted kidney transplantation (MIVAKT) (2007). *J Surg Res* Vol 141, pp 204-10.

Wolf JSJ, Tchetgen MB & Merion RM (1998). Hand-assisted laparoscopic live donor nephrectomy. *Urology*, Vol 52, No 5, pp 885-87.

7

Obesity and Kidney Transplantation

Alex Chang[1], Susan Hou[1] and Holly Kramer[1,2]
[1]*Loyola University Medical Center, Department of Medicine, Division of Nephrology and Hypertension*
[2]*Department of Preventive Medicine and Epidemiology, USA*

1. Introduction

Worldwide, countries continue to face an epidemic of obesity, the number one risk factor for diabetes and hypertension. Obesity likely mediates, at least in part, the majority of kidney disease among industrialized societies. Due to the rising prevalence of obesity, the incidence of chronic kidney disease (CKD) and end-stage kidney disease (ESKD) will likely not decrease over the next several decades, but may in fact increase. The impact of obesity is especially important for kidney transplantation because many obese individuals are precluded from kidney transplantation due to concerns over the potential medical and surgical complications associated with their body habitus. Because higher BMI appears to be associated with decreased mortality among patients receiving dialysis, clinicians may be reluctant to counsel obese patients to lose weight. To understand the impact of obesity on transplantation, the discussion needs to begin with a review of how obesity impacts mortality in populations with CKD. This chapter will then discuss trends in obesity among adults receiving dialysis, controversies surrounding the preclusion of morbidly obese individuals from transplantation, and behavior modifications and surgical interventions and their respective risks and benefits for obesity management.

2. BMI and mortality in the general population

Body mass index (BMI) (the weight in kilograms divided by the square of the height in meters) has been widely used to estimate overweight and obesity. Weight indexed for height was first used by life insurance companies to estimate life expectancy in the early part of the twentieth century (1, 2). In 1997, the World Health Organization (WHO) created categories for underweight (BMI<18.5 kg/m^2), overweight (BMI 25.0-29.9 kg/m^2), and obesity stages I (BMI 30.0-34.9 kg/m^2) , II (BMI 35.0-39.9 kg/m^2), and III (≥40 kg/m^2) (Table 1) (3). Controversy exists as to whether these BMI categories are applicable for assessing mortality risk in all age and racial/ethnic groups. However, in the general U.S. population, studies have consistently shown that a BMI ≥ 35 kg/m^2 heightens mortality risk in young and middle-aged individuals (4-6) but this risk declines with advancing age (7). A meta-analysis of studies limited to adults 65 years or older concluded that federal guidelines for ideal weight (BMI 18.7-25 kg/m^2) may be too restrictive for populations over the age of 70 years due to lack of evidence that overweight in the elderly confers excess mortality risk (8).

BMI	(kg/m²)
Underweight	<18.5
Normal	18.5-24.9
Overweight	25.0-29.9
Class I Obesity	30.0-34.9
Class II Obesity	35.0-39.9
Class III Obesity	≥40
Waist circumference	**(cm)**
Increased risk	Men ≤ 102 Women ≤ 88
Decreased risk	Men >102 Women >88

*Adapted from World Health Organization 1998 guidelines for obesity classification (3)

Table 1. Classification of Underweight, Overweight, and Obesity by BMI and Waist Circumference*

3. Abdominal obesity in the general population

The indexing of weight for height (BMI) includes fat mass and fat-free mass and provides no information about body composition or regional adiposity. Abdominal fat remains a strong predictor of mortality even after adjustment for sensitive measures of total body fat. In fact, the increased cardiovascular risk associated with obesity is mainly mediated by abdominal fat (9). Visceral adipose tissue produces cytokines including tumor necrosis factor alpha, which can cause insulin resistance by the suppression of adiponectin. Abdominal obesity can amplify this problem by the high influx of portal fatty acids, cytokines, and hormones into the liver from omental adipocytes, resulting in increased hepatic synthesis of apolipoprotein B and very low density lipids (10). Although abdominal fat can be measured directly by using dual-energy X-ray absorptiometry, computed tomography, or magnetic resonance imaging, waist circumference correlates highly with abdominal fat and can be measured easily and fairly reliably (11-13). The definition of abdominal adiposity (waist circumference ≥102 cm in men and ≥88 cm in women) is based on a Scottish study which found that this threshold for waist circumference effectively identified obese (BMI ≥30kg/m²) individuals in addition to adults with BMI < 30 kg/m² in the setting of a high waist/hip ratio (Table 1) (14). While waist circumference thresholds for abdominal adiposity may differ by racial/ethnic groups (i.e. > 87cm and > 83cm in Japanese men and women, respectively) (15), individuals with abdominal adiposity are more likely to have hypertension, diabetes, dyslipidemia, and the metabolic syndrome than individuals without abdominal adiposity, even after adjusting for BMI class (16, 17). Furthermore, abdominal adiposity is associated with increased mortality risk regardless of BMI or racial/ethnic group (16-18).

4. Obesity trends in CKD stages 1-5

Rates of obesity worldwide have increased dramatically over the past 20 years. In the U.S., prevalence of obesity has doubled from 15 to 30% while morbid obesity prevalence increased by four-fold (19). Overall, obesity trends in adults with ESKD mirror those in the general population. Not surprisingly, during years 1995-2002, the mean BMI among patients initiating dialysis increased from 25.7 to 27.5 kg/m^2 (20). The percentage of incident ESKD patients who had stage II obesity (BMI>35 kg/m^2) during this timeframe increased from 9.4% to 15.4%. Likewise, the percentage of patients listed for kidney transplantation who were obese (BMI≥30kg/m^2) increased from 11.6% to 25.1% between the years 1987 and 2001 (21).

5. Adiposity measures and mortality in adults with CKD

Using BMI measures as a proxy of adiposity in CKD patients may not account for differences in body composition or muscle wasting. Indeed, studies using BMI to study adverse outcomes in the CKD population have shown conflicting results from the general population (22-24). Similarly, in studies of adults with CKD who are not receiving dialysis, BMI has not been found to be an independent predictor of cardiovascular disease or all-cause mortality (25,26). To examine associations between abdominal adiposity as measured by the waist-hip ratio (WHR) and BMI with cardiovascular events, Elsayed et al pooled data from the Atherosclerosis Risk in Communities Study and the Cardiovascular Health (ARIC) Study (27). A total of 1,669 adults with CKD were followed for a mean of 9.3 years. Mean age was 70.3 years and mean estimated glomerular filtration rate (eGFR) was 51.1 ml/min/m^2. The highest WHR group had a 36% increased hazard of cardiovascular events compared to the lowest WHR group. Obesity (BMI>30 kg/m^2) was not associated with cardiovascular events when compared to those with an ideal BMI (18.5-24.9 kg/m^2).

Among adults receiving dialysis, numerous studies have reported a survival benefit with higher BMI compared to BMI in the ideal (18.5-24.9 kg/m^2) and low (< 18.5 kg/m^2) range (28-31). It has been posited that fat may play a protective role in these patients who often suffer from protein-energy malnutrition and inflammation (28). However, BMI represents both muscle mass and abdominal and peripheral fat. Higher muscle mass reflects better physical functioning, which is extremely important for predicting mortality in patients with co-morbid conditions such as ESKD. An Italian study of 537 dialysis patients examined associations of waist circumference, waist-to-hip ratio (WHR), and BMI with cardiovascular and total mortality (32). The inverse relationship between BMI and mortality was reaffirmed whereas waist circumference and WHR were directly associated with increased cardiovascular and total mortality. After adjustment for cardiovascular risk factors, every 10-cm higher waist circumference conferred an excess 26% risk for death and an excess 38% risk for cardiovascular death (32). The association between BMI and mortality in patients receiving dialysis has also been shown to be modified by muscle mass as reflected by 24-hour creatinine excretion (33).

Few studies have examined the link between adiposity measures and mortality in adult kidney transplant recipients. Kovedsky examined BMI and waist circumference in 993 kidney transplant recipients in Hungary (34). Mean age was 50.9 years, 21% were diabetic, and mean eGFR rate was 50.9 ml/min/1.73 m^2. Individuals with higher BMI or waist circumference were more likely to be diabetic, less likely to smoke, and more likely to have had delayed graft function. While risk of mortality declined with higher BMI, a 15 cm higher waist circumference was associated with greater than 2-fold increase in all-cause mortality after adjustment for BMI (34).

In summary, BMI may be inadequate by itself to assess mortality risk associated with adiposity. Waist circumference reflects visceral adiposity burden and is directly associated with mortality among individuals with co-morbid conditions such as ESKD while BMI appears to be inversely related to mortality (30-32, 34). Many centers currently exclude patients with BMI >35 kg/m^2 from kidney transplantation until they are able to lose weight (35, 36). Use of waist circumference in the evaluation of kidney transplant candidates may provide more accurate information regarding the pre- and post-transplantation risks associated with obesity.

6. Access to kidney transplantation and barriers due to obesity

Obesity is currently an important barrier keeping many individuals from being listed for kidney transplantation (37). A study of the UNOS database from 1995-2006 evaluated the association between BMI and time to transplantation (38). Individuals with severe obesity (BMI 35-40 kg/m^2) and morbid obesity (BMI 40-60 kg/m^2) at time of initial listing were 28% and 44% less likely, respectively, to receive a deceased-donor kidney transplant compared to individuals with an ideal BMI (18.5-24.9 kg/m^2) (38). This study could not account for the number of obese individuals who were never listed at all due to their weight, and likely underestimates the impact obesity may have on access to transplantation. Indeed, 15% of transplant centers did not list a single severely obese (BMI 35-40 kg/m^2) patient during the 11-year period of the study (38). While this study cannot prove causality, it seems likely that body habitus is a major deciding factor when determining whether a person may be listed for transplantation. Certainly, economic pressures favor kidney transplantation for "low-risk" non-obese patients in which complication rates and hospital stay may be lower. Moreover, obesity is considered a reversible risk factor, and losing weight prior to transplant is thought to be beneficial, especially considering how common weight gain is after kidney transplantation (37). Obese kidney transplant recipients are at increased risk for short-term complications including delayed wound healing, longer surgical times, and delayed graft function (39, 40). Data on whether obese transplant recipients are at higher risk for long-term adverse outcomes remains controversial, but the majority of larger studies suggest poorer long-term outcomes among obese individuals compared to non-obese individuals (40-42).

The decision by some transplant centers to use BMI thresholds for the exclusion of patients from kidney transplantation should consider both societal and individual level concerns. From an individual-level perspective, kidney transplantation offers a clear survival benefit over dialysis regardless of obesity status (43,44). Among obese adults receiving dialysis for ESKD during years 1995-1999, both living and deceased donor kidney transplant recipients had decreased mortality risk of 61% and 77%, respectively, compared to those remaining on the kidney transplant waiting list. Due to the excess surgical risks and graft failure among obese individuals, one option would be to limit opportunities for cadaveric kidneys. However, evidence for this is contentious. Excluding obese individuals due to increased risk ignores the fact that co-morbid conditions such as diabetes pose similar risk as obesity yet these conditions do not preclude transplantation (40). Transplantation centers should also consider the extra time an obese patient spends on dialysis while trying to lose weight in order to be listed for transplantation. Unfortunately, weight loss is usually unsuccessful for individuals with severe obesity (45).

7. Obese kidney transplant patients

7.1 Post-operative complications

For all surgical procedures, obesity can complicate the post-operative period with delayed wound healing, increased rates of ventral hernias, and longer operating times and hospitalizations. In transplant recipients, obesity is also associated with heightened risk of infections, and post-transplant diabetes (49-53). One single-center study which included 2013 adult kidney transplants performed between 1984 and 1998, superficial or deep wound infections occurred in 4.8%, whereas 3.6% developed either a fascial dehiscence or hernia of the wound (54). Those with BMI ≥ 30 kg/m^2 had a 340% increased risk for a wound infection and 182% increased risk for a fascial dehiscence or incisional hernia compared to those with BMI < 30 kg/m^2.

Delayed graft function (DGF), defined as the need for dialysis therapy in the first week after kidney transplantation, places a recipient at increased risk for chronic rejection and decreased graft survival. Only a minority of single-center studies have shown that obesity increases risk for decreased graft survival after kidney transplantation (46-53) but this may be due to small sample sizes in these single-center studies. In a large study which included 51,927 kidney transplant recipients, severe obesity (BMI > 35 kg/m^2) was associated with a 51% increased risk of DGF compared to the transplant recipients with a BMI between 22-24 kg/m^2 (41). These findings were supported by a study which included data from 27,377 kidney transplant recipients (40).

Overall mortality, regardless of obesity status, is substantially reduced with kidney transplantation (43,44). However, compared to non-obese kidney transplant recipients, obese transplant recipients appear to have an increased risk of graft loss although not all studies agree (39-56). Overall, BMI > 35 kg/m^2 appears to increase graft failure risk by approximately 20-30% compared to recipients who are not obese while no excess risk is seen among transplant recipients with a BMI between 30-35 kg/m^2 (40,41). The magnitude of the association between morbid obesity and graft failure is similar to the increased risk of graft failure associated with diabetes (40). Overall mortality after kidney transplantation does not appear to be associated with obesity itself. However, obese patients may have co-morbid conditions which influence survival (40).

7.2 Weight loss interventions for obese adults with CKD

7.2.1 Who should lose weight

The management of obesity requires identification of individuals who will benefit from weight loss. All obese patients (BMI ≥ 30 kg/m^2) should be counseled to modify their lifestyles (diet and physical activity) to induce weight loss but goals must be individualized (57). In adults with CKD, abdominal obesity, measured by waist circumference should be considered an indication for weight loss considering the increased risk of cardiovascular and total mortality associated with increased waist circumference (27, 32, 34). Weight loss in patients with diabetic and non-diabetic kidney diseases has been shown to reduce proteinuria (58, 59). However, there is a paucity of data regarding the long-term outcomes of intentional weight loss in adults with CKD. Perhaps the strongest evidence supporting weight loss in this population comes from surgical intervention studies in the morbidly obese. Successful weight loss dramatically improves blood pressure, proteinuria, and in some cases, stabilizes GFR (60-63). However, surgical interventions for obesity carry significant risks as discussed later.

Regardless of the small survival benefits associated with obesity observed among patients receiving dialysis, kidney transplantation greatly improves longevity and survival is substantially higher among obese kidney transplant recipients compared to individuals remaining on the waiting list (38). In fact, obesity should be considered the most important modifiable mortality risk factor if a patient receiving dialysis is not listed for kidney transplantation solely due to obesity (45). Weight loss goals for obese patients receiving dialysis who are seeking kidney transplantation must be assessed individually and goals should account for the obesity-related co-morbid conditions and nutritional status of that individual. Moreover, interventions should also account for the patient's body composition because increasing muscle mass may improve overall fitness and survival (31, 45).

7.2.2 Weight gain after kidney transplantation

Weight gain after kidney transplantation is very common, with studies showing increased weight between 8-14 kg one year post-transplant (37, 39, 64). Johnson et al showed that a 10% weight gain correlated with increased serum cholesterol and triglyceride levels which may heighten cardiovascular risk (49, 65). In a study of 3,899 white Australian and New Zealand adults, weight gain of 10% to 19.9% during the first year after transplantation and stable weight (0% to 4.9% gain) during the second year after transplantation were associated with the best outcomes while weight loss over the first two years after transplantation was associated with the worst outcomes (66). A 20% weight gain above the pre-transplant weight during the first year with continued weight gain during the second year after transplantation was associated with increased graft loss and mortality compared to transplant recipients who maintained their weight after the second year.

Certain individuals may be at higher risk for excessive weight gain after kidney transplantation than others. Certainly the improved appetite and sense of well-being may lead to augmented caloric intake. A study of renal transplant recipients from a racially diverse center between 1983 and 1998 reported that African Americans were at higher risk for weight gain (67), and these results have been supported by several other studies (47, 49, 50, 64). Part of this race disparity may be due to socioeconomic status because accounting for income level attenuates the association between race and weight gain after kidney transplantation (64). Weight gain patterns after transplantation seem to mirror the general population as the majority of studies have shown that younger age, female sex and low income-status increase the probability of weight gain (47, 49, 50, 64). Patients who are obese at the time of kidney transplantation appear to have similar (67) or greater weight gain (47, 64) compared to non-obese kidney transplant recipients.

Immunosuppressant medications have varying adverse cardiovascular risk profiles. Corticosteroids can cause excessive weight gain and redistribution of fat to undesired areas (face and back) as well as worsen blood pressure, glucose and lipid metabolism (68). Overall, steroid doses used for kidney transplantation are much lower than in the past with some transplant protocols minimizing or avoiding steroid use. However, minimization or avoidance of steroid use in kidney transplantation must be counterbalanced with adequate immunosuppression, which often requires lymphocyte depleting agents or anti-IL2 strategies coupled with the use of other immunosuppressive medications (69). One study examined 95 kidney transplant recipients enrolled in National Institutes of Health clinical transplant trials (70). Regardless of therapy received, weight increased by 5 kg (not BMI) on average among all patients at one year post-transplant. Another small retrospective study compared patterns of weight gain among 301 kidney transplant recipients receiving chronic corticosteroid therapy to patients who had early corticosteroid withdrawal (within 7 days post-transplant) (71). A 33% lower rate of weight gain among the early corticosteroid withdrawal group was observed. In contrast, a Dutch study which included 123 patients found no difference in one year post-transplant weight gain between patients who were and were not maintained on low dose steroids (72). In a study of 334 transplant patients at a single institution, average weight gain in patients treated with a steroid taper to 10 mg/day over the course of a year was 28.5% lower compared to the group in whom the steroid dose was tapered to 5mg/day at 6 months (73). The benefits of corticosteroid-sparing regimens on weight gain as well as long-term outcomes are yet uncertain and deserve further study.

7.3 Weight management before and after kidney transplantation

7.3.1 Lifestyle modifications

A multidisciplinary approach to weight management is necessary to maximize weight loss. This approach should utilize all members of the kidney transplant or CKD team including dieticians, nurses, psychologists, social workers and physicians. These members should work together to identify specific needs, motivations, and barriers for each individual patient who requires weight loss. For most patients, a combined approach including diet, exercise and behavior modifications, similar to methods used in the general population, should be applied. Preclusion of kidney transplantation due to obesity generally focuses on BMI thresholds > 35 kg/m^2. Patients with this level of obesity will frequently fail traditional methods for weight loss and surgical interventions should be considered after a trial of lifestyle changes. In the following paragraphs, we describe traditional dietary changes for weight loss and the benefits of exercise in patients with CKD. This is then followed by a discussion of the risks and benefits of weight loss drugs and bariatric surgery.

7.3.2 Dietary interventions for patients not receiving dialysis

Dietary modification remains the most important component of any weight loss intervention and dietary interventions have been shown to be effective in ameliorating weight gain after kidney transplantation (74-76). As weight gain is quite common after kidney transplantation, dietary counseling prior to kidney transplantation with frequent follow-up after transplantation should be done. To aid in developing a plan, a diet history should be obtained and patients can take part in this plan by keeping a food diary for several days. Review of medications that may contribute to weight gain should be completed. While numerous diets exist, none can be universally recommended for patients with CKD including the kidney transplant recipient (77). A conservative approach is to restrict caloric intake by approximately 500 kcal/day, which in the absence of physical activity changes, will lead to a weight loss of 1 pound per week (74). More restrictive diets (<1,200 kcal/day) require more intensive monitoring of the nutritional status and well-being of the patient.

With the exception of protein intake, there are no exact recommendations for specific nutrient and dietary composition for patients with CKD. The American Heart Association guidelines for a healthy lifestyle provide no specific recommendations for diet and state that the exact percentage of carbohydrates, proteins, and fat within a given meal will not in itself influence weight management (78). Addressing portion size and reducing energy intake to less than energy expenditure is the only reliable way to facilitate weight loss (78). High protein diets for weight loss are quite popular and can be successful for some individuals, but data on long-term safety is lacking (79). High protein diets should be avoided in adults with CKD due to concerns that higher protein intake can accelerate loss of GFR (80). Accordingly, the National Kidney Foundation-Kidney Disease Outcomes Quality Initiative (NKF-KDOQI) guidelines recommend that protein intake not exceed 0.8g/kg/day with 50 to 75% of the protein derived from lean poultry, fish, and vegetables (81). This level of protein intake is substantially lower than the average protein intake in many individuals in the U.S. and other countries where protein intake may exceed 1.2 gm/kg/day. Diets such as the Dietary Approaches to Stop Hypertension (DASH) diet emphasize the consumption of fresh fruits and vegetables, whole grains, and low dairy while minimizing red meat intake, sodium intake and processed foods. The DASH diet may provide additional benefits beyond those associated with weight loss (82). However, the DASH diet contains higher levels of protein (1.4 g/kg/d), potassium (4500mg/d), and phosphorus (1.7g/d) than recommended by the NKF-KDOQI guidelines for the CKD patient (74). Specific nutritional recommendations for CKD and kidney transplant recipients remain poorly defined, and more research needs to be done to better define an optimal diet before making specific recommendations. Thus, diet interventions for the CKD patient must be individualized and focus should be on portion size reduction. Identification of excess snacking times (e.g. night time) and intake of nutrient poor yet high calorie foods will help the individual patient reduce their caloric intake. In general, the weight loss goals should not exceed 1 pound per week.

7.3.3 Dietary interventions for patients receiving dialysis

Studies to support dietary recommendations for patients receiving dialysis to promote weight loss are substantially limited. Current guidelines for patients receiving dialysis recommend protein intake of 1.2g/kg/day and 30 to 35 kcal/kg/day for stable patients (81). However, in order to lose weight, obese patients must reduce caloric consumption to less than caloric expenditure. Nutritional plans should be individualized to ensure that the unique nutritional requirements of patients receiving dialysis are met. Food diaries and dietary histories can be used to help identify sources of empty calories. There is no strong evidence to suggest any particular dietary intervention to promote weight loss in patients receiving dialysis. One conservative approach is to start with 25 kcal/kg/d based on the adjusted body weight (ideal body weight - [dry total body weight - ideal body weight]/4) and then adjustments can be made based on the patient's weight loss (45). However, this method is not as reliable as using direct measures of resting energy expenditure to determine caloric needs. Additional research is needed to determine safe and effective interventions for weight loss in this patient population.

7.3.4 Dietary interventions for kidney transplant recipients

Several studies have examined dietary interventions to ameliorate weight gain after kidney transplantation. One single-center study gave 11 consecutive kidney transplant recipients individualized, intensive dietary advice for the first 4 months after transplantation (76). These individuals were then compared to 22 patients who received kidney transplants 4 years prior to the study and had not received dietary advice post-transplantation. Baseline characteristics of the two groups were similar with mean BMI of about 24 kg/m^2 in both groups. The group who received dietary advice showed no statistically significant change in weigh four months after transplantation compared to their pre-transplant weight. In contrast, the group with no dietary intervention had a significant weight gain of 7kg four months after transplantation and

11.8 kg at one year after transplantation (76). Another study enrolled 34 overweight and obese (mean BMI 33 kg/m^2) kidney transplant recipients who were highly motivated to lose weight in a weight loss program (83). During the initial visit, the negative impact of obesity after kidney transplantation was discussed and participants wrote down and reviewed a detailed 3-day history of their own dietary habits but no dietary advice was given. After six months of follow-up, only 27% of those in the weight loss program had weight gain compared to 80% of controls (83). While these two studies were not randomized controlled clinical trials, the study results support a beneficial role for dietary counseling after kidney transplantation. Transplant centers should utilize an approach whereby all potential kidney transplant recipients receive some individualized counseling on lifestyle (diet and physical activity) both before and after kidney transplantation. The use of dietary histories and food diaries are encouraged because it will enable the patient to participate in the development of plans to facilitate changing their own dietary habits.

8. Exercise

Increasing physical activity may promote modest weight loss and improve physical functioning. Patients with CKD are overall a sedentary population with markedly reduced peak maximal oxygen and reduced physical functioning compared to individuals with normal kidney function (84, 85). A study of ambulatory patients new to dialysis found that physical activity scores for these patients were below the 5th percentile of healthy individuals and estimated that 95% of patients initiating dialysis have very low fitness levels (84). Decreased physical activity is associated with excess mortality in adults with CKD (85, 86). Exercise in patients with CKD improves functional aerobic capacity, muscular strength, and blood pressure (87, 88). However, currently there is insufficient evidence to make specific exercise recommendations for patients with CKD. In addition, the co-existence of multiple co-morbid conditions in this patient population limits the capacity to exercise. In any case, considering the poor physical functioning demonstrated in the majority of patients receiving dialysis, exercise should be encouraged if possible (84). Low-to-moderate-intensity aerobic exercise three times per week should be recommended to all patients able to do so, just as it is recommended for the general population (89). The risk of cardiac events during exercise has not been quantified in patients with CKD, but the risks are likely no greater than those occurring during diagnostic tests for cardiovascular disease (3.6 myocardial infarctions per 10,000 tests) (90, 91).

9. Pharmacologic agents for weight loss

Dietary change remains difficult for the majority of individuals and some patients may request weight loss medications to augment weight loss. It should be noted that weight loss medications will only modestly improve weight loss and these drugs are frequently accompanied by substantial side effects. These possible risks and benefits must be discussed with the patient when considering the use of weight loss medications. Moreover, the safety of any weight loss drug should be strongly scrutinized given that two weight loss medications, sibutramine and rimonabant, were removed from the U.S. and European markets due to concerns about heightened risk of cardiovascular disease and suicide, respectively (92, 93). This illustrates the need for extreme caution with any weight loss medication.

In the U.S., the only medication currently approved by the FDA for long-term use is orlistat, which can promote modest weight loss but is accompanied by frequent gastrointestinal side effects. Short-term agents that are FDA-approved such as phentermine or diethylpropion should be avoided in kidney transplant recipients or individuals with CKD due to associated conditions such as hypertension, and cardiovascular disease risk. Thus, the only weight loss medication that potentially could be safe in populations with CKD is orlistat. Orlistat reversibly inhibits gastric and pancreatic lipases and blocks approximately 30% of gastrointestinal absorption of triglycerides. Only a small amount of orlistat is systemically absorbed with 800 mg of orlistat daily yielding minimal plasma concentrations of the drug (94). A small non-randomized trial of orlistat was conducted among patients with stages 3-5 CKD (95). These participants followed a low-fat renal-specific diet, and exercise was encouraged (95). Orlistat was given at the standard dose of 120 mg three times daily and patients were followed for two years. An average of 8.3 kg weight loss was noted and this loss occurred mostly during the initial six month period of the study. However, the weight loss was maintained after two years of follow-up. Gastrointestinal adverse events were common including flatulence, diarrhea, and fatty stools, with 43% reporting at least one side effect in the initial month of therapy. After six months of orlistat use, only 10% reported side effects (95). Thus, orlistat augments weight loss, but only modestly.

Among kidney transplant recipients, orlistat use may complicate the immunosuppressant regimen. Orlistat interferes with cyclosporine absorption because cyclosporine is highly lipid-soluble. To prevent this issue, orlistat should not be taken within a two-hour window of taking cyclosporine and cyclosporine levels should be closely monitored (96, 97). Another concern is the increased risk of oxalate nephropathy with this drug. Although rare, acute kidney injury due to renal oxalosis has been reported in an adult with CKD taking orlistat for weight loss (98). Patients should also be advised that fat intake must be limited to less than 30% of total calories otherwise the patient may experience fecal incontinence. Fat-soluble vitamin deficiencies can also occur with use of orlistat and it is recommended that patients be supplemented with fat-soluble vitamins when taking orlistat (99).

Other pharmacologic agents such as serotonin reuptake inhibitors and buproprion are not approved for long-term use of weight maintenance in the general population, and have not been well-studied in adults with CKD. Over-the-counter dietary supplements should also be discouraged due to a dearth of evidence regarding efficacy, safety, and possible interactions with immunosuppressive medications.

10. Surgical options

Surgical options for weight management should only be considered after lifestyle interventions fail to yield adequate weight loss. These surgical options include procedures that divert food from the stomach into lower parts of the gastrointestinal tract to limit food absorption and reduce the size of the stomach leading to early satiety (Roux-en-Y diversion) and gastric banding (100). An adjustable gastric band placed around the upper part of the stomach may be inflated or deflated by injecting or removing saline through a port underneath the skin (100). Given the procedure is performed by an experienced surgeon, mortality risk is < 2% with gastric banding and approximately 3% with gastric diversion procedures. However, mortality risk may be higher in patients with a BMI≥ 50 kg/m^2 (101, 102). Regardless of the type of procedure, the majority of weight loss occurs during the first year after surgery with greater weight loss consistently occurring with gastric diversion procedures (70.1%) vs. gastric banding (47.5%) (101, 102). Advantages of gastric banding include less hospitalization time and fewer short-term complications (see Table 2) (103). However, long-term complications of gastric banding are higher than gastric diversion procedures albeit less severe. For instance, intragastric band erosion is caused by chronic ischemia of the gastric wall due to the constrictive effects of the band. The gastric band can also migrate and lead to severe abdominal pain and vomiting. A recent report of long-term followup at a center in Belgium reported that approximately 1 out of every 3 patients who underwent gastric banding experienced gastric band erosion with almost half required band removal (104).

	Roux-en-Y Gastric Bypass	Laparoscopic Adjustable Gastric Banding
Mortality	<1%	<1%
Resolution of type 2 diabetes	++	+
Maintenance of weight loss after 2 years	+++	+
Length of hospitalization	2-8 days	1-3 days
Short-term complications	More common	Less common
Long-term complications	Less common, but more serious (i.e. bowel obstruction, marginal ulcer, incisional hernia, nutrient deficiency)	More common, but less serious (i.e. band slippage with pouch dilation, band erosion, port problems)
Reoperation rates§	10-20%	20-60%
Vitamin deficiencies (B vitamins, fat soluble vitamins)	++ (may require substantial supplementation)	+ (often corrected with multivitamin supplement)

*Adapted from Tice et al. (102)
§Reoperation rates from studies with long-term follow-up >24 months (102, 121-123)
Table 2. Comparison of Roux-en-Y Gastric Bypass and Laparoscopic Adjustable Gastric Banding*

Patients receiving dialysis may obtain substantial weight loss allowing for kidney transplantation (105-107), but information on risk and long-term benefits remains limited. Using Medicare claims data during years 1991-2004 linked with the United States Renal Data System, investigators evaluated post-bariatric surgery mortality risk and outcomes (108). On average, patients lost 30-60% of their total pre-surgery body weight. Overall 30-day mortality risk was similar for patients listed for a kidney transplant and for kidney transplant recipients (3.5%). Allograft failure was reported in a patient 30 days after the kidney transplant (108). The largest single-center series of kidney transplant patients reported outcomes for 10 kidney transplant recipients who underwent gastric bypass surgery for excessive weight gain leading to morbid obesity after transplantation (109).

Mean age was 44 years and the gastric bypass surgeries occurred on average 5.3 years after transplantation. In this group, there were no fatalities within the first 30 days after bariatric surgery and patients on average lost 70.5% of their excess weight above ideal weight (109).

Clearly, the substantial weight loss after bariatric surgery can lead to resolution of diabetes and less need for blood pressure lowering medications in adults without CKD. In fact, 98% and 48% of adults with obesity and diabetes no longer have type 2 diabetes two years after undergoing gastric diversion and gastric banding, respectively, for obesity management (102). Other obesity related co-morbid conditions may resolve as well such as fatty liver, hypercholesterolemia and sleep apnea (101). These long-term benefits likely apply to patients with CKD, but the surgical risks may be heightened in this population. Gastric band erosion has been reported in a kidney transplant recipient treated with gastric banding for weight management (110). While these surgical complications are not unique to the transplant population, the presence of immunosuppressant agents could worsen the side effects of bariatric surgery.

Nutritional deficiencies are common after bariatric surgery for weight loss and this may be complicated by poor nutritional choices of the individual patient. Patients may become deficient in iron, calcium, B vitamins and fat soluble vitamins (101). An important complication of gastric bypass surgery includes increased oxalate absorption due to decreased intestinal absorption of fatty acids, and this could lead to kidney stones, renal oxalosis, acute kidney injury, allograft loss and even oxalate-induced anemia (111-115). The Roux-en-Y surgery results in a smaller gastric pouch which may not produce as much acid, and as a result, the higher stomach pH and the smaller surface area of both stomach and small intestine may impact the absorption of some drugs (116, 117). It should be noted that increased cyclosporine dosing may be required after gastric diversion procedures (117). The pharmacokinetics of tacrolimus, mycophenolate, and sirolimus may also change after gastric diversion, and higher doses of several immunosuppressants may be needed after gastric bypass (116). Obese patients often require lower doses of cyclosporine per body weight compared to lean recipients (118, 119) and dosing for cyclosporine based on ideal body weight is recommended (118-120). Given the excessive weight loss which occurs rapidly after bariatric surgery, levels of immunosuppressant drugs including mycophenolate mofetil, should be followed closely after gastric bypass surgery, especially during the first 18 months after bariatric surgery.

Due to the lack of information on long-term consequences of bariatric surgery, no specific recommendations can be made for patients with CKD or kidney transplant recipients. Thus, the decision to utilize bariatric surgery for weight management needs to be individualized. Most importantly, clinicians must ensure that these patients are informed of the associated risks before they proceed with surgical interventions for obesity management.

Regardless of obesity status, kidney transplantation is associated with improved survival and decreased morbidity compared to dialysis. Thus, obesity may be viewed as the most important modifiable mortality risk factor for patients precluded from kidney transplantation due to obesity status. Weight management should include a multi-disciplinary approach with dietary advice on caloric restriction and encouragement to increase physical activity. Patients should actively take part in the development of the obesity management plan (e.g. keep food diary). If lifestyle interventions fail to yield adequate weight loss, then surgical options should be considered. Clinicians should discuss frankly the potential risk of bariatric surgery for weight management. Transplant centers should also incorporate dietary counseling both before and after kidney transplantation to ameliorate weight gain after transplantation which may heighten cardiovascular risk. Future research should address the use of both BMI and waist circumference to improve risk stratification and obesity interventions for patients before and after kidney transplantation.

11. References

Metropolitan Life Insurance Company. New weight standards for men and women. Stat Bull Metropol Life Insur Co 1959;40:1–4.

Kuczmarski RJ, Flegal KM. Criteria for definition of overweight in transition: background and recommendations for the united states. Am J Clin Nutr. 2000 Nov;72(5):1074-81.

WHO: Obesity: Preventing and managing the global epidemic: Report of a WHO Consultation on Obesity, Geneva, June 3-5, 1997. Geneva, Switzerland, World Health Organization, 1998.

Adams KF, Schatzkin A, Harris TB, Kipnis V, Mouw T, Ballard-Barbash R, et al. Overweight, obesity, and mortality in a large prospective cohort of persons 50 to 71 years old. N Engl J Med. 2006 Aug 24;355(8):763-78.

Fontaine KR, Redden DT, Wang C, Westfall AO, Allison DB. Years of life lost due to obesity. JAMA. 2003 Jan 8;289(2):187-93.

Peeters A, Barendregt JJ, Willekens F, Mackenbach JP, Al Mamun A, Bonneux L, et al. Obesity in adulthood and its consequences for life expectancy: A life-table analysis. Ann Intern Med. 2003 Jan 7;138(1):24-32.

Stevens J, Cai J, Pamuk ER, Williamson DF, Thun MJ, Wood JL. The effect of age on the association between body-mass index and mortality. N Engl J Med. 1998 Jan 1;338(1):1-7.

Heiat A, Vaccarino V, Krumholz HM. An evidence-based assessment of federal guidelines for overweight and obesity as they apply to elderly persons. Arch Intern Med. 2001 May 14;161(9):1194-203.

Bigaard J, Frederiksen K, Tjonneland A, Thomsen BL, Overvad K, Heitmann BL, et al. Waist circumference and body composition in relation to all-cause mortality in middle-aged men and women. Int J Obes (Lond). 2005 Jul;29(7):778-84.

Haslam DW, James WP. Obesity. Lancet. 2005 Oct 1;366(9492):1197-209.

Rankinen T, Kim SY, Perusse L, Despres JP, Bouchard C. The prediction of abdominal visceral fat level from body composition and anthropometry: ROC analysis. Int J Obes Relat Metab Disord. 1999 Aug;23(8):801-9.

Reeder BA, Senthilselvan A, Despres JP, Angel A, Liu L, Wang H, et al. The association of cardiovascular disease risk factors with abdominal obesity in canada. canadian heart health surveys research group. CMAJ. 1997 Jul 1;157 Suppl 1:S39-45.

Pouliot MC, Despres JP, Lemieux S, Moorjani S, Bouchard C, Tremblay A, et al. Waist circumference and abdominal sagittal diameter: Best simple anthropometric indexes of abdominal visceral adipose tissue accumulation and related cardiovascular risk in men and women. Am J Cardiol. 1994 Mar 1;73(7):460-8.

Lean ME, Han TS, Morrison CE. Waist circumference as a measure for indicating need for weight management. BMJ. 1995 Jul 15;311(6998):158-61.

Narisawa S, Nakamura K, Kato K, Yamada K, Sasaki J, Yamamoto M. Appropriate waist circumference cutoff values for persons with multiple cardiovascular risk factors in japan: A large cross-sectional study. J Epidemiol. 2008;18(1):37-42.

Janssen I, Katzmarzyk PT, Ross R. Body mass index, waist circumference, and health risk: Evidence in support of current national institutes of health guidelines. Arch Intern Med. 2002 Oct 14;162(18):2074-9.

Balkau B, Deanfield JE, Despres JP, Bassand JP, Fox KA, Smith SC,Jr, et al. International day for the evaluation of abdominal obesity (IDEA): A study of waist circumference, cardiovascular disease, and diabetes mellitus in 168,000 primary care patients in 63 countries. Circulation. 2007 Oct 23;116(17):1942-51.

Koster A, Leitzmann MF, Schatzkin A, Mouw T, Adams KF, van Eijk JT, et al. Waist circumference and mortality. Am J Epidemiol. 2008 Jun 15;167(12):1465-75.

Mokdad AH, Ford ES, Bowman BA, Dietz WH, Vinicor F, Bales VS, et al. Prevalence of obesity, diabetes, and obesity-related health risk factors, 2001. JAMA. 2003 Jan 1;289(1):76-9.

Kramer HJ, Saranathan A, Luke A, Durazo-Arvizu RA, Guichan C, Hou S, et al. Increasing body mass index and obesity in the incident ESRD population. J Am Soc Nephrol. 2006 May;17(5):1453-9.

Friedman AN, Miskulin DC, Rosenberg IH, Levey AS. Demographics and trends in overweight and obesity in patients at time of kidney transplantation. Am J Kidney Dis. 2003 Feb;41(2):480-7.

Kalantar-Zadeh K, Kopple JD. Obesity paradox in patients on maintenance dialysis. Contrib Nephrol. 2006;151:57-69.

Kalantar-Zadeh K, Kopple JD, Kilpatrick RD, McAllister CJ, Shinaberger CS, Gjertson DW, et al. Association of morbid obesity and weight change over time with cardiovascular survival in hemodialysis population. Am J Kidney Dis. 2005 Sep;46(3):489-500.

Kovesdy CP, Czira ME, Rudas A, Ujszaszi A, Rosivall L, Novak M, et al. Body mass index, waist circumference and mortality in kidney transplant recipients. Am J Transplant. 2010 Dec;10(12):2644-51.

Madero M, Sarnak MJ, Wang X, Sceppa CC, Greene T, Beck GJ, et al. Body mass index and mortality in CKD. Am J Kidney Dis. 2007 Sep;50(3):404-11.

Kwan BC, Murtaugh MA, Beddhu S. Associations of body size with metabolic syndrome and mortality in moderate chronic kidney disease. Clin J Am Soc Nephrol. 2007 Sep;2(5):992-8.

Elsayed EF, Tighiouart H, Weiner DE, Griffith J, Salem D, Levey AS, et al. Waist-to-hip ratio and body mass index as risk factors for cardiovascular events in CKD. Am J Kidney Dis. 2008 Jul;52(1):49-57.

Kalantar-Zadeh K, Kopple JD. Obesity paradox in patients on maintenance dialysis. Contrib Nephrol. 2006;151:57-69.

Kalantar-Zadeh K, Kopple JD, Kilpatrick RD, McAllister CJ, Shinaberger CS, Gjertson DW, et al. Association of morbid obesity and weight change over time with cardiovascular survival in hemodialysis population. Am J Kidney Dis. 2005 Sep;46(3):489-500.

Kalantar-Zadeh K, Kuwae N, Wu DY, Shantouf RS, Fouque D, Anker SD, et al. Associations of body fat and its changes over time with quality of life and prospective mortality in hemodialysis patients. Am J Clin Nutr. 2006 Feb;83(2):202- 10.

Johansen KL, Young B, Kaysen GA, Chertow GM. Association of body size with outcomes among patients beginning dialysis. Am J Clin Nutr. 2004 Aug;80(2):324- 32.

Postorino M, Marino C, Tripepi G, Zoccali C, CREDIT (Calabria Registry of Dialysis and Transplantation) Working Group. Abdominal obesity and all-cause and cardiovascular mortality in end-stage renal disease. J Am Coll Cardiol. 2009 Apr 14;53(15):1265-72.

Beddhu S, Pappas LM, Ramkumar N, Samore M. Effects of body size and body composition on survival in hemodialysis patients. J Am Soc Nephrol. 2003 Sep;14(9):2366-72.

Kovesdy CP, Czira ME, Rudas A, Ujszaszi A, Rosivall L, Novak M, et al. Body mass index, waist circumference and mortality in kidney transplant recipients. Am J Transplant. 2010 Dec;10(12):2644-51.

Holley JL, Monaghan J, Byer B, Bronsther O. An examination of the renal transplant evaluation process focusing on cost and the reasons for patient exclusion. Am J Kidney Dis. 1998 Oct;32(4):567-74.

Scandling JD. Kidney transplant candidate evaluation. Semin Dial. 2005 Nov-Dec;18(6):487-94.

Potluri K, Hou S. Obesity in kidney transplant recipients and candidates. Am J Kidney Dis. 2010 Jul;56(1):143-56.

Segev DL, Simpkins CE, Thompson RE, Locke JE, Warren DS, Montgomery RA. Obesity impacts access to kidney transplantation. J Am Soc Nephrol. 2008 Feb;19(2):349-55.

Johnson DW, Isbel NM, Brown AM, Kay TD, Franzen K, Hawley CM, et al. The effect of obesity on renal transplant outcomes. Transplantation. 2002 Sep 15;74(5):675-81.

Gore JL, Pham PT, Danovitch GM, Wilkinson AH, Rosenthal JT, Lipshutz GS, et al. Obesity and outcome following renal transplantation. Am J Transplant. 2006 Feb;6(2):357-63.

Meier-Kriesche HU, Arndorfer JA, Kaplan B. The impact of body mass index on renal transplant outcomes: A significant independent risk factor for graft failure and patient death. Transplantation. 2002 Jan 15;73(1):70-4.

Chang SH, Coates PT, McDonald SP. Effects of body mass index at transplant on outcomes of kidney transplantation. Transplantation. 2007 Oct 27;84(8):981-7.

Pelletier SJ, Maraschio MA, Schaubel DE, Dykstra DM, Punch JD, Wolfe RA, et al. Survival benefit of kidney and liver transplantation for obese patients on the waiting list. Clin Transpl. 2003:77-88.

Glanton CW, Kao TC, Cruess D, Agodoa LY, Abbott KC. Impact of renal transplantation on survival in end-stage renal disease patients with elevated body mass index. Kidney Int. 2003 Feb;63(2):647-53.

Kramer H, Tuttle KR, Leehey D, Luke A, Durazo-Arvizu R, Shoham D, et al. Obesity management in adults with CKD. Am J Kidney Dis. 2009 Jan;53(1):151-65.

Bennett WM, McEvoy KM, Henell KR, Valente JF, Douzdjian V. Morbid obesity does not preclude successful renal transplantation. Clin Transplant. 2004 Feb;18(1):89-93.

Drafts HH, Anjum MR, Wynn JJ, Mulloy LL, Bowley JN, Humphries AL. The impact of pre-transplant obesity on renal transplant outcomes. Clin Transplant. 1997 Oct;11(5 Pt 2):493-6.

Howard RJ, Thai VB, Patton PR, Hemming AW, Reed AI, Van der Werf WJ, et al.

Obesity does not portend a bad outcome for kidney transplant recipients. Transplantation. 2002 Jan 15;73(1):53-5.

Johnson CP, Gallagher-Lepak S, Zhu YR, Porth C, Kelber S, Roza AM, et al. Factors influencing weight gain after renal transplantation. Transplantation. 1993 Oct;56(4):822-7.

Merion RM, Twork AM, Rosenberg L, Ham JM, Burtch GD, Turcotte JG, et al. Obesity and renal transplantation. Surg Gynecol Obstet. 1991 May;172(5):367-76.

Modlin CS, Flechner SM, Goormastic M, Goldfarb DA, Papajcik D, Mastroianni B, et al. Should obese patients lose weight before receiving a kidney transplant? Transplantation. 1997 Aug 27;64(4):599-604.

Marks WH, Florence LS, Chapman PH, Precht AF, Perkinson DT. Morbid obesity is not a contraindication to kidney transplantation. Am J Surg. 2004 May;187(5):635-8.

Yamamoto S, Hanley E, Hahn AB, Isenberg A, Singh TP, Cohen D, et al. The impact of obesity in renal transplantation: An analysis of paired cadaver kidneys. Clin Transplant. 2002 Aug;16(4):252-6.

Halme L, Eklund B, Salmela K. Obesity and renal transplantation. Transplant Proc. 1995 Dec;27(6):3444-5.

Holley JL, Shapiro R, Lopatin WB, Tzakis AG, Hakala TR, Starzl TE. Obesity as a risk factor following cadaveric renal transplantation. Transplantation. 1990 Feb; 49(2): 387-9.

Meier-Kriesche HU, Vaghela M, Thambuganipalle R, Friedman G, Jacobs M, Kaplan B. The effect of body mass index on long-term renal allograft survival. Transplantation. 1999 Nov 15;68(9):1294-7.

Snow V, Barry P, Fitterman N, Qaseem A, Weiss K, Clinical Efficacy Assessment Subcommittee of t5he American College of Physicians. Pharmacologic and surgical management of obesity in primary care: A clinical practice guideline from the american college of physicians. Ann Intern Med. 2005 Apr 5;142(7):525-31.

Morales E, Valero MA, Leon M, Hernandez E, Praga M. Beneficial effects of weight loss in overweight patients with chronic proteinuric nephropathies. Am J Kidney Dis. 2003 Feb;41(2):319-27.

Praga M, Hernandez E, Andres A, Leon M, Ruilope LM, Rodicio JL. Effects of body-weight loss and captopril treatment on proteinuria associated with obesity. Nephron. 1995;70(1):35-41.

Palomar R, Fernandez-Fresnedo G, Dominguez-Diez A, Lopez-Deogracias M, Olmedo F, Martin de Francisco AL, et al. Effects of weight loss after biliopancreatic diversion on metabolism and cardiovascular profile. Obes Surg. 2005 Jun-Jul;15(6):794-8.

Navarro-Diaz M, Serra A, Romero R, Bonet J, Bayes B, Homs M, et al. Effect of drastic weight loss after bariatric surgery on renal parameters in extremely obese patients: Long-term follow-up. J Am Soc Nephrol. 2006 Dec;17(12 Suppl 3):S213-7.

Serra A, Granada ML, Romero R, Bayes B, Canton A, Bonet J, et al. The effect of bariatric surgery on adipocytokines, renal parameters and other cardiovascular risk factors in severe and very severe obesity: 1-year follow-up. Clin Nutr. 2006 Jun;25(3):400-8.

Chagnac A, Weinstein T, Herman M, Hirsh J, Gafter U, Ori Y. The effects of weight loss on renal function in patients with severe obesity. J Am Soc Nephrol. 2003 Jun;14(6):1480-6.

Clunk JM, Lin CY, Curtis JJ. Variables affecting weight gain in renal transplant recipients. Am J Kidney Dis. 2001 Aug;38(2):349-53.

Kasiske BL. Cardiovascular disease after renal transplantation. Semin Nephrol. 2000 Mar;20(2):176-87.

Chang SH, McDonald SP. Post-kidney transplant weight change as marker of poor survival outcomes. Transplantation. 2008 May 27;85(10):1443-8.

Baum CL, Thielke K, Westin E, Kogan E, Cicalese L, Benedetti E. Predictors of weight gain and cardiovascular risk in a cohort of racially diverse kidney transplant recipients. Nutrition. 2002 Feb;18(2):139-46.

Marcen R. Immunosuppressive drugs in kidney transplantation: Impact on patient survival, and incidence of cardiovascular disease, malignancy and infection. Drugs. 2009 Nov 12;69(16):2227-43.

Augustine JJ, Hricik DE. Steroid sparing in kidney transplantation: Changing paradigms, improving outcomes, and remaining questions. Clin J Am Soc Nephrol. 2006 Sep;1(5):1080-9.

Elster EA, Leeser DB, Morrissette C, Pepek JM, Quiko A, Hale DA, et al. Obesity following kidney transplantation and steroid avoidance immunosuppression. Clin Transplant. 2008 May-Jun;22(3):354-9.

Rogers CC, Alloway RR, Buell JF, Boardman R, Alexander JW, Cardi M, et al. Body weight alterations under early corticosteroid withdrawal and chronic corticosteroid therapy with modern immunosuppression. Transplantation. 2005 Jul 15;80(1):26-33.

van den Ham EC, Kooman JP, Christiaans MH, Nieman FH, van Hooff JP. Weight changes after renal transplantation: A comparison between patients on 5-mg maintenance steroid therapy and those on steroid-free immunosuppressive therapy. Transpl Int. 2003 May;16(5):300-6.

Marcic S, kramer H, luke A, holt DR, hou SH. risk factors for weight gain following renal transplantation. abstract presented at 37th annual meeting of the american society of nephrology; october 29-november 1, 2004; st. louis, MO. .

Eckel RH. Clinical practice. nonsurgical management of obesity in adults. N Engl J Med. 2008 May 1;358(18):1941-50.

Guida B, Trio R, Laccetti R, Nastasi A, Salvi E, Perrino NR, et al. Role of dietary intervention on metabolic abnormalities and nutritional status after renal transplantation. Nephrol Dial Transplant. 2007 Nov;22(11):3304-10.

Patel MG. The effect of dietary intervention on weight gains after renal transplantation. J Ren Nutr. 1998 Jul;8(3):137-41.

Packard DP, Milton JE, Shuler LA, Short RA, Tuttle KR. Implications of chronic kidney disease for dietary treatment in cardiovascular disease. J Ren Nutr. 2006 Jul;16(3):259-68.

Lichtenstein AH, appel LJ, brands M, et al, for the American Heart Association Nutrition Committee: Diet and lifestyle recommendations revision 2006: A scientific statement from the American Heart Association Nutrition Committee [erratum in Circulation 114:E629, 2006]. Circulation 114:82-96, 2006.

Kennedy ET, Bowman SA, Spence JT, Freedman M, King J. Popular diets: Correlation to health, nutrition, and obesity. J Am Diet Assoc. 2001 Apr;101(4):411-20.

Levey AS, Adler S, Caggiula AW, England BK, Greene T, Hunsicker LG, et al. Effects of dietary protein restriction on the progression of advanced renal disease in the modification of diet in renal disease study. Am J Kidney Dis. 1996 May;27(5):652- 63.

National kidney foundation: K/DOQI clinical practice guidelines for nutrition in chronic renal failure.am JKidney dis 35:S1-S140, 2000 (suppl 2).

Appel LJ, Moore TJ, Obarzanek E, Vollmer WM, Svetkey LP, Sacks FM, et al. A clinical trial of the effects of dietary patterns on blood pressure. DASH collaborative research group. N Engl J Med. 1997 Apr 17;336(16):1117-24.

Jezior D, Krajewska M, Madziarska K, Regulska-Ilow B, Ilow R, Janczak D, et al. Weight reduction in renal transplant recipients program: The first successes. Transplant Proc. 2007 Nov;39(9):2769-71.

Johansen KL, Kutner NG, Young B, Chertow GM. Association of body size with health status in patients beginning dialysis. Am J Clin Nutr. 2006 Mar;83(3):543-9.

Johansen KL. Exercise and chronic kidney disease: Current recommendations. Sports Med. 2005;35(6):485-99.

Beddhu S, Baird BC, Zitterkoph J, Neilson J, Greene T. Physical activity and mortality in chronic kidney disease (NHANES III). Clin J Am Soc Nephrol. 2009 Dec;4(12):1901- 6.

Moinuddin I, Leehey DJ. A comparison of aerobic exercise and resistance training in patients with and without chronic kidney disease. Adv Chronic Kidney Dis. 2008 Jan;15(1):83-96.

Boyce ML, Robergs RA, Avasthi PS, Roldan C, Foster A, Montner P, et al. Exercise training by individuals with predialysis renal failure: Cardiorespiratory endurance, hypertension, and renal function. Am J Kidney Dis. 1997 Aug;30(2):180-92.

Office of the US surgeon general. physical activity and health a report of the surgeon general. washington, DC: US department of health and human services, national center for chronic disease prevention and health promotion, 1996. .

Copley JB, Lindberg JS. The risks of exercise. Adv Ren Replace Ther. 1999 Apr;6(2):165-71.

Haskell WL. Cardiovascular complications during exercise training of cardiac patients. Circulation. 1978 May;57(5):920-4.

FDA. FDA drug safety communication: FDA recommends against the continued use of Meridia (sibutramine). http://www.fda.gov/Drugs/DrugSafety/PostmarketDrugSafetyInformationforPa tientsandProviders/ucm191652.htm (accessed March 26, 2011).

European Medicines Agency. Public statement on Zimulti: Withdrawal of the marketing authorisation in the European Union. http://www.ema.europa.eu/ema/index.jsp?curl=pages/news_and_events/news/ 2009/11/news_detail_000125.jsp&jsenabled=true (accessed March 26, 2011).

Henness S, Perry CM. Orlistat: A review of its use in the management of obesity. Drugs. 2006;66(12):1625-56.

MacLaughlin HL, Cook SA, Kariyawasam D, Roseke M, van Niekerk M, Macdougall IC. Nonrandomized trial of weight loss with orlistat, nutrition education, diet, and exercise in obese patients with CKD: 2-year follow-up. Am J Kidney Dis. 2010 Jan;55(1):69-76.

Zhi J, Moore R, Kanitra L, Mulligan TE. Pharmacokinetic evaluation of the possible interaction between selected concomitant medications and orlistat at steady state in healthy subjects. J Clin Pharmacol. 2002 Sep;42(9):1011-9.

Nagele H, Petersen B, Bonacker U, Rodiger W. Effect of orlistat on blood cyclosporin concentration in an obese heart transplant patient. Eur J Clin Pharmacol. 1999 Nov;55(9):667-9.

Singh A, Sarkar SR, Gaber LW, Perazella MA. Acute oxalate nephropathy associated with orlistat, a gastrointestinal lipase inhibitor. Am J Kidney Dis. 2007 Jan;49(1):153-7. Finer N, James WP, Kopelman PG, Lean ME, Williams G. One-year treatment of obesity: A randomized, double-blind, placebo-controlled, multicentre study of orlistat, a gastrointestinal lipase inhibitor. Int J Obes Relat Metab Disord. 2000 Mar;24(3):306-13.

Phurrough S, salive M, brechner R, tillman K, harrison S, O'Connor D: Decision memo for bariatric surgery for the treatment of morbid obesity 2006. available at http://www.cms.hhs.gov/mcd/viewdecisionmemo.asp ?id_160. accessed march 22, 2011.

Bouldin MJ, Ross LA, Sumrall CD, Loustalot FV, Low AK, Land KK. The effect of obesity surgery on obesity comorbidity. Am J Med Sci. 2006 Apr;331(4):183-93.

Buchwald H, Avidor Y, Braunwald E, Jensen MD, Pories W, Fahrbach K, et al. Bariatric surgery: A systematic review and meta-analysis. JAMA. 2004 Oct 13;292(14):1724- 37.

Tice JA, Karliner L, Walsh J, Petersen AJ, Feldman MD. Gastric banding or bypass? A systematic review comparing the two most popular bariatric procedures. Am J Med. 2008 Oct;121(10):885-93.

Himpens J, Cadiere GB, Bazi M, Vouche M, Cadiere B, Dapri G. Long-term outcomes of laparoscopic adjustable gastric banding. Arch Surg. 2011 Mar 21.

Koshy AN, Coombes JS, Wilkinson S, Fassett RG. Laparoscopic gastric banding surgery performed in obese dialysis patients prior to kidney transplantation. Am J Kidney Dis. 2008 Oct;52(4):e15-7.

Newcombe V, Blanch A, Slater GH, Szold A, Fielding GA. Laparoscopic adjustable gastric banding prior to renal transplantation. Obes Surg. 2005 Apr;15(4):567-70.

Takata MC, Campos GM, Ciovica R, Rabl C, Rogers SJ, Cello JP, et al. Laparoscopic bariatric surgery improves candidacy in morbidly obese patients awaiting transplantation. Surg Obes Relat Dis. 2008 Mar-Apr;4(2):159,64; discussion 164-5.

Modanlou KA, Muthyala U, Xiao H, Schnitzler MA, Salvalaggio PR, Brennan DC, et al. Bariatric surgery among kidney transplant candidates and recipients: Analysis of the united states renal data system and literature review. Transplantation. 2009 Apr 27;87(8):1167-73.

Alexander JW, Goodman H. Gastric bypass in chronic renal failure and renal transplant. Nutr Clin Pract. 2007 Feb;22(1):16-21.

Buch KE, El-Sabrout R, Butt KM. Complications of laparoscopic gastric banding in renal transplant recipients: A case study. Transplant Proc. 2006 Nov;38(9):3109-11.

Asplin JR, Coe FL. Hyperoxaluria in kidney stone formers treated with modern bariatric surgery. J Urol. 2007 Feb;177(2):565-9.

Nelson WK, Houghton SG, Milliner DS, Lieske JC, Sarr MG. Enteric hyperoxaluria, nephrolithiasis, and oxalate nephropathy: Potentially serious and unappreciated complications of roux-en-Y gastric bypass. Surg Obes Relat Dis. 2005 Sep-Oct;1(5):481-5.

Nasr SH, D'Agati VD, Said SM, Stokes MB, Largoza MV, Radhakrishnan J, et al. Oxalate nephropathy complicating roux-en-Y gastric bypass: An underrecognized cause of irreversible renal failure. Clin J Am Soc Nephrol. 2008 Nov;3(6):1676-83.

Sinha MK, Collazo-Clavell ML, Rule A, Milliner DS, Nelson W, Sarr MG, et al. Hyperoxaluric nephrolithiasis is a complication of roux-en-Y gastric bypass surgery. Kidney Int. 2007 Jul;72(1):100-7.

Bernhardt WM, Schefold JC, Weichert W, Rudolph B, Frei U, Groneberg DA, et al. Amelioration of anemia after kidney transplantation in severe secondary oxalosis. Clin Nephrol. 2006 Mar;65(3):216-21.

Rogers CC, Alloway RR, Alexander JW, Cardi M, Trofe J, Vinks AA. Pharmacokinetics of mycophenolic acid, tacrolimus and sirolimus after gastric bypass surgery in end- stage renal disease and transplant patients: A pilot study. Clin Transplant. 2008 May-Jun;22(3):281-91.

Alexander JW, Goodman HR, Gersin K, Cardi M, Austin J, Goel S, et al. Gastric bypass in morbidly obese patients with chronic renal failure and kidney transplant. Transplantation. 2004 Aug 15;78(3):469-74.

Orofino L, Pascual J, Quereda C, Burgos J, Marcen R, Ortuno J. Influence of overweight on survival of kidney transplant. Nephrol Dial Transplant. 1997 Apr;12(4):855.

Kasap B, Soylu A, Turkmen M, Kavukcu S, Bora S, Gulay H. Effect of obesity and overweight on cyclosporine blood levels and renal functions in renal adolescent recipients. Transplant Proc. 2006 Mar;38(2):463-5.

Flechner SM, Kolbeinsson ME, Tam J, Lum B. The impact of body weight on cyclosporine pharmacokinetics in renal transplant recipients. Transplantation. 1989 May;47(5):806-10.

Rodrigo E, de Cos MA, Sanchez B, Ruiz JC, Pinera C, Fernandez-Fresnedo G, et al. High initial blood levels of tacrolimus in overweight renal transplant recipients. Transplant Proc. 2005 Apr;37(3):1453-4.

Sjöström L, Narbro K, Sjöström CD, Karason K, et al. Swedish Obese Subjects Study. Effects of bariatric surgery on mortality in Swedish obese subjects. N Engl J Med. 2007 Aug 23;357(8):741-52.

Suter M, Calmes JM, Paroz A, Giusti V. A 10-year experience with laparoscopic gastric banding for morbid obesity: high long-term complication and failure rates. Obes Surg. 2006 Jul;16(7):829-35.

Mittermair RP, Obermüller S, Perathoner A, Sieb M, Aigner F, Margreiter R. Results and complications after Swedish adjustable gastric banding-10 years experience. Obes Surg. 2009 Dec;19(12):1636-41.

8

Proactive Management Approach in Prevention of Kidney Transplantation

Levent B. Kidak

Izmir Bozyaka Training and Research Hospital
Hospital and Health Care Institutions Management
Deputy of Head Physician, Izmir,
Turkey

1. Introduction

Chronic kidney disease (CKD) is a serious health problem that increases both in terms of prevalence and importance all around the world. However, while the number of patients is steadily increasing, not enough organs are available for transplantation and the gap between the patients who need transplantation and the number of existing donors has widened considerably. In order to address the problem of the increased demand for kidneys, we need to review the real issues underlying the existing situation. Is the problem related to the insufficient number of donors? Or are there too many diseased kidneys? If we can accurately define the problem referred to as the "organ shortage", a major step towards the solution can be achieved. The goal of this chapter is to discuss an applicable strategy that aims to reduce or prevent kidney transplantations using a proactive management approach that includes medical as well as managerial strategies.

2. Proactive management approach

Proactive management is based on preventing a mistake before it happens being one step ahead of that mistake. The concept of proactive means taking action before an event happens; and proactive management is an approach based on designing the desired future and the managerial environment in the said future. Proactive management approach is frequently used in management field to change the course of existing conditions deliberately or create new conditions. The essence in this approach which requires developing new paths and strategies to shape the future for organisations and services is long term gains. (Charles, 2008; Kocel, 2005).

Above all, proactive management represents a philosophy, understanding and a belief. This philosophy and belief do not follow after the events but instead shape events by predicting and having an impact on the future. Proactive management or mainly proactive planning approach is to review and explore strategies that enable us to foresee future events (Teixidor, 2006). The beginning of proactive management, i.e. planning is to understand that we have to to look into the future. Planning stage requires to understand that there are opportunities to be used or certain events which may interfere with the structure are about to happen. Planning is the main tool of proactive behaviour. Especially to achieve such an understanding in long term strategic planning, it should be clearly defined as to with what goals the organisation is established, what the organisation plans to do and where the organisation wants to see itself (Kocel, 2005).

Whereas reactive management is defined as a working and management style to look for solutions for the problems already encountered. Reactive management approach means to react to the conditions already encountered, to search to find what needs to be done to adapt to the conditions encountered. Most of the reactive approaches or reactive actions are based on the practices of reactive planning algorithm after the problem happens. The major disadvantage of these processes is that they also include the flexibility which may change the processes assuring the quality of the services. Reactive approach is generally used in situations where the degree of uncertainty is high or there is no information regarding the uncertainty (Teixidor, 2006)

Proactive approach is beyond being dull and over analytical. It is a starting point for change and creativeness. As a result of reactive approach managers become too busy running from crisis to crisis and give a wrong impression that they are constantly working. In reality this situation should be seen as an indication that the management has lost the control. Proactive management includes tools, methods and applications which enable the replacement of reactive managerial habits with a dynamic management style that can actually respond to needs. Proactive approach is related with critical work behaviours for success; it is to develop assertive goals, to frequently review these goals, to develop open policies, to focus on preventing problems, to inquire why work is done in a certain way instead of defending blindly the way in that the work is done (Procen, 2010).

Proactive approach is always more preferred than reactive approach. In proactive approach, it is necessary to monitor the conditions closely to foresee possible developments and to make changes within the organisation. Proactive managerial approach enables organisations to make necessary arrangements so that they could be the least affected by the conditions that they may face in the future. In that sense, developing an early warning system for individuals and organisations is an effective method (Toland, 2007). Early warning system increases the awareness of individuals and at the same time creates a database contributing to the decision making process of organisations while defining paths and strategies.

Although this approach corresponds to preventive medicine approach, this is also a managerial approach which includes calculating risks and challenges in advance, making predictions and developing strategies accordingly. Due to the above qualities, it is used in certain fields of healthcare services such as monitoring and preventing some chronic diseases such as diabetics, cardiac failures and obesity (MacStravic, 2008; Daleiden-Burns & Stiles, 2007). This approach has started to be used also in activating databases in healthcare services and reducing health expenditures of social security organisations (Overhage, 2008; Richardson, 1997).

3. Kidney transplantation and proactive management approach

3.1 Definition

Chronic kidney disease (CKD) is a nephrological syndrome characterised by chronic, progressive and irreversible nephron loss resulting from multiple etiologies. Chronic kidney disease is one of the most important public health issues in Turkey and in the world. Nowadays, the number of people suffering from chronic kidney disease is increasing (Levey, 2007; Obrador & Pereira, 2010).

3.2 Importance

As of the end of 2008, there were 60,592 patients with chronic kidney disease in Turkey. Of these patients 13,346 were added to the total figure within the same year (TSN, 2009). These patients need dialysis treatment or kidney transplantation. 54,700 chronic kidney disease patients were on dialysis treatment and at the same time hoping for kidney transplantation. According to the data of the Ministry of Health, only 2502 of these patients received kidney transplants in 2010. Every year, 110 of 1000 End Stage Renal Disease (ESRD) patients lose their lives waiting for kidney transplantation; and 4506 patients lost their lives in 2008 (TSN, 2009; MHT, 2011). As of the end of 2007, there were 527,283 ESRD patients in the USA. Of these patients 111,000 were included in the ESRD programme in 2007 (Obrador & Pereira, 2010). According to the yearly report of the U.S. Organ Procurement and Transplantation Network and the Scientific Registry of Transplant Recipients, in 2007 16,120 patients and in 2008 16,067 patients of the above received kidney transplantation. In the USA 87,812 ESRD patients lost their lives in 2007. One, two and five year life expectancy of dialysis patients is 81, 65 and 34 percent respectively (Obrador & Pereira, 2010).

CKD is a condition which in addition to causing loss of lives, creates serious social problems for patients especially for paediatric patients, patients' families and the society as with many chronic diseases (Richardson, 1997; Şirin et al., 1995). For adult patients, in addition to economical, social and psychological problems, an important loss of working time is assigned. Children with CKD have growth failure, and their education is hampered and severe psychological problems emerge in their families (Karakavak, 2006; Falkenstein, 2004). CKD does not only cause loss of lives and social losses but also with a yearly expenditure of USD 25,000 per patient, and although relatively less, a yearly expenditure of USD 10,000 for patients who have undergone kidney transplantation, it also causes major economic losses (Kapuagası, 2010). In the USA the total of the costs of ESRD treatment programmes is estimated to be USD 28 billion based on the number of patients in 2010 (Obrador & Pereira, 2010). Such economic consequences of ESRD cause problems in appropriation and use of the resources allocated for healthcare service (El Nahas & Bello, 2005).

3.3 Etiology and reasons

There are certain risk factors leading to the occurrence of CKD. Generally, history of diabetes mellitus, cardiovascular disease, hypertension, hyperlipidemia, obesity, metabolic syndrome, smoking, HIV or hepatitis C virus infection, and malignancy are among risk factors for CKD. In addition to those, family history of CKD, advanced age and treatment with potentially nephrotoxic drugs are other risk factors. Among these risk factors diabetes mellitus, high blood pressure and cardiovascular diseases are the ones which require the most attention to prevent the occurrence of CKD (Obrador & Pereira, 2010).

In the report prepared by The Turkish Society of Nephrology (TSN, 2009) in Turkey, in haemodialysis patients, diabetes mellitus and high blood pressure ranked in the top two among the risk factors of CKD. In addition to these, glomerulonephritis, polycystic kidney diseases, pyelonephritis, amyloidosis and other diseases are also among the risk factors. The frequency and ratios of these risk factors are shown in Table 1.

When the etiology of chronic renal failure in children is examined, the chief ethiologies are found to be vesico ureteral reflux (VUR) and recurrent urinary tract infection (25.9%), then primary glomerulonephritis (18.4%), other known causes (15.1%) and congenital urologic anomalies (excluding VUR) (13.4%) (TSN, 2009). Urinary tract infection (UTI) known to be the most common cause of CKD is usually a preventable disease coming second after respiratory tract infections among childhood infections. According to the studies, UTI is currently an important etiology of CKD even in the developed countries (Warady & Chadha, 2007). Except some congenital diseases, early diagnosis and suitable treatment of almost all anomalies and of UTI and monitoring results can prevent permanent and dangerous results. Additionally children are especially susceptible to permanent kidney damage (ISM, 2005).

Diseases	N	%
Diabetes mellitus	10762	27.9
Type 1 DM	*1761*	4.6
Type 2 DM	*9001*	23.3
Hypertension	10177	26.4
Glomerulonephritis	3343	8.7
Polycystic kidney diseases	1707	4.4
Pyelonephritis	1616	4.2
Amyloidosis	793	2.1
Renal vascular disease	477	1.2
Other	3005	7.8
Unknown etiology	6210	16.1
Missing data	514	1.3
Total	38604	100.0

Table 1. Distribution of chronic HD patients followed, according to etiology.
National Hemodialysis, Transplantation and Nephrology Registry Report of Turkey (TSN, 2009).

Today it is known that every year, an average of 60 per million people are diagnosed with CKD in Turkey and we know that these patients consult a physician at a very late stage (Kocak, 1993). In the study, the urinary tract disease found in 543 (3.2 %) children coming to clinics for regular vaccinations without any complaints indicates that this is a disease progressing without any symptoms (Kıdak, 2010). In other studies, it is expressed that urinary tract disease constitutes a major health problem due to the reasons that its clinical symptoms can sometimes be very inconspicuous, that it is difficult to obtain valid urine samples and reach to a definitive diagnosis, has a high recurrence rate, is frequently coinciding with urogenital system anomalies, and that it leads to permanent kidney failure in the long term (El Nahas & Bello 2005; Ardissino et al. 2003; Prodjosudjadi, 2006; ISM, 2005).
Consequently, CKD is generally an insidious disease. Most patients are diagnosed with a kidney disease during routine examinations performed without any symptom or sign. Some of the etiologies of CKD are treatable diseases if they are diagnosed at early stages; thus CKD can be prevented or delayed. The most frequently seen and easily detected indicator of kidney damage is proteinuira (ISM, 2005).

3.4 Treatment

There are currently two main strategies to be followed for the treatment of CKD patients diagnosed with ESRD (El Nahas & Bello, 2005; Warady, 2007). These are;

- Dialysis and
- Kidney transplantation.

A good and regular dialysis treatment process is the first strategy to follow. Dialysis treatment which is the treatment method of ESRD is performed to improve the general condition of a patient, to restore water-electrolyte balance and to remove uremic toxins accumulated in the body. When we consider the 10 % possibility for CKD patients to undergo organ transplantation, the importance of dialysis in treatment of patients becomes apparent. Under good circumstances, the life expectancy of the patient can be 10 years in average and sometimes, though seldom, this can go up to 25 years (Kocak, 1993).

Kidney transplantation is the second strategy serving to far less number of patients and with which patients continue to hope for kidney transplantation waiting in the organ waiting lists. Advances in medical technology, improvements in surgical techniques and developments in post operative medications have made organ transplantation an effective and powerful treatment (Fuzzati, 2005). After successful kidney transplantations there remains no need for dialysis treatment and patients become independent. Therefore interest, on reasonable grounds, on human tissue and organ transplantations is continuously increasing.

The goal of these two strategies is to improve quality of life of patients and provide more permanent solutions to patients with transplantation of organs obtained through organ donation. However both strategies serving effectively to the ESRD patients are reactive approaches based on providing solutions after the problem has occurred. In other words, as in most reactive behaviour, actions are carried out after the problem has occurred based on a reactive planning algorithm.

3.5 Problem

Although the number of donors has been constantly increasing in all European countries, this said number is still not sufficient to meet existing donor kidney needs (Fuzzati, 2005). There has been a growing gap between the frequency ESRD in Turkey and in the world and organ donation (Fuzzati, 2005; Ateş, 1998). New alternative solutions are needed for "shortage of donor organs" problem which is still growing in the world. To solve this problem, scientists have been working on both epidemiology of the disease in terms of frequency and diagnosis and treatment management (Ardissino et al., 2003; El Nahas & Bello, 2005; Prodjosudjadi 2006; Warady & Chadha, 2007). In these studies, there is strong evidence that CKD can be screened and treated using simple laboratory tests. It is also indicated that with the same tests, cardiovascular risks causing CKD are lowered, the progression of renal diseases is slowed down, complications are delayed or eliminated (Kıdak, 2010; Levey, 2007). Therefore, in addition to the existing two strategies, new strategies to solve organ shortage problem are needed.

In order to make real and true assessment about CKD incidence and prevalence, epidemiologists and clinicians have been working on different population groups management (Ardissino et al., 2003; El Nahas & Bello, 2005; Warady & Chadha, 2007). Within this scope, protective medicine has been approached with a different understanding all around the world since it has been understood that only a medical perspective is not sufficient for healthcare issues which are increasing in numbers and becoming more complex and contribution of healthcare management sciences is also needed. Donor organ need, besides being a medical problem to be solved, is also a healthcare management problem and managerial solution options should also be considered. Here at this point proactive management approach comes to the scene (MacStravic, 2008; Overhage, 2008).

In some relevant studies conducted, efforts to slow down the progress of CKD and improve clinical results were evaluated and costs of such services were assessed. It is indicated that early diagnosis of CKD and early treatment of patients reduce the costs of the disease and improve clinical results (Jabs & Warady, 1999). At the same time, it is also concluded that early diagnosis diminishes the need for organ transplantation. The proactive management approach may lower the incidence rate of the disease, slow progress of the disease, and therefore improve clinical results and economic aspects of the disease (Khan & Amedia, 2008). In Pereira's study about renal anaemia management period, the importance of early diagnosis and aggressive treatment of anaemia which causes a serious mortality and morbidity in CKD is emphasized (Pereira, 2001). These studies demonstrate that proactive management approach is highly considered for the early diagnosis and treatment of kidney diseases.

3.6 Solution proposal - Proactive management approach in prevention of kidney transplantation

This chapter aims to contribute to the prevention of ESRD and hence decrease the number of kidney transplantations with proactive management approach. In proactive management approach, problems or uncertainties present in the development of ESRD must be defined. It will be advisable to identify what level of performance weaknesses or risks cause uncertainties or problems.

It is known that 10 % of ESRD patients have the chance of organ transplantation, that the disease develops and progress insidiously and most patients consult to a physician at later stages of the disease. When some diseases causing ESRD are detected at an earlier stage, they can be treated thus kidney disease can be prevented or delayed. In light of this information, the importance of the proactive approach becomes apparent. Since proactive approach means taking actions before the event, it is clearly understood that it is of vital importance to detect the signs of the insidious disease before it becomes apparent and monitor the cases. Proactive management of the disease represents an approach based on a desire for a future which will prevent the increase of the number of ESRD patients and on designing the future environment. The goal here is to establish the management structure which identifies risks not after but before patients become sick and takes necessary precautions.

What needs to be done is strategic analysis and this analysis is the starting point of proactive management. It is the stage where problems are defined again, strategies are developed and proactive planning is made (Dincer, 2005). Some basic questions are needed to be asked to make the analysis necessary at this stage (Teixidor, 2006). The first question to be asked in this regard is "what should we do to understand this uncertainty or problem?" This question is the basic question to identify and analyze characteristics of the origins of the problems causing ESRD. The second question is "how can we examine the uncertainty or the problem with proactive approach?" Proactive and reactive approaches address essentially the most prominent and the biggest problems. Identifying and defining problems in a healthy and accurate way will act as a guide not only for implementation but also for controlling activities. Some problems such as determining the implementation time can be solved very easily. Third question is "how can we understand whether the model is suitable and healthy?" The aim of this question is to prevent differences between goals and objectives although they are defined in a suitable and healthy manner and the implementation. Fourth question is "can the problem be identified and solved scientifically?" This question can help us to make progress with solving the problem and also contribute to defining the limits and boundaries of activities. And fifth question is "what are the benefits of the approach and how can it be improved?" This final question is directly related with the basics of research and development activities (Teixidor, 2006).

In this respect, the existing problem should be redefined, the right question should be found and asked. With reactive approach, donor organ need is accepted as the main problem and organ donation is encouraged to be increased thus corrective actions can be taken. However, unless we address the real problems which render organs dysfunctional, donor organ need will grow despite increasing organ transplantations. Is the existing organ need a problem or a consequence of another problem? We need to identify what the problem is and for what we should look for solutions.

According to proactive management approach, the main question here is why there are so many organ failures. When we look into the problem with this approach one of the important options to improve the existing situation of organ transplantation is to lower the need for donor organs. Therefore, it is understood that there are critical processes in this field, which should be managed with proactive management approach; and the first of these processes is to determine the factors causing organ failure and to look for solutions. In other words, the purpose here is to minimise organ failures or to prevent organs from becoming dysfunctional.

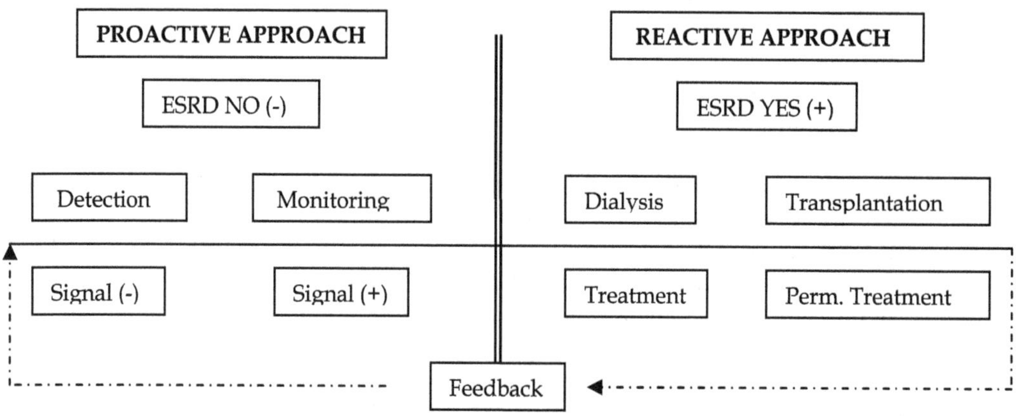

Fig. 1. ESRD in proactive and reactive approach processes

Proactive management approach, as seen in the above Figure 1 focuses on the stage before the disease develops. "Modern medicine" which includes preventive medicine can be considered as the common point between the approach and healthcare services. Accordingly, three main strategic plans; namely primary, secondary and tertiary prevention, can be made in relation to the proactive management of ESRD. These are (Irgil, 2006);

- Primary prevention level is to define risk factors for ESRD, control and monitor signals, and to prevent the disease before it starts and develops. Activities can be oriented to individuals or to the society. Special preventive measures for the diseases are included in this group.
- Secondary prevention level is early detection and treatment of symptoms and diseases causing ESRD and to reduce the number of severe cases. With this method, serious progression of the disease can be monitored, minimised or slowed down. It is a strategy applicable to the diseases which can be diagnosed at early stages and against which there are effective treatments.

- Tertiary prevention level is to prevent the progression of already developed diseases and its complications. It is to mitigate the problems caused by the disease. It enables to improve the life quality by preventing the progression of especially chronic diseases.

The main strategy of proactive management is to systematically investigate signals of the disease in otherwise healthy people before ESRD occurs and to monitor cases giving positive signs more closely taking risk factors into consideration. CKD gives out some signals before reaching to the disease stage. If these signals are detected early, evaluated correctly and necessary measures are taken, it is believed that the existing situation which could be described as the "organ shortage" can be improved and be more problem free. It is assumed that proactive management approach with early diagnosis of insidious kidney diseases, investigation of reasons, slowing progression and prevention of complications has a major effect on the prevention of future negative consequences. With the implementation of this approach, a third strategy could be added to the existing two strategies to solve the problem. Then, these three strategies are; to increase organ donation for more organ supply, to improve the life quality of existing patients by treating them and to work with proactive management approach to lower the need for donor organs.

4. Proactive management algorithm in prevention of kidney transplantation

Healthcare institutions are compelled to deal with diseases which develop as a result of common health risks that, for various reasons, are not evaluated correctly. Proactive methods and strategies are developed to prevent before it becomes a disease. Therefore, the importance of immediate implementation of such methods and strategies which can make the provision of healthcare services effective is clear. Otherwise, or if no new strategy is developed, more resources will be allocated for these services; organ shortage and this vicious circle will become increasingly problematic. In other words, since available structures and resources are not used effectively and efficiently, people who may be prevented from developing ESRD or who should not die of ESRD will continue to die.

In order to the healthcare services to be effective in a social sense i.e. to make the desired changes in the health status of the society, the healthcare services should have certain qualities. It would be useful to take such qualities into consideration when micro and macro planning, organising and delivering the healthcare services. Management in organisations are shaped according to the different structures in the organisation hierarchy. As seen in the Figure 2, there are 3 main management levels in an organisation. These are called senior management level, middle management level and lower management level. Each management level carries out different managerial activities. Accordingly, senior level managers are responsible for strategic management, middle level managers are responsible for functional and tactical management and lower level managers are responsible for operational and program management. There is a close relation among the plans made at these three management levels. Senior level plans are binding decisions for lower level plans. Plans of senior level management should provide guidance for lower level plans whereas lower management level plans should support senior level plans (Dincer, 2004). Plans made at these three levels should constitute a whole connected in terms of the goals and the activities of all units. Plan implementations should not conflict with each other. Realisation of strategic plans is possible only with the realisation of lower level plans. As the management level rises, scope of planning widens.

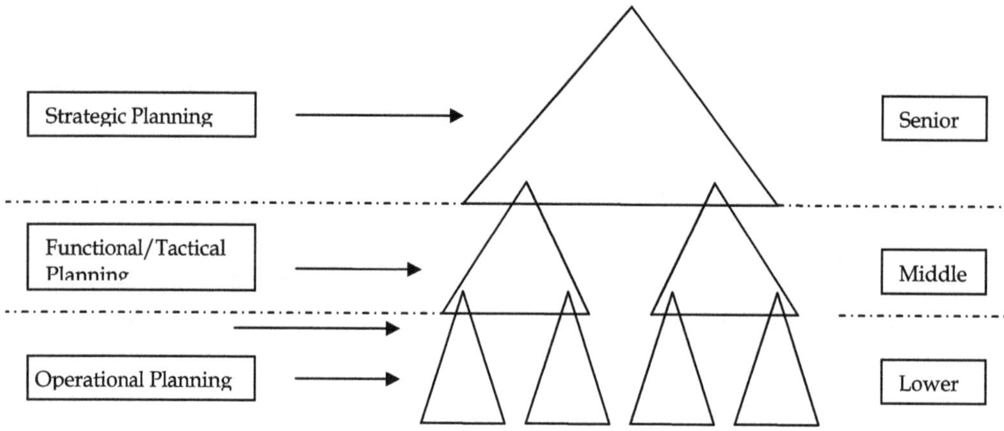

Fig. 2. Types of planning and organisation levels in proactive management (Kocel, 2005)

In line with the above information, ESRD prevention planning and implementation organisation is required through proactive management approach according to the management levels of the healthcare services. Healthy design of this stage plays an important role in the efficiency and success of implementation. Converting strategies into action plans requires suitable organisational structure. Organisation structure refers to differentiating of activities and work as vertical, horizontal and spatial to prevent and reduce ESRD. At the end of this differentiation, activities need to be coordinated. Differentiation is the process in which activities are described for each to management level and for each healthcare institution. These descriptions should be compatible with the characteristics of the work, people and institutions and goals of the organisation (Kocel, 2005). Therefore, to organise the implementation of reduction and prevention plan of ESRD using proactive management;

- Work to be carried out,
- Authorities and responsibilities of the individuals and organisations which carry out the work,
- Knowledge and skills necessary for the individuals and organisations which carry out the work should be defined.

To structure this implementation organisation; exogen factors such as goals, departments, necessary equipment, and endogen factors such as qualifications of employees and environmental factors are used. Senior management should link these factors with each other and define the structure. The structure achieved as a result of this process should be described with an organisation chart. At the same time main responsibilities, duties and authorisation relations which constitute this structure should be explained in a written document called the handbook (Kocel, 2005).

4.1 Proactive management algorithm in the health care organisation for prevention of ESRD

The management levels in the healthcare services organisation are respectively; senior management level is the Ministry of Health, middle management level is Local Health Directorates and lower level management is the management of local healthcare institutions. Each of these three main management levels should carry out different managerial activities within proactive management of ESRD. Therefore in the organisation of healthcare services to prevent and mitigate ESRD activities, authorities and responsibilities, duties of individuals and organisations together with necessary information and competencies should be defined for all management levels. According to the above explained information, decision and planning types of the healthcare management regarding this implementation should be as following:

1. **Senior of Health Management - Ministry of Health:** Strategic planning and new politics
2. **Local Health Directorate**: Functional planning and tactics
3. **Primary Secondary and Tertiary Health Care Facilities - Family Physicians and Hospitals:** Detection and monitoring of ESRD candidates, treatments of patients for prevention of ESRD.

The first step in the algorithm is the integrated strategy of the senior management (Ministry of Health) which manages various institutions and various services. The senior management should develop new policies to prevent ESRD. The Local Health Directorates coordinating and organising activities of healthcare institutions in provinces should determine tactics to implement strategies. Lower management levels which are the management units to carry out activities for individuals and patients should develop implementation plans. Healthcare institutions in all three levels should carry out the activities assigned to them. At first, due to the reasons such as possible lack of information in the primary level healthcare institutions, terminology confusion, difficulties in the recording system, a coordinated work should be planned together with primary, secondary and tertiary health care levels. These activities which will be explained in detail later are shown collectively in Table 2. The study of Teixidor (2006) was referred to while preparing this table.

Ministry of Health Strategic Plannings	**Local Health Directorate Functional and Tactical Plannings**	**Health Care Institutions Operational Plannings**
• Strategic goals and objectives • Vision and mission • Population data (General) • Social and environmental conditions • Medical and technologic developments • Disease information and data • Regional/specific qualities • International aspect • Government regulations • Laws and legal factors • Financial issues • Clinical experiences	• Information flow • Personnel training • Population information (Local) • Capacities of institutions *-Primary* *-Secondary and Tertiary level* • Material supply • Demands of patients and patient relatives • Budgeting	• Business processes • Time plans • Continuity of resources • Quality of resources • Recording system • Collecting of data • Control systems

Table 2. Contents of plan types according to the management levels

4.2 Senior of health management – the Ministry of Health: Strategic planning and new politics

The first stage of proactive management is to identify long term goals which are a part of the strategic planning. This is done by the senior management of the organisation. The most important feature of strategic planning is the time period set forth and the operational activities covered. A strategic plan maintains its qualities to the extent that the time period is prolonged and the plan deals with the organisation in its entirety (Kocel, 2005). The strategic planning under the responsibility of the senior management involves mainly identifying and solving problems in the external environment. Answering the questions about where the organisation will be in the long run, strategic planning is the process in which activities to determine the direction are defined.

"New" ways and strategies should be developed using proactive management approach to shape the future for ESRD on behalf of the healthcare services. Such "new" ways and strategies should be developed by the senior management. Therefore the main activity that the senior management (Ministry of Health) should carry out is strategic analysis which is the starting point of proactive management. At this point, the problem of kidney failure should be redefined, strategies should be developed and proactive plans including new policies should be prepared.

The main duties of the Ministry of Health are to protect individuals' and the society's health and to make, implement and enforce plans and programs covering the entire country for this purpose; to take all kinds of measures, establish necessary organisations or oversee that such organisations are established (Eren, 1985). Goals and objectives should be defined under the scope of prevention of ESRD; the defined vision and mission should be explained to all relevant units and institutions. Information about the present condition of the disease should be monitored and evaluated together with the epidemiologic result of the disease. Future path of the disease should be foreseen using suitable techniques and alternative plans should be prepared. Financial resources should be reviewed to make necessary allocations for the implementation. Medical technology that can prevent the disease should be explored, appropriate techniques should be identified. Characteristics and structure of the population should be studied to ascertain whether there are any local differences. Structural arrangements required for the success of the implementation should be made, legal and statutory requirements should be complied with. These are explained below (Teixidor, 2006; Kocel, 2005; Dincer, 2004);

- Vision and mission: This could be summarised as the way the senior management expresses its opinions about ESRD. What the basic services to prevent ESRD are, which patient groups are offered which services in which institutions, what the main technologies to be used in these institutions are, what the opinions are about the incidence and prevalence of the disease and what kind of image is desired should be identified. All these should be kept in writing and distributed to relevant people, mainly health care providers and institutions. Thus, health care providers will understand why they do what they do, use initiative and decide better about how they can contribute to this service. To achieve these, the senior management should combine existing realities with anticipated conditions to design a future hoped for ESRD. The senior management should visualise its vision regarding this disease, and express its dreams about the future outlook of the disease. The senior management should also define the "game plan" to prevent ESRD and to reduce the number of kidney transplantations.
- Strategic goals and objectives: Goals and objectives of the management play a central role both in decision making and planning. "New" methods should be developed using proactive management approach to shape the future of ESRD on behalf of the

healthcare services. The goals and objectives involving these new methods and strategies can be defined as the strategy to change the conditions. Change in ESRD can be achieved not through better treating patients but through changing the conditions of the existing situation. At this stage, the organisation should decide, in a given period of time, what and how much they want to achieve or where they want to be with regard to ESRD. The number of people screened for ESRD, the number of patients treated, the number of ESRD cases prevented, the desired incidence and prevalence rates, the number of personnel to be employed in a given time, for example 5 years later and the number of training programmes in this period of time should be determined. The most important principle of setting goals and objectives is that the goals are measurable, that they indicate necessary actions and have a time dimension.

- Population data (General): Is to analyse the structure of the population constituting the society. These analyses cover the age, sex, education, economic condition, place of residence etc and other characteristics of the population. Data obtained from these analyses enable managers to make accurate projections, to take proactive actions. This data allows them to identify the risks related with the changes that will happen to the structure of the population, and allows them to take necessary measures in advance. On the other hand, a population structure which can be defined, calculated and estimated will mitigate the risks included in the decision of the senior management. Thus, data about the structure of the population stands out as a secure way for resource planning of the future (Drucker, 2003).
- Social and environmental conditions: Changes and developments in social and environmental conditions are one of the most important determining factors in strategic planning decisions and implementation. Continuous changing of the environment and long time horizon of strategic planning further increases the uncertainty in the environment and emphasises its importance for the organisation. Threats and opportunities introduced by ESRD are evaluated in this context forming the decision focus of the senior management.
- Medical and technologic developments: Medical and technological developments are the fastest changing factors in the healthcare services. What is meant here by technology is the tools and equipment-devices together with the information and processes which are used in the operations. Medical materials, methods and processes used in screening, treatment and monitoring of ESRD, changes and improvements in the devices used should be followed closely. The existing structure and development potential of the technology both in the country and abroad should be identified. In order to do this, in which areas of activities the research and development funds are focused should be established.
- Disease information and data: People with ESRD risk nationwide should be identified, common characteristics of the patients diagnosed with ESRD should be established, results of medical treatments should be monitored, costs of the disease should be calculated, mortality rates and incidence and prevalence rates should be estimated. By investigating the epidemiology of the disease it will be easier to find the reasons of the problem, and parameters to be monitored in controlling activities will be identified. Researches regarding the etiology of the disease which is explained in this chapter and in other studies should be followed; parameters applied to the model should be established.
- Regional/specific characteristics: Tracking regional distribution of ESRD disease, related factors and characteristics is useful in mapping population with risk factors of

this disease and layering risk factors. The prevalence of the disease in certain regions, whether the distribution in cities and towns is clustered in certain areas should be investigated. Demographic characteristics of ESRD patients according to regions should be identified and reported to the concerned local health directorates (Varol, 2009). Infrastructures of the health care services in the regions should be examined, and compared with the regional characteristics of the disease.

- International aspect: Social and economic problems occurred due to ESRD and organ shortage problem should be monitored together in the international arena. The dimensions of the relevant social and economic problems experienced in the developed and developing countries at certain times should be explained. Perhaps if this problem continues to increase, ESRD approaches of all countries will have to be redesigned. Developments and changes with regard to the diagnosis, treatment and monitoring of the disease at the international level are of particular concern to senior managements.
- Government regulations: Governments and ministries are executive authorities. They are responsible for implementing the budget and the programme. Government regulations have strategic influence on defining working conditions about the strategic planning of the implementation, provision of materials and resources, deciding about motivational elements such as rewards, incentives. Furthermore, to increase the efficiency of the implementation, individuals and organisations which will be affected by the model should be informed, suggestions coming from these individuals and institutions should be received and evaluated, a structure to include suitable ones into the regulations should be created.
- Political and legal factors: Political tendencies and legal regulations at both national and international levels may change in time. Such regulations have effects on the success of the implementation of the government and local authorities. With political and legal regulations, in addition to the efforts to further the implementation, development strategies should continue to be created. Furthermore, strategic, political and legal developments in different platforms should be explored. It is advisable to build cooperation between different institutions such as education and social services and create separate mechanisms and structures for these institutions.
- Financial issues: Success of the implementation requires the provision of financial resources reserved for the planned services. And this depends on the balances in the financial structure. The important element here is that the activities planned to prevent ESRD and reduce the number of kidney transplantations should above all achieve the desired results. The beginning, development and maturation stages of the implementation should be defined. Implementation activities are affected by the changes in these stages. Changes in the financial requirements deemed necessary for these stages should be identified and met. Furthermore, the amount saved from the existing expenditures as a result of the implementation should be established and monitored; the possibility of these savings returning to other investment areas in the healthcare services should be investigated.
- Clinical experiences: Clinical studies both national and international should be followed; the applicability of the innovations achieved through research and development activities, their suitability to the country's conditions, financial effectiveness should be monitored comparing long term results. Hence, existing associations (e.g. TSN) should be actively effective; they should support and improve

clinical studies not only about organ transplantation and dialysis but also to prevent ESRD nationwide. Or new structures for which clinical studies have been completed at all three stages to prevent and monitor this disease can be created.

4.3 Local health directorate: Functional plannings and tactics

Local health directorates are responsible for planning and delivering functional and tactical planning services, making human resources and finance related decisions. A directorate makes the connection between strategic plans and operational plans. It is focused more on increasing the efficiency of the resources. At this level, plans are closer to implementation stage and the directorate provides coordination of activities. At this stage, cooperation between organisations, collaboration and mutual support become prominent. The effect of existing organisation on the success of the planned new strategies and new activities should be evaluated. These plans about the synergy of inter-organisational harmony and skills allow to build a connection between the strengths and weaknesses of the organisation and the desired objectives (Dincer, 2005).

- Information flow: Information flow should be addressed in two main groups. The first is the information flow among the levels of the healthcare services, and the second is the information flow among the healthcare management levels. Thus an information flow effectively established between healthcare institutions will enable individuals and organisations to easily reach to information. Cooperation and sharing that ensure an information flow via the internet among the primary, secondary and tertiary level healthcare services will also increase the value of the present infrastructure of the organisation. This structure will allow the problems and opportunities which could not previously be noticed to be seen. With the strengthening of the information flow both between organisations and between organisations and individuals more synergy will be created and the information flow between the levels of healthcare services will become healthier.

  The local health directorates play an effective role in providing information flow between the healthcare management levels. The key role of the Directorates stems from the fact that there is a continuous information and data flow coming from healthcare institutions and they are the local authorities to evaluate such information. Relevant branches of the directorates should monitor and control the results of the implementation comparing them with the plans and goals. The implementation status of the plans and early detection and correcting possible deviations from the plans are vital for the success of the implementation. The local health directorates should periodically report data and information they receive in a predefined format to the senior management (Ministry of Health). This reporting may allow the senior management to follow the implementation. Therefore strategic plans can be controlled and updated.

  Provision of information flow will enable the information flow between primary healthcare institutions which are one of the most important bases of the implementation and hospitals. In order to achieve this there should be a computer network ready to be used. An effective computer network is as vital as the blood circulation in a body in terms of sharing information and generating new information; it will strengthen the connection between the local healthcare directorates and the senior management in addition to the above institutions.

- Personnel training: In this category, teams consisting of doctors and nurses working in the primary level institutions should receive training. Training materials should be prepared by nephrologists, urologists, other clinicians and relevant healthcare services managers. The training materials should consist of intelligible work flow algorithms and be of standard quality nationwide. Trainings of personnel in groups of predefined numbers in a province should be given, if applicable, by expert teams working in the same province. Here the training activities should include operational activities as well as the information about the importance of clinical substructure, registration system, provision of communication and information flow.
- Population information (Local): With the demographic information about the local population, data providing a basis for the planning of the implementation can be prepared. Population and its characteristics registered with primary healthcare institutions or family physicians in that region should be identified. Risk groups in male, female, infant, children and senior population over 60 years of age registered with the primary healthcare institutions which represent the basis for ESRD screening should be identified. To contribute to the ESRD screening activities, information about changes of residence and household density should be obtained.
- Institution capacity: In this category, primary, secondary and tertiary healthcare services for reducing kidney transplantation and preventing ESRD in line with proactive approach should be explained; capacities and roles of these healthcare institutions should be defined.
  - Primary healthcare institutions: The number of primary health care institutions and family physicians in the province should be reviewed. Those who execute the programme at the primary level are family physicians. Therefore, first the quality of accuracy and content of the data of population registered with family physicians should be controlled; problems, if any, should be solved. Additionally, physical structure, number of rooms, laboratory infrastructure, availability, number of employees and their qualifications, consumables and the condition of equipment of institutions, daily, monthly and yearly number of patients in a routine schedule should be reviewed. The number of people to be screened in a given period of time within the capacity of each family practice should be specified. Computer network providing information flow and data processing programme to be used, connections with other people and institutions should be checked.
  - Second and tertiary health care institutions: The purpose of determining hospital capacities is to define their limits in terms of providing treatment to all diagnosed patients. Hospital personnel medically and administratively responsible for the programme should be identified. Number of specialist physicians in the relevant specialty, number of nurses, the quality of laboratory and specific tests, necessary equipment and devices, number of beds and yearly number of patients and number of operations of secondary healthcare institutions in a province should be reviewed. Furthermore, localisations of hospitals should be reviewed to determine with which primary healthcare institutions they are connected. Tertiary health care training and research hospitals should be designated for the patients who require further research and treatment. Yet, the number of nephrologists, paediatric nephrologists and other specialists and other assets of these institutions should be

established. In order to implement strategic plans, number of estimated patients and capacity targets should be identified to provide treatment to all diagnosed patients. It should to determine compatibility with the functional plans. At the same time a structure to provide information flow should be established.

- Provision of materials: Infrastructure of the institutions at all three levels should be examined. Human force, materials, devices, equipment and information flow infrastructure should be reviewed. Personnel shortage, if any, should be solved, and employees should be equipped with necessary information through trainings. Consumables for all institutions, especially urine testing strips, urine collection containers etc should be supplied continuously for primary health care providers.
- Demands of patients and patient relatives: The main goal of the implementation is ESRD patients thus their demands are important. Increase of patients' awareness, their opinions about the medical and support services provided changes of the preferences of patients along the process and factors affecting those have an influence on the understanding and sensitivity of the managers towards patients' demands. Demands and wishes of patients which may be expressed during diagnosis, examination or treatment stages are vital to uncover and solve existing problems. Identifying the problems experienced by patients and their relatives and by those who were treated in the past play an important role for the success of the implementation. Demands and expectations of patients have an impact on the screening monitoring and treatment plans of ESRD and creating algorithms. Identifying medical and social needs of patients will improve patient satisfaction and contribute to faster and lower cost treatment and recovery of patients.
- Budgeting: is to express the plans and the anticipated results in numbers. This activity involves measuring and calculating in numbers and expressing in monetary terms all the activities such as human force, working hours, devices and equipments used etc. Budgeting shows the outcome of the model, what kind of earnings there will be and what level of resources is needed. Obtaining and using the resources economically, effectively and efficiently is necessary to evaluate the performance of the implementation model. It also enables the implementation to be transparent, its accountability to be maintained. Budgeting enables that the results of the applied strategy can be reviewed with different perspectives and the reasons behind can be studied.

4.4 Primary secondary and tertiary health care facilities-family physicians and hospitals: Operational planning, detection and monitoring of ESRD candidates, treatments of patients for ESRD

Multi-level health care services model is used to provide health care services. Multi level health care services refer to providing services which are complementary to each other. This classification involves primary health care services, secondary health care services and tertiary health care services (Hayran, 1998; Kartal, 2004). The main purpose of having multi-level health care services is to enable people to have the right kind of services at the right place. This multi-level structure of health care services ensures that the services provided are efficient and effective and prevents unnecessary utilisation of resources (Belek, 2001). There should be an integrity between the levels of health care services and these services should be provided in coordination. The one which is the most available one to the public and the most frequently used among health care services is the primary health care service. In an effective health care system there should be a relation between the levels. In most of the countries, people are first required to use primary health care services. Provided that primary health care providers find it suitable and necessary, other levels, namely secondary and tertiary can be utilised (Kavuncubası, 2000).

Operational planning is to plan implementation activities. This is the stage which comes after the plans are prepared in line with the objectives, approved according to the operational conditions, and the alternatives to be implemented are identified. Implementation plans should be prepared in a more detailed manner; how and by whom, where and when each activity to reach the goal will be carried out should be explained. At the same time, implementation plans should describe the structure of the organisation and should also include coordination activities (Gözlükaya, 2007).

The purpose of operational planning is to screen patients with ESRD risk, to treat and monitor ESRD patients. Therefore, provision of health care services requires an effort which involves and coordinates all three levels. At this stage, primary, secondary and tertiary prevention principles explained in the proactive management of ESRD are appropriately coordinated between the three levels of health care services.

The success of the implementation depends on the power of the infrastructure of the health care services organisation. Suitability of the organisation's structure, accessibility level of the services, effectiveness of the communication and correspondence systems, technologic advantages of the organisation, cooperation and coordination, qualifications and motivation of human resources, the quality of the materials, devices and equipment used, and maintenance of continuity are the main elements defining the strength of the infrastructure. Success will be achieved within the existing activities of the health care institutions, with the help of the compatibility of the existing resources and structures with the resources necessary for the implementation aimed with proactive approach.

4.4.1 Primary health care facilities: (Family physicians, health centres)

Primary health care services involve the services which combine and provide preventive health care services together with home care and outpatient health care services. These are the health care services which are designed in a way that people can easily access to and use. Healthcare institutions providing these services are the basic and important service facilities which people refer to first. These services are provided in facilities which are positioned and designed to be in locations where people in that area can easily reach to. Primary health care services are considered to be the main starting point in defining health plans and policies of countries, and achieving health care goals (Rico, 2003). These services, depending on the individual country, are provided either in family practices or in clinics.

Primary health care institutions constitute the basis of proactive management implementation with regard to prevention of ESRD due to their availability throughout the country, accessibility and personal data infrastructure. Special preventive measures for diseases are planned in these institutions. The purpose here is to screen and control predefined signals of the risk factors of ESRD, to prevent the disease before it develops. Planned activities should be designed, in addition to addressing individuals and the society, to detect otherwise healthy people who have underlying risk factors without showing any signs or symptoms. Screening and monitoring the symptoms and the diseases defined in the algorithm should be made in these institutions which have an integrated service approach.

- Business processes: Processes and work flows regarding the activities carried out in primary health care. Certain norms should be created for these. Designing business processes allows the distribution of strategic and tactical plans to lower level units and people. In addition to business processes, short term programme objectives or personal success goals should be defined.
- Time planning: Time planning helps to steer the strength of the organisation towards goals and objectives. Time planning is one of the critical processes determining the contribution of the activities for the efficiency. In order to do this, the plan should be kept under control and necessary monitoring should be made to detect any problem. With the help of a schedule, each responsible person can both create his/her own plan and define and track cooperative work activities with other people With time planning; activities for ESRD which are important and not urgent can be identified; those that are vital and have the priority can be emphasised and prioritised.
- Continuity of resources: The final objective of screening and monitoring activities of ESRD is to continue their existence. Availability and continuity of the model depends on the success of the results. Existence and continuity of the resources is also closely related with the success and improvement of the model.
- Quality of resources: Quality of the resources used in ESRD screening has an important role in the implementation of the model. Improving the quality and the features of the resources consisting of materials, equipment and devices is important for successful results and to lower the costs.
- Recording system: Developments in patient recording system contribute significantly to the improvement of the health care services provided during ESRD screening and monitoring activities. The recording system combines physician's records, laboratory records and health care providers' records in all three levels. Here, it should be stressed that the hidden quality of the primary health care services is the recording system.
- Collecting data: Since ESRD is one of the most important public health problems, healthcare data systems are the biggest data sources for this kind of screening monitoring activities. Today, owing to the developments in information systems and communication technologies a lot of medical and health care data can be stored in digital media and are easily accessible. Information systems created with the purpose of collecting, processing and sharing data contain demographic information, disease and treatment condition, tests made, invoicing and administrative information about patients (Yıldırım, 2007).
- Control systems: Control systems are used to control the conformity of the results achieved through the implementation model with the planned outcomes and whether the anticipated success has been achieved. Control process is closely related with the other functions of the model, notably planning. This process which determines the conformity of the strategic plans and plans of implementation with the current situation should be conducted in a very delicate manner and control techniques suitable for the plans should be used.

Urine samples of those coming to primary health care institutions should be tested for leucocytes, nitrite, albumin, protein, blood and glucose parameters using simple analysis techniques (strip); in the event that any of the parameters is found positive, these findings should be subjected to further testing (Kıdak, 2010; Levey, 2007). Since primary health care institutions are the first to accept people, they act as gate keepers, filters for secondary health care institutions (Willems, 2001). Therefore, screening should first be carried out in primary health care institutions; positive cases diagnosed by health care personnel working in these institutions should be referred to secondary and tertiary health care institutions. Gate keeping means that primary health care physicians have the authority to control the access of patients to other levels of the health care system and that patients could access to secondary and tertiary health care services only by referrals of primary health care physicians (Guy, 2001). Therefore, patients with values outside the normal ranges should be planned to be referred to nephrology clinics of consultant hospitals (centres) of the model for further tests and treatment. Screenings can be made during check-ups of healthy people or when they come to health care institutions for other reasons. Positive cases found during these checks should be referred to higher level institutions and results and feedback should be tracked again by primary health care institutions.

The important point to be emphasized in this chapter is the effective role primary health care institutions play in reducing the number of kidney transplantations. This role is basically the result of the integrated/holistic perspective already present in primary health care services. The efficiency level of the role is directly linked to the strength of the primary health care services infrastructure. The stronger this infrastructure is the more efficient the model will work and ease the workload of secondary and tertiary health care institutions.

4.4.2 Secondary and tertiary health care facilities (hospitals)

Secondary health care services consist of inpatient and outpatient health care services including examination, diagnosis, treatment and rehabilitation. They are hospital-based services. They are also referred to as secondary level or therapeutic health care services. The main function of a hospital should be to provide inpatient treatments; outpatient clinic services are not their main services. Secondary health care services in which more advanced technologies are used are evaluated in two groups; outpatient and inpatient therapeutic health care services (DPT, 1989). Tertiary health care institutions, in addition to secondary health care services, are the places where high end medical technologies are used, diseases requiring research to diagnose and treat are intended to be treated. These hospitals are advanced treatment centres where cutting edge medical technologies are used. These mostly include university hospitals, training and research hospitals and specialty hospitals. Therapeutic health care services provided in secondary and tertiary levels involve situations where diseases are treated. These services consist of medical and complementary medical services.

In secondary and tertiary health care institutions early diagnosis and treatment of signs and symptoms leading to ESRD and mitigating severe conditions should be aimed. Monitoring, minimising and delaying the progress of the diseases which can be diagnosed at early stages and be treated effectively should be aimed. Thus, positive cases diagnosed in primary health care institutions should be referred to secondary and tertiary health care institutions (hospitals). Here, people with CKD risk should be identified and monitored for CKD and progression of ESRD in patients diagnosed with CKD should be halted or retarded. Especially patients with diabetes, cardiovascular diseases, high blood pressure, hyperlipidemia, malignancy etc should be closely monitored (Obrador & Pereira, 2010). Urine samples received by health care centres should be tested again with urine test strips and urine microscopy for pyuria and/or nitrite positive. Urine cultures should be taken directly from asymptomatic patients; and from symptomatic patients and patients in whose urine culture samples growth is detected, urine cultures should be taken with catheters.

In hospitals, patients who have developed the disease earlier should be treated to prevent progression and complications. The goal here is to prevent problems caused by the disease and to improve the quality of life by preventing especially the progression of chronic diseases.

4.4.3 Evaluation and sharing of data

One of the most important stages of proactive management implementation is the stage of data collection, evaluation and converting into information. The main purpose of this stage is to develop an early warning and monitoring system. The information obtained will support control activities (measuring the level of goal achievement). The information should be used in updating organisational goals and developing new strategies.

Some of the important elements of the proactive management approach are to develop proactive monitoring tools, activate recording system and improve data flow process (Daleiden-Burns & Stiles, 2007). For this purpose in order to collect necessary information from all three levels, tracking forms which include and detail all data should be created and distributed to the institutions. Clinical examination and laboratory test results on these forms together with monthly activity reports of the institutions should be sent to the Local Health Directorates (relevant department) in electronic format and data should be systematically evaluated. The database created will assist decision makers to make more accurate decisions when defining strategies and goals. On one side, organisational information is produced and shared and on the other side this will contribute to transforming the entire organisation into a **learning organisation.**

In light of this information, despite the negative situation described above, it is observed that most of the present problems can be solved even with the available resources. The existing health care service infrastructure allows developments and improvements to be effected on health care services without necessitating large scale changes. The efficiency and effectiveness of health care services regarding screening and monitoring of ESRD should be improved. With such new strategies existing resources can be utilised more effectively, and with the prevention of ESRD without increasing the resources an improvement in efficiency will be achieved.

5. Application of proactive management model and its results

Up to that part of chapter, theoretical frame work of proactive management approach to prevent ESRD was explained. A summary of the study wchich described the implemented proactive management model is given in last part of the Chapter. This study was published with the title "Decreasing the need for kidney transplantation through proactive management" in Journal of Nobel Medicus in 2010.

In order to prevent ESRD, a program has been started in 2005 in the city of Izmir, Turkey. The aim of this program was to determine the incidence of UTIs in children and diagnose kidney anomalies at an early stage. Also the objective of this program was to start treating the affected children immediately and prevent the occurence of permanent kidney damage. This program, under the leadership of Healt Authority in Izmir city, academicians and specialists in pediatric nephrology that working in two training and research hospitals were included in this study. This study includes all the primary care facilities within the boundaries of the city of Izmir with 239 (91%) health centers and 25 (9%) maternity and child health and family planning centers. The program has been planned and realized for a period of one year between 2005 and 2006. The target grup of the study consisted of all the children within the city limits who applied to these healthcare facilities for inoculation. The most appropriate and efficacious period to reach the target age group has been chosen as the rubella vaccination scheduled at the 9th month, and the diphtheria, pertussis and tetanus boosters together with the polio booster at the 16th month. The population of Izmir is 3.5 million people and the population at the age of 0 is around 45 thousand.

In this study, teams from each facility consisting of a physician and a nurse or midwife (responsible of the laboratuar) have been given a training. The training material has been prepared by the teams serving at the children's nephrology clinics of the related hospitals and the same team also completed the training of the 528 employees in groups of 50. The urine samples of the children applying to primary care facilities have been tested for leukocytes, nitrites, proteins, blood and glucose parameters using a strip. If one of these parameters were positive, the cases have been taken under further examination. The cases outside the normal values are planned to be referred to the pediatric nephrology clinics of the advising (central) hospitals of the project for further analysis and treatment. The urine samples of the cases referred to the centers have been re-analysed using strips and urine microscopy, and bag and urine cultures have been taken from the asymptomatic patients positive for pyuria and/or nitrites. The symptomatic patients and those whose bag and urine cultures showed evidence of multiplication have been taken catheterized culture specimens for the final diagnosis of the UTI. Data collection forms have been designed, printed and distributed for the documentation of the project. Every month, all the urine test results documented with these forms have been sent digitally to the ACSAP Department of the Local Health Authority and assessed using frequency analysis.

Within the one year period when the study was conducted, 16908 children in Izmir aged 0-30 months have been assessed for urinary tract infections. Of these 9080 (53.7%) were male and 7828 (46.3%) were female. Their mean age was 15.6±13.4 months with a median value of 12 months; and the age distribution was 0 to 30 months. During the first evaluations made in the primary care facilities using a urine strip, the samples taken from 14098 (83.4%) children were assessed as normal, whereas 2810 (14.8%) samples tested positive for findings. The 302 (1.8%) children who tested positive have been treated in the primary health facilities, 2508 (14.8%) children have been referred to screening centers for further analysis. Among these children referred to the centers, 1096 (44%) reached the screening centers, whereas 1412 (56%) did not. 490 (44.7%) of the 1096 cases evaluated further in the screening centers have been assessed as normal while 543 (49.5%) of them were classified as pathological. 483 (44.1%) of these cases had UTI, 32 (2.9%) proteinuria, 28 (2.6%) hematuria and 27 (2.5%) urogenital anomalies. 27 (2.5%) patients having UTI together with a urogenital anomaly have been detected. Among the patients in this last group, 63 (5.8%) have discontinued investigations after the first examination (Table 3).

Evaluated Children	Number	Ratio (%)	Further Evaluation	Number	Ratio (%)
Total	16908	100.0	Total	1096	100
Normal	14098	83.4	Normal	490	44.7
Abnormal (Positive finding)	2810	16.6	Pathological	543	49.5
-Treated	*302*	*1.8*	*-UTI*	*483*	*44.1*
-Referred to hospital	*2508*	*14.8*	*-Proteinuria*	*32*	*2.9*
			-Hematuria	*28*	*2.6*
			Discontinued	63	5.8

Table 3. Results of the evaluated cases and the cases after further evaluation

The most important result of this study is the revelation of the fact that the urinary tract disease detected in 543 children (3.2%) who had no complaints at all and had applied to the local healthcare facility only for vaccination, has been demonstrated to be a disease progressing insidiously without giving any evidence. The main issue here is that most of these cases are preventable cases of UTI (483). This number is 2.8% of all the children screened. According to the study findings, there have been a significant number of cases without any complaints or clinical evidence. Of course not all of the detected cases shall develop CKD; but still, unless they are treated appropriately, all of them are candidates for CKD.

This study constitutes an important example for the training, solidification and application of the infrastructure, and the collection and evaluation of the data throughout the three steps in healthcare services. Evaluation of the targeted number of children and complete training supports this view. As in this study, the primary, secondary and tertiary health services may be supplementary and complementary for each other even in a highly technical subject like organ transplantation. The study has also shown that the health system must be managed with a multidisciplinary approach for a more effective and productive use of the sources allocated to healthcare services.

Another finding of the study, that only 1069 of all the cases that tested positive in primary care facilities applied to screening centers and that some of the cases discontinued tests and treatment after the initial application to the centers indicates the shortcomings of this cooperative effort that must be worked on. In additionally, this study pointed out that proactive monitoring systems as a vital part of this proactive management approach must therefore be formed with the registration system activated and the data flow process improved.

6. Conclusion

Evidently, the application of screening and prevention programs in order to reduce the need for kidney transplants arises as a basic necessity. Therefore, through the proactive management approach involving early diagnosis and screening programs, preventable etiologies of ESRD such as UTIs, diabetes mellitus, hypertension, etc beneath the visible part of the iceberg can be diagnosed and treated at an early stage and the number of the ESRD cases may be reduced. The early diagnosis and screening techniques must be in a way applicable in primary care facilities. This screening test must be integrated into the routine healthcare. This method will help reduce the number of the patients undergoing dialysis and waiting for an organ transplant, making comprehensive social and economic improvement possible.

7. Acknowledgments

I would like to thank Dr. Nese Nohutcu, Chief of ACSAP Department; Ass. Prof. Mustafa Bak, Chief of Pediatric Nephrology; Ass. Prof. Nejat Aksu, Pediatric Nephrology Specialist; and their teams and the primary healthcare staff in the city of Izmir for their contributions to the screening program of UTIs in children. Also, I would like to thank Ass. Prof. Nazif Erkan General Surgery for his contribution.

8. References

Ardissino, G.; Daccò, V. Testa, S. Bonaudo, R. Appiani, A. C. Taioli, E. Marra, G. Edefonti, A. & Sereni, F. (2003). Epidemiology of Chronic Renal Failure in Children: Data From the ItalKid Project, *Official Journal of the American Academy of Pediatrics*, Pediatrics; 111; pp. 382-387. ISSN: Print, 0031-4005; Online, 1098-4275

Ates, E.; Erkasap, S. Ihtiyar, E. Yılmaz, S. & Kiper, H. (1998). Böbrek Transplantasyonu Için Donör Havuzunun Genişletilmesinde Bir Kavram: Non-Heart Beatıng Donor Bir Yıllık Retrospektif Inceleme, *Türk Nefroloji Dializ ve Transplantasyon Dergisi* ; 1: pp. 32-34. ISSN 1300-7718

Belek, I. (2001), *Sosyal Devletin Çöküşü ve Sağlığın Ekonomi Politiği*, Sorun Yayınları, Istanbul. ISBN: 975-431-039-4

Charles, S. (2011). Proaktif Yönetim: Yenilik & Strateji, Sabancı Universty, Executive Development Unit, Penn State University, ABD, 17.02.2011, Available from www.su-edu.com.

Daleiden-Burns, A. & Stiles, P. (2007). Proactive Monitoring: Implications Of Implantable Devices For Future Heart Failure Management. *Critical Care Nursing Q*. Oct-Dec;30(4): pp.321-8. ISSN: 08879303 EISSN: 15505111

Dincer, Ö. (2004). *Stratejik Yönetim ve Işletme Politikası*, Beta Basım Dağıtım, Istanbul. ISBN: 9789754865547

DPT, (1989), Türkiye Sağlık Sektörü Masterplan Etüdü Mevcut Durum Raporu, Price Waterhouse, Ankara.

Drucker, P. (2003). *On the profession of management*. The Harvard Business Review Book Series, Boston. ISBN 1-59139-322-1

El Nahas, A. M. & Bello, A. K. (2005). Chronic Kidney Disease: The Global Challenge, *Lancet*, 365: pp. 331-40.

Varol, E. Varol, S. & Tokgözlü, A. (2009). Isparta Ilinde Koroner Arter Ektazisinin Demografik Özellikleri ve Hastalığın Bölgesel Dağılımının Coğrafi Bilgi Sistemleri Ile Gösterilmesi, *S.D.Ü. Tıp Fak. Derg*, 16(1)/ pp. 11-15. ISSN 1300-7416

Falkenstein, K. (2004). Proactive Psychosocial Management Of Children And Their Families With Chronic Liver Disease Awaiting Transplant, *Pediatric Transplantation,* Jun;8(3): pp. 205-7. Print ISSN: 1397-3142 Online ISSN: 1399-3046

Fuzzati, R. Faltings, B. & Calisti M. (2005). Organ Transplantation Management, Swiss Federal Institute of Technology Lausanne, EPFL Technical Report IC/2005/022, Switzerland.

Obrador, G. T. & Pereira, B.J.G. (2010). Epidemiology Of Chronic Kidney Disease And Screening Recommendations, UpToDate Available from: http://www.uptodate.com

Gözlükaya, T. (2007). Yerel Yönetimler Ve Stratejik Planlama: Modeller Ve Uygulama Örnekleri, Pamukkale Üniversitesi, Y. Lisans Tezi.

Guy, M.H.J. (2001). How Do Primary Health Care Systems Compare Across Western Europe, *The Pharmaceutical Journal*; 267; pp. 269-73.

Hayran, O. & Sur H. (1998). *Sağlık Hizmetleri El Kitabı Örgütlenme Finansman Yönetim Mevzuat,* Çevik Matbaası, Istanbul.

Irgil, E. (2006). Sağlığı Koruma, Uludağ Üniversitesi Halk Sağlığı ABD, 2005-2006 Eğitim Programı ve Ders Notları, 11.02.2011, Available from: http://halk-sagligi.uludag.edu.tr/EGITIM.HTM

ISM, Izmir Il Sağlık Müdürlüğü (2005). Izmir Ili 5 Yaş Altı Çocuklarda Idrar Yolu Enfeksiyonlarının Kontrolü Programı, AÇSAP Departman.

Jabs, K. & Warady, B.A. (1999). The Impact Of The Dialysis Outcomes Quality Initiative Guidelines On The Care Of The Pediatric End-Stage Renal Disease Patient, *Advances in Renal Replacement Theraphy,* Jan;6(1): pp. 97-106.

Kapuağası, A. (2010). Sağlık Bakanlığı Tedavi Hizmetleri Genel Müdürlüğü, 27. Ulusal Nefroloji, Hipertansiyon, Diyaliz ve Transplantasyon Kongresi, *Sağlık Dergisi,* 10/22/2010. Available from: http://www.aymedilac.com/tr_haber/haberdetay.asp?hid=5

Karakavak, G. & Çırak, Y. (2006). Kronik Hastalıklı Çocuğu Olan Annelerin Yaşadığı Duygular, *İnönü Üniversitesi Eğitim Fakültesi Dergisi* Cilt: 7 Sayı:12 Güz, pp. 95-112. ISSN: 1300 - 2899

Kartal, M. & Mollahaliloğlu, S. (2004). OECD Sağlık Hesapları Sistemine Göre Türkiye Ulusal Sağlık Hesapları 1999 - 2000, T.C. Sağlık Bakanlığı Refik Saydam Hıfzıssıhha Merkezi Başkanlığı, Ankara.

Kavuncubaşı, Ş. (2000), *Hastane ve Sağlık Yönetimi,* Siyasal Kitabevi, Ankara. ISBN: 975735151-2

Khan, S. & Amedia, C.A. Jr. (2008). Economic Burden Of Chronic Kidney Disease. *Journal of Evaluation in Clinical Practice,* Mar 24, Epub ahead of print ISSN 1356-1294

Kıdak, L.B. (2010). Decreasing The Need For Kidney Transplantation Through Proactive Management, Journal of Nobel Medicus, 16, 6(1): pp. 61-67. ISSN 1305-2381

Kocak, H. (1993). *Doku ve Organ Transplantasyonları,* Haberal M.A., (ed). Haberal Eğitim Vakfı, Ankara.

Kocel T. (2005). *İşletme Yöneticiliği, Yönetim ve Organizasyonlarda Davranış Klasik-Modern-Çağdaş ve Güncel Yaklaşımlar,* Arıkan Bas. Yay. Dağ. Ltd. Şti, 2005 Istanbul. ISBN 9756145447

Levey, A.S.; Atkins, R. Coresh, J. Cohen, E.P. Collins, A.J. Eckardt, K.U. Nahas, M.E. Jaber, B.L, Jadoul, M. Levin, A. Powe, N.R. Rossert, J. Wheeler, D.C. Lameire, N. & Eknoyan, G. (2007). Chronic Kidney Disease As A Global Public Health Problem: Approaches and Initiatives–A Position Statement From Kidney Disease Improving Global Outcomes. *SO Kidney Int.* 72(3): pp. 247-59.

Levin, A. (2001). Identification Of Patients And Risk Factors In Chronic Kidney Disease--Evaluating Risk Factors And Therapeutic Strategies, Nephrology Dialysis Transplantation. *Oxford Journals, Medicine,* 16 Suppl 7: pp. 57-60.

MacStravic, S. (2008). The Real Potential In Proactive Health Management, *Marketing Health Services,* Spring; 28(1): pp. 44. ISSN: 1094-1304

MHT (The Ministry Of Health Of Turkey) (2011). Health Statistics Yearbook 2010, Refik Saydam Hygiene Center Presidency, School of Public Health, Ankara.

Overhage, J.M. (2008). Proactive Medicine. The Benefits Of An EMR In Locations Without One, *Modern Healthcare,* Feb 4;38(5): pp. 24.

Pelczarski, K.M. (2007). Take A Proactive Approach To Bariatric Patient Needs, *Material Management in Health Care,* Jun;16(6): pp. 24-6. ISSN: 1059-4531

Pereira, B.J. (2001). Management Of Chronic Renal Insufficiency: A Call For A Proactive Approach, *Nephrology News and Issues,* Feb;15(3):32, pp. 35-39. ISSN: 0896-1263

Yıldırım, P.; Uludağ, M. & Görür, A. (2008). Hastane Bilgi Sistemlerinde Veri Madenciliği, *X. Akademik Bilişim Konferansı,* Çanakkale Onsekiz Mart Üniversitesi, Çanakkale, 30 Ocak - 01 Şubat 2007

Procen. (2010). Egitim ve Danısmanlık Hizmetleri, 18.02.2011, Available from: http://www.procen.com.tr/altisigma5.htm

Prodjosudjadi, W. (2006). Incidence, Prevalence, Treatment and Cost of End-Stage Renal Disease in Indonesia, *Ethn Dis.* Spring;16(2 Suppl 2):S2- pp. 14-6. pISSN = 1049-510X

TSN (Turkish Society of Nephrology) (2009). 2008 Registry of The Nephrology, Dialysis and Transplantation in Turkey, Istanbul.

Richardson, R.C. (1997). Discipline And Children With Chronic Illnesses: Strategies To Promote Positive Patient Outcomes, *ANNA J.* 1997 Feb;24(1): pp. 35-40. ISSN:8750-0779

Rico, A.; Saltman, R. & Boerma, W. (2003). Organizational Restructuring in European Health Systems: The Role of Primary Care, *Social Policy and Administration;* 37 (6): pp. 592-608. Online ISSN 1467-9515

Süleymanlar, G. (2007). Kronik Böbrek Hastalığı ve Yetmezliği: Tanımı, Evreleri ve Epidemiyolojisi, *Turkiye Klinikleri J Int Med Sci,* 3(38): pp. 1-7. ISSN: 1300-0292

Şirin, A.; Emre, S. Alpay, H. Nayır, A. Bilge, I. & Tanman, F. (1995). Etiology of Chronic Renal Failure in Turkish Children, *Pediatric Nephrology,* Volume, 9, No:5, pp. 549-552. pISSN 0931-041X online ISSN 1432-198X

Teixidor, A.B. (2006). Proactive Management Of Uncertainty To Improve Scheduling Robustness In Process Industries, A thesis submitted for the degree of Doctor Universitat Politµecnica de Catalunya Barcelona.

The U.S. Organ Procurement and Transplantation Network and the Scientific Registry of Transplant Recipients the 2009 OPTN/SRTR Annual Report: Transplant Data 1999-2008.

Toland, C. Meenan, C. Warnock, M. & Nagy, P. (2007). Proactively Monitoring Departmental Clinical IT Systems With An Open Source Availability System. *J Digit Imaging*. Nov; 20 Suppl 1: pp.119-24. ISSN 0897-1889

Warady, B. A. & Chadha, V. (2007). Chronic Kidney Disease In Children: The Global Perspective, *Pediatric Nephrology* 22: 1999–2009. ISSN 0931-041X

Willems, D. L. (2001). Balancing Rationalities: Gatekeeping In Health Care. *Journal of Medical Ethics*; 27: pp. 25-9. ISSN 0306-6800

9

Surgical Complications of Renal Transplantation

Marcelo Ferreira Cassini, Murilo Ferreira de Andrade
and Silvio Tucci Junior
Ribeirão Preto Medical School,
São Paulo University
Brazil

1. Introduction

In the early era of kidney transplant, surgical complications were a major cause of graft loss. Between 1960 and 1980, the estimated incidence was around 20%. With the improvement of surgical techniques, the frequency of these complications has dropped significantly and this subject until then common in the medical literature came to be seldom discussed (Botto V, 1993; Hernandez D, 2006). Currently, it is estimated that in large transplant centers the incidence of surgical complications is less than 5%. In general, the results of renal transplantation have improved primarily as a consequence of advances in medical and immunosuppressive therapy and progress in surgical techniques. Posttransplant urologic complications are unusual, with the range of 2.5% to 27% in most series, and can cause significant morbidity and mortality (Zargar MA, 2005; Dalgic A, 2006) Results have improved over the past decade as a direct application of less invasive endourologic diagnostic and therapeutic techniques of the surgical complications (Streem SS, 1994).

However, the etiologies are the most common technical problems and association with immunological complications. Surgical complications after renal transplantation can be classified mainly as vascular (arterial and venous thrombosis, renal arterial stenosis, lymphocele, hemorrhage) and urologic (ureteral obstruction, vesicoureteral reflux, urinary fistula), although other types of complications are not uncommon, like graft's rupture and hematoma. These complications can occur early in the intra-operative, immediate postoperative period or later, and imply in increase morbidity, hospitalization and costs (Humar A, 2005).

Urologic complications are the most common surgical complication after renal transplantation, causing significant morbidity and mortality. Recently, the incidence of urologic complications after renal transplantation has decreased to 2.5% to 12.5% (Emiroglu R, 2001). Unfortunately, there is a still higher incidence of technical complications in pediatric recipients, reaching approximately 20% with an associated 58% and 74% graft survival rates for cadaveric and living-related transplantation (Salvatierra O Jr, 1997; US Renal Data System, 1996). Urologic complications represent an important cause of morbidity, delaying normal graft functioning, and in some cases leading graft loss and/or patient death (Beyga ZT, 1998; Colfry AJ Jr, 1974; Mundy AR, 1981; Hakim NS, 1994).

The most frequent urological complications after kidney transplantation involves the ureterovesical anastomosis (fistula, stenosis and reflux), with a frequency ranging from 5% to 10% in different séries.

2. Urologic complications

2.1 Urinary fistula

This is the leakage of urine from the collecting system. It can occur at the level of the bladder, ureter or renal calices. The leakage of urine can be collected around the graft, move to the retroperitoneum, scrotum or may manifest through the incision. His average prevalence in many studies is around 5.7%. In general, most urinary leaks are the results of ureteral problems, failure of ureterovesical anastomosis or ischemia and necrosis of the distal ureteral stump.

Like the majority of surgeons now employ an extravesical ureteroneocystostomy technique for implantation of the ureter, there are shorter ureter and decreased likelihood of ischemia, and a limited cystostomy that rarely leads to leakage from the bladder (Gibbins WS, 1992; Thrasher JB, 1990).

Clinical presentation:

In most cases, there is constant discharge of clear liquid (yellow citrus) through the drain, in the immediate postoperative period, and sometimes the flow through the drain can even surpass the diuresis the urinary catheter.

When later, after removal of the tubular drain, there may be bulging store kidney with extension into the perineum and scrotum or decreased urine output with maintenance of renal function. Unexplained graft dysfunction, pelvic fluid collection, fever, graft tenderness, an lower extremity edema can also occur (Streen SB, 1994).

Early urinary leaks can be divided into two types: the first usually occurs within the first 1 to 4 days and is almost always related to technical problems with the implantation. In this case, the ureter has usually pulled out of a tunnel caused by excessive tension at the anastomosis. This complication appears to be more common with the extravesical ureteroneocystostomies (Streen SB, 1994). Some authors have recommended use of a ureteral stent to lessen the likelihood of this complication (Gibbins WS, 1992). The second type of early ureteral leak, usually presents between 5 and 10 days, is associated with distal ureteral ischemia, which may be a consequence of injury during the donor nephectomy, technical causes such as tunnel hematoma or distal stripping of the blood supply (Rosenthal JT, 1994).

Diagnosis:

For being the most common surgical complication of kidney transplantation, urinary fistula is easily diagnosed. In doubtful cases, where there is need to exclude the lymphocele as main differential diagnosis, biochemical analysis of the liquid is characterized by having elevated levels of creatinine, urea and potassium. In the lymphocele, creatinine should be similar of blood. Urinary leak are often suspected because of increased drainage from the wound. Radiographic tests of help include an abdominal ultrasound and nuclear renal scan. The ultrasound is nonspecific for evaluating patients with suspected urinary fistula after kidney transplantation. It will only reveal a fluid collection (anechoic image) around the graft. A renal scan demonstrating extravasation (figures 1.1, 1.2) is the most sensitive method to differentiate a urine leak from other fluid collections such lymphoceles or hematomas (Bretan PN Jr, 1989). A cystogram should be performed if a bladder leak is suspected.

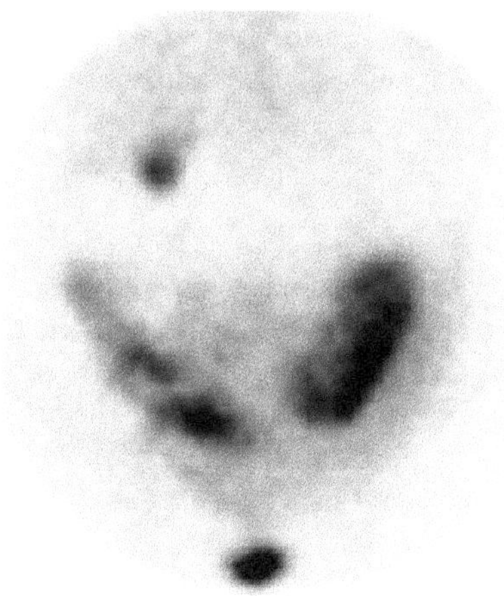

Fig. 1.1. Renal scan with contrast early extravasation (urinary fistula).

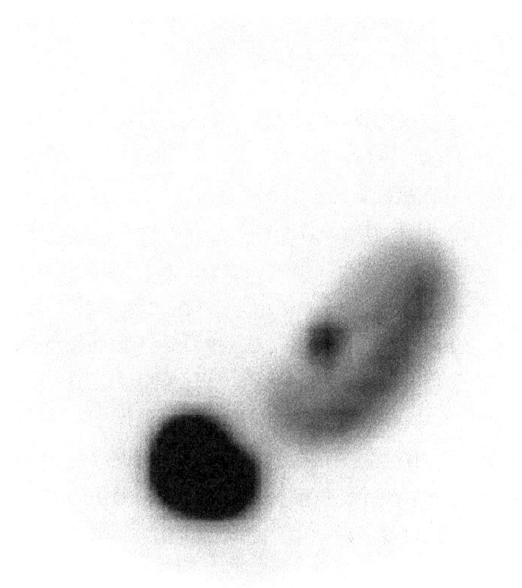

Fig. 1.2. Late renal scan without contrast extravasation (no fistula).

In the evaluation of transplant patients, nuclear medicine can contribute in the earliest complications that may arise in the period immediately following transplantation, as in the late complications and complications of surgical nature. A landmark study, conducted an initial assessment within the first 72 hours of surgery, is important so that we can better assess possible changes in the course of evolution. Studies with DTPA or MAG3 are the ones who will advise on the vascular phase and functional phase, and excretory phase, all parameters of the utmost importance in the evaluation of the graft (Kahan BD, 1989; Luk SH, 1999).

As surgical complications of kidney transplantation, the urinary fistulas are observed by scintigraphy an accumulation of the radiotracer outside the kidney (Luk SH, 1999). In cases of hematoma, other surgical complication, shows an area of low concentration of the tracer near the kidney, which may cause displacement of large structures such as vessels, ureter, bladder and collecting system obstruction. The diuretic renogram may help elucidate this issue, because the transplanted kidney has the same performance as a native kidney scintigraphy.

Management of the urinary fistula:

Disruption of urinary tract in a renal transplant patient or graft dysfunction requires rapid diagnosis and treatment. Ureteral leakage needs careful and accurate diagnosis of the exact cause and site. It is important to know if the problem has a physical cause such a leak or an obstruction and is not associated with an acute rejection episode that required specific treatment (Streen SB, 1994; Rosenthal JT, 1994).

Surgical treatment has to be performed in all patients except those presenting with minimal extravasation at the ureteral reimplantation site and clinically stable. This group was initially treated by urinary drainage. In cases of unfavorable outcome after clinical treatment, surgery is indicated. Surgery is the initial aproach for big extravasation or when leaks arising from the mid or upper ureter were suspected. We use the same incision of the transplant to access the fistulae. The type of surgical reconstruction is based on the intraoperative evaluation of the extent of the ureteral necrosis and local and systemic condition of the patient at the time of surgery. Primary reconstruction with the ureter of the recipient or a new ureteral reimplantation are performed preferentially when local and systemic condition allowed; if local or systemic infection are present and the patient is clinically unstable an ureteral ligature associated to a nephrostomy can be performed. Ureteral stenting alone is used exceptionally. All patients received prophylactic or therapeutic antibiotic according to the antibiogram of the collected fluid (Mazzucchi E, 2006).

The need for immediate open operative surgical intervention has been replaced, to a large extent, by early endourologic intervention (Banowsky LHW, 1991). The placement of a percutaneous nephrostomy can divert a leak or relieve obstruction and allow more definitive diagnosis. As described by Streem et al., endourologic management can select patients for whom the likelihood of successful nonoperative management is good. In a few cases, percutaneous access can offer long-term treatment with chronic stent management. Percutaneous techniques like nephrostomy associated to antegrade ureteral stenting works in 40% of a much selected group of patients presenting with small fistulae from the distal ureter (Campbell SC, 1993).

Early open surgery is our preferred approach. Our policy is to perform primary urinary tract reconstruction whenever local and systemic condition allows. Termino-lateral anastomosis of the graft ureter or pelvis with the ureter of the recipient can be used as technique for the correction of urinary leaks. Some groups use termino-terminal anastomosis with the ureter of the recipient (Salomon L, 1999) with good results but can results in ureterohydronephrosis of the native kidney after ureter ligation for reconstruction. Ureteroneocystostomy "de novo" is used for reimplantation defects or for small distal ureteral necrosis and can fail in many cases due to necrosis extension or incomplete ureteral and bladder wall resection during surgery. Ureteral reimplantation remains an important option for urinary fistulae management. Ureteral ligature and nephrostomy is performed when there is gross infection of the fossa or when the patient presents in sepsis. There is also described, in cases of infected urinary fistulas and to prevent distal ureteral ligature and nephrostomy, the introduction of a Foley's catheter throught the bladder wall. The catheter's balloon is inflated at the transplanted renal pelvis to occlude the pyeloureteral junction and dry the region of the fistula (Suaid HJ, 2010).

Recurrences are due to insufficient ureter resection, leaving an ischemic stump extension of the process after the surgery or inadequate anastomosis. We recommend always leaving a double J stent in these cases in order to reduce recurrences but stents do not work if the necrosis extends. Recurrences were always managed surgically and an anastomosis with the ureter of the recipient was the first choice. Some patients can need a third procedure due to a new recurrence showing that the necrosis can extend after surgery and that extensive resection of the ureter is frequently necessary.
Mortality directly related to the fistula or to its correction was high in the early transplantation era (Dreikom K, 1992) and nowadays is reported to range from 0 to 8% (Salomon L, 1999). These better results are due to an earlier and more aggressive approach, reduction in the amount of corticosteroids in the immunosuppressive regimen and to better antibiotics and clinical support. The increase in the experience with these cases can still improve such results.
Routine ureteral stenting, to avoid urinary fistula, does not reduce significantly your incidence and its use is recommended only in special cases (contracted bladder, difficult anastomosis) (Campbell SC, 1993; Salomon L, 1999). In our center the modified Gregoir technique has been the procedure of choice in the last 35 years and the incidence of ureteral complications has been low.

2.2 Ureteral obstruction

Ureteral obstruction and ureteral leakage are the most common urinary complication after renal transplantation (Azhar, Hassanain et al. 2010). The incidence related in literature varies from 3 to 8% (Fontana, Bertocchi et al.; Smith, Windsperger et al.; Kaskarelis, Koukoulaki et al. 2008). Obstruction may occur during the early postoperative course due to blood clots, ureteral malrotation or kinking, tight submucosal tunnel, unsuspected donor calculus (Poullain, Devevey et al. 2010) or perigraft fluid collection (Kahan and Ponticelli 2000; Campbell, Wein et al. 2007). Late ureteral obstructions generally after the first month or even at years posttransplant are secondary to chronic ischemia which leads to chronic fibrosis and strictures. Other cause includes compressive limphoceles or pelvic masses, ureteral lithiasis and rarely obstruction by ureteral carcinoma (Huurman, Baranski et al. 2008) or fungus ball (Vuruskan, Ersoy et al. 2005).
The clinical presentation includes pain over the surgical site, decreased urine volume leading to oligoanuria and rise in blood pressure secondary to impaired renal function. Diagnostic tests shows gradual rise in serum creatinine. The ultrasound demonstrates pyelocaliectasis (fig. 2.1) or ureteropyelocaliectasis (fig. 2.2) in most of cases. Nuclear scintigraphy is less sensitive because the obstructed kidney also displays impaired radionuclide uptake, a sign often present in allograft rejection. When the diagnosis is unclear the antegrade pyelogram must be performed, because is an accurate method to define anatomically the site, degree of obstruction (Kahan and Ponticelli 2000).
The treatment must be instituted as early as possible to avoid loss of renal graft function. Initially the nephrostomy by puncture must be done to ensure the patency of the kidney and restore renal function to normal. The definitive treatment of the obstruction is oriented according to the etiology. Stenosis ureteral at the site of bladder reimplantation is more common and can be addressed by several endourology techniques such as ureteral meatotomy or percutaneous ureteral dilation with balloon followed by angioplasty and implant of stent at the ureters. Such techniques are at acceptable levels of success especially

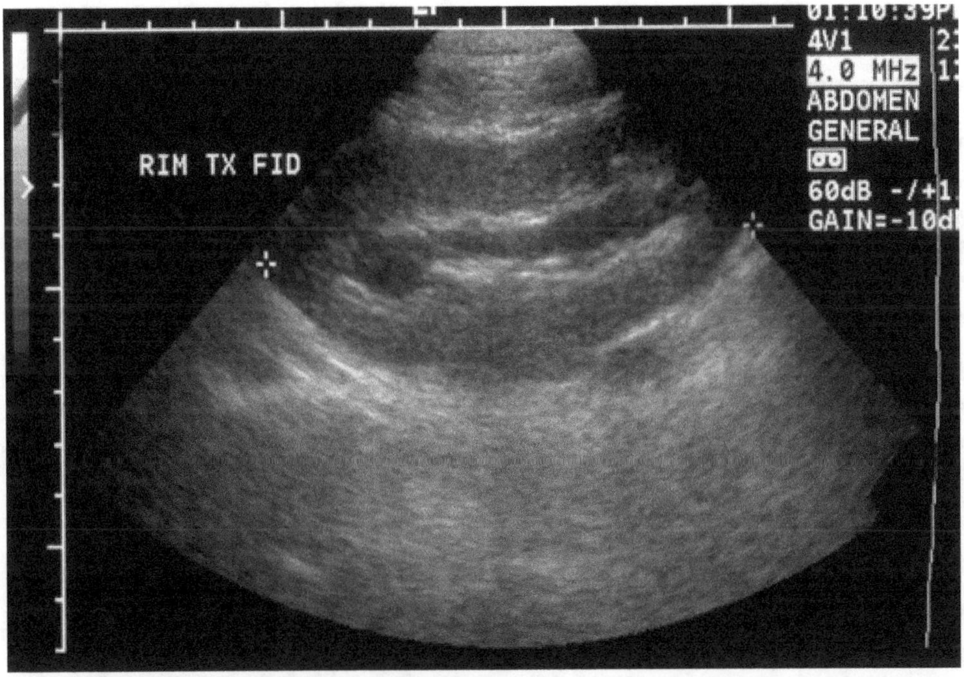

Fig. 2.1. Ultrasound with moderate hidronefrosis.

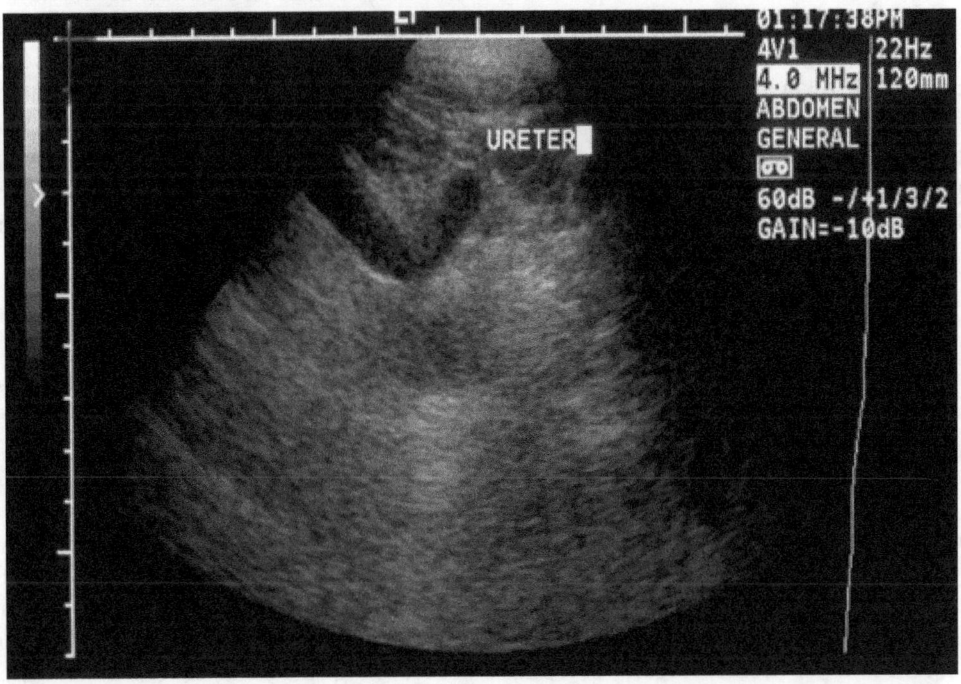

Fig. 2.2. Ultrasound of transplant kidney with ureteroectasis secundary to distal ureteral obstruction.

when treat small lesions (Burgos, Bueno et al. 2009). However, open surgery with reconstruction of the excretory pathway is still considered the gold standard. In distal ureteral obstructions or when there is redundant ureter, we can review the ureteroneocystostomy by extravesical Lich-Gregoir modified techniques (Campos Freire, de Goes et al. 1974) or intravesical (Politano-Leadbetter, 1958).

When there are multiple, long stenosis of the ureter or even poor vascularization, it is necessary to perform the anastomosis of the renal pelvis with the host ureter (ureteropyelostomy) or the ureter with the host ureter (ureteroureterostomy). However, the last technique has a higher rate of stenosis. When the native ureters cannot be used, the "Boari flap" should be done joining the short ureteral stump or the renal donor pelvis, allowing an adequate distance to the bladder. This allows tunneling the flap under the ureter, decreasing reflux and bacterial contamination during episodes of infection at the lower urinary tract. Extreme situations may require a pyelovesicostomy with anastomosis the donor urinary pelvis directly to the bladder. In this circumstance there is direct transmission of voiding pressure to the urinary collecting system as well as any urinary infection, leading to chronic pyelonephritis and deteriorating renal graft (Kahan and Ponticelli 2000).

3. Vascular complications

Although theoretically there is greater risk of surgical complications associated with living donors and recipients of kidneys with multiple arteries, in actuality it has not been considered more as a problem in laparoscopic (VLP) or open nephrectomy. This, indeed, is standard procedure in many transplant centers, (Wilson CH, 2005; Hsu TH, 2003) showing no significant adverse effects on the function and graft survival in VDL nephrectomies without or with hand assistance which may lead to higher vascular extension. (Saidi R, 2009; Hoda MR, 2010; Hoda MR, 2011) However, there is need for close attention to the anatomy of the donor due to the possibility of having two or more arteries and veins, or early arterial bifurcation (Benedetti E, 1995; Mazzucchi E, 2005; Harper JD, 2010). Furthermore, knowledge of microsurgical techniques for careful arterial graft reconstruction with multiple arteries and is essential for the reduction of vascular complications in these situations (Saidi R, 2009; Beckmann JH, 2008).

4. Arterial renal thrombosis

The most worrisome of vascular complications, it occurs in about 1% of all kidney transplants (Penny MJ, 1994; Bakir N, 1996) arterial thrombosis can reach values lower or higher in different series (Salehipour M, 2009).

Usually results from technical difficulties in removing the organ or implant. In nephrectomy and perfusion injury may occur in the endothelial layer, facilitating the process of thrombosis. The anastomoses of small vessels or of very different sizes or twisting or bending pressure are other predisposing factors for thrombosis, making demand for assessing the floor space of the kidney as well as proper positioning of the graft at surgery. With some frequency, there is a need to adjust the length of the renal artery to avoid kinking of the same. A technical care is obliquely sectioning the end of the renal artery (espatulating), which can reduce the risk of thrombosis and stenosis. Another factor to consider is the quality of the receiver because the arterial embolization of atheromatous plaques predispose to thrombosis. Lesions in the endothelial artery caused by vascular clamp during anastomosis should also be considered (Gang S, 2009). Other situations of greater risk for vascular complications are patients receiving three or four kidney transplants, hyperacute rejection, and antiphospholipid antibodies (Gang S, 2009; Baños JLG 2005).

In children, either as donors or as recipients, renal transplantation deserves special attention, or some authors recommend the exclusion of donors under the age of 3 years and the best use of infusion solutions to reduce vascular complications and increase survival rates graft (Irtan S, 2010).

Clinical presentation and diagnosis:

The hallmark of renal artery thrombosis is the absence of blood perfusion of the parenchyma, which can still be identified intra-operatively. In the postoperative period the most common clinical presentation is the sudden interruption of urinary flow, without pain in the graft. Obstruction should be excluded from the catheter by blood clots. The renal perfusion should be evaluated by DMSA renal scintigraphy, by ultrasound Doppler, and even with arteriography, if needed (Nezami N, 2007).

The immediate surgical exploration may allow in a few cases, revascularization and recovery of the graft, especially if the diagnosis of arterial thrombosis is done before closing the incision. The loss of the graft is the most common consequence and nephrectomy should be performed (fig. 3.3).

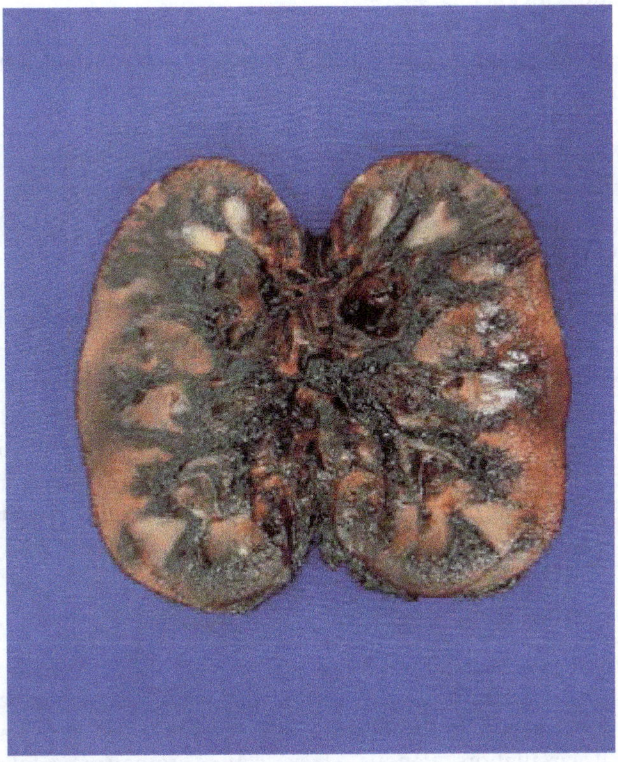

Fig. 3.3. Nephectomy: Arterial Renal Thrombosis.

5. Renal artery stenosis

The prevalence of renal artery stenosis is around 2% to 10% (mean 3.7%) (Benoit G, 1990). Clinical picture is suggested by onset severe hypertension post-renal transplant, dysfunction or presence of acute renal failure with prolonged NTA. With a peak onset at six months, renal artery stenosis can manifest itself as early as two days and as late as two years after transplantation. Stenoses located in the line of anastomosis, especially in termino-terminal anastomosis, the most frequent etiologic factor is technical failure. Other etiologic factors are largely the same that lead to arterial thrombosis, but acting with less intensity.

Clinical picture and diagnosis:

The suspicion must always occur when a transplant patient started with a progressive decline of renal function, heart murmur audible (or increasing its intensity) in the graft site and hypertension refractory to medical treatment. The diagnosis may be suggested by non-invasive techniques such as ultrasound associated with (color) Doppler (sensitivity 87 to 94%, specificity 86 to 100%). Doppler ultrasound is useful as screening and may show an increased blood flow velocity > 6 kHz12 (Nezami N, 2007).

The arteriography still remains the gold standard for diagnosis of arterial stenosis renal (Rengel M, 1998) The degree of stenosis is considered significant when more than 50% of the arterial lumen. Recently, gadolinium-enhanced MRI has allowed a noninvasive and efficacy comparable to that of renal arteriography convencional (Thornton MJ, 1999). The test with captopril, with plasma renin may be a method in the diagnosis of renal artery stenosis of kidney transplantado (Glicklich D, 1990).

The therapy depends on the location and degree of stenosis. Conservative treatment can be used in cases of mild stenosis in which blood pressure is controlled with medication and serum creatinine level remained stable.

Invasive procedures are indicated when blood pressure is not controllable by medication, there is progressive worsening of renal function or when noninvasive tests suggest the progression of stenosis. In this situation, diagnostic arteriography is indicated in combination with transluminal angioplasty and "stenting" (fig. 4.1, 4.2) (Leertouwer TC, 2000). This technique allows restoring renal perfusion in most cases and its effectiveness is confirmed immediately by a second angiography (Ghaffari S, 2009).

Intraluminal balloon dilatation with stenting is the preferred therapy for most patients, especially recommended in cases of localized stenosis and distant > 1 cm of the anastomosis. Surgery is reserved for lesions involving the anastomosis, or the surrounding area, and in cases of early artery stenosis renal (Benoit G, 1990). Other surgical procedures are indicated when the stenosis is severe and unsuitable for angioplasty or else, in this failure. Surgical techniques include reviewing local resection of the stricture and reanastomosis, may or may not be used autologous grafts (saphenous vein) or heterologous (Teflon) in the form of a patch graft or bypass, with success rates ranging between 63 to 92% (Bruno S, 2004), (fig. 4.3).

6. Renal vein thrombosis

The renal vein thrombosis is uncommon but serious complication, with incidence ranging between 0.9 and 4.5%, usually occurring in the first week after transplantation and with great potential for graft loss (Giustacchini P, 2002). Because the transplanted kidney does not have collateral circulation, venous stasis causes impairment of blood flow and consequent loss of function.

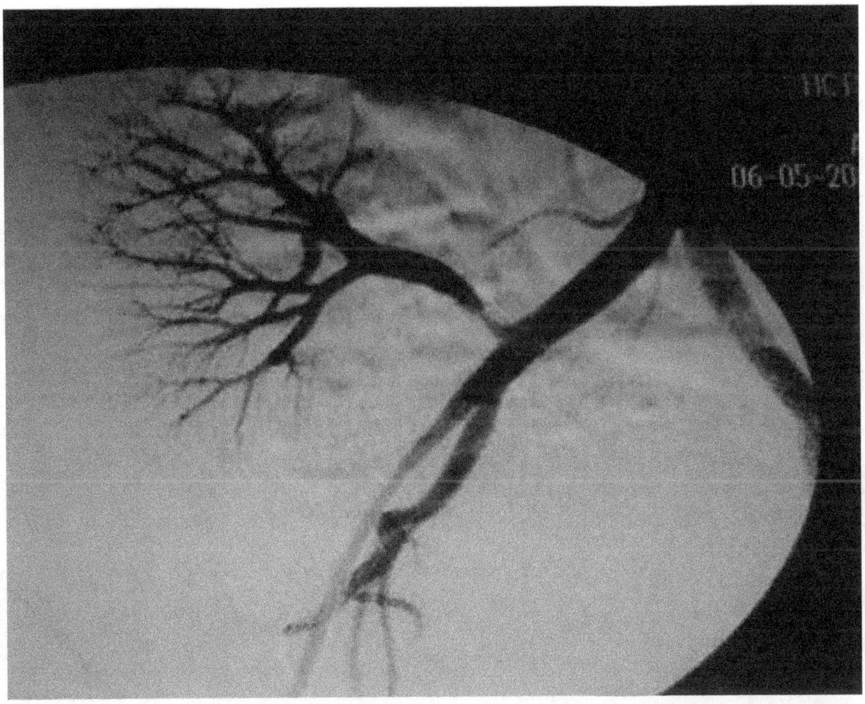

Fig. 4.1. Arteriography (post-transplant) showing a renal stenosis artery.

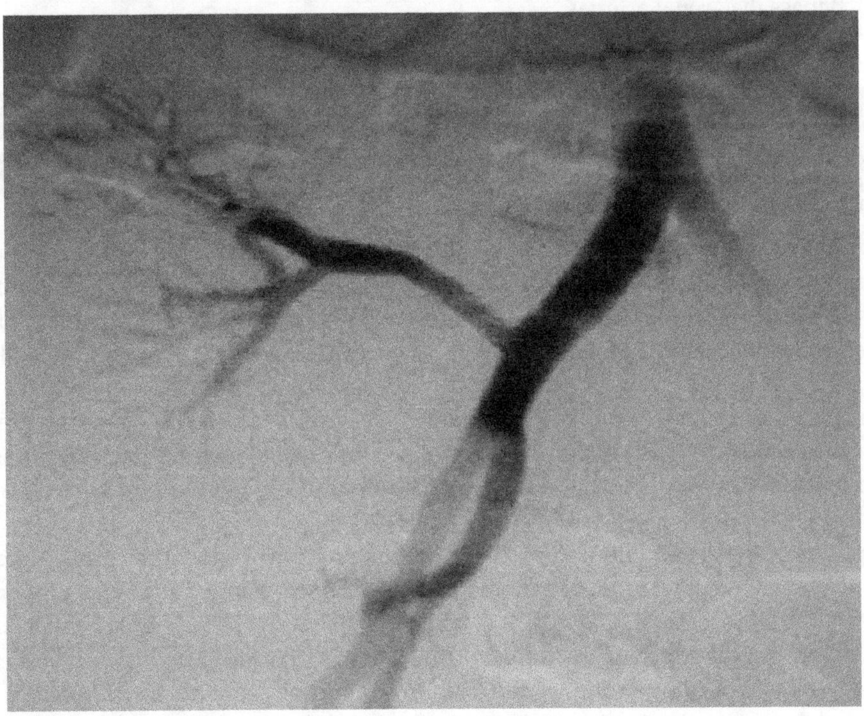

Fig. 4.2. Result after "stent" angioplasty.

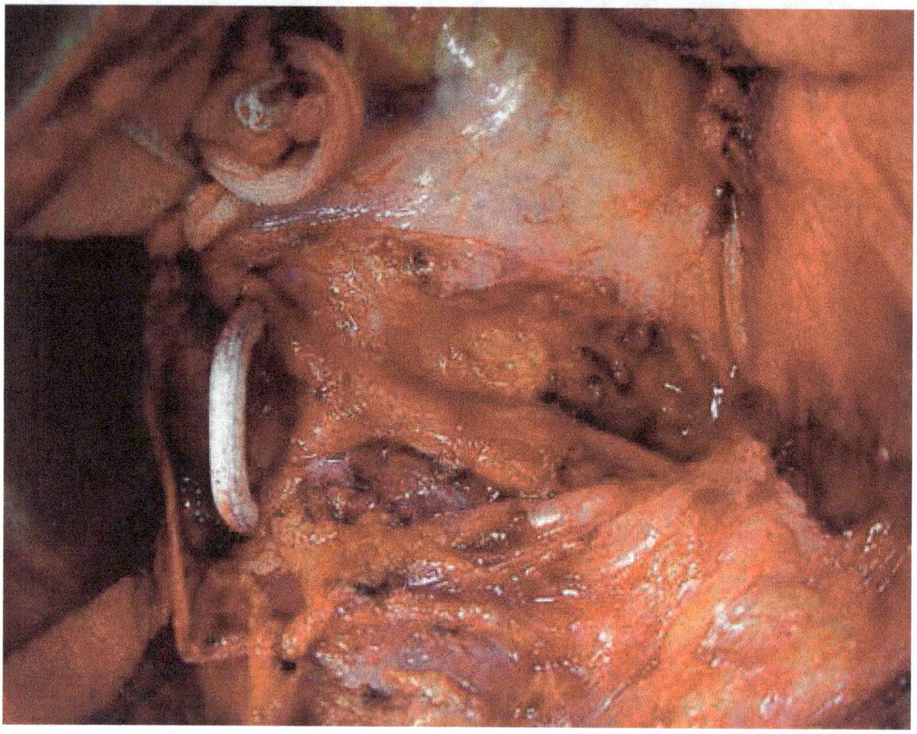

Fig. 4.3. Bypass iliac-renal arteries.

As causative agents related are: angulation of the renal vein or anastomotic stricture, dehydration, venous compression by lymphocele or hematoma, progression of ipsilateral iliofemoral thrombophlebitis should also be considered. Late cases of renal vein thrombosis have been associated with recurrence of membranous nephropathy, (Carrasco A, 2008).

Clinical presentation and diagnosis:

The symptoms is nonspecific as the sudden onset of hematuria, oliguria or anuria, accompanied by local pain and swelling of the graft. There may also increase the diameter of the ipsilateral lower limb deep venous thrombosis associated. The evaluation of renal Doppler ultrasound confirms the increase in renal volume and absence of venous flow. In the arterial can be seen reverse diastolic flow. Although it has been reported that early surgical exploration and thrombectomy allow the preservation of the graft in cases with renal vein thrombosis, but usually the kidney is no longer viable at the time of surgical exploration due to the spread intrarenal venous thrombus and prolonged hypertension. In most cases the nephrectomy is performed (Fathi T, 2007).

A complication associated with renal vein thrombosis is the rupture of the graft, which may cause hemorrhage and large hematoma perinephric (confirmed by ultrasonography), together with signs of hypovolemia and circulatory shock. Physical examination usually reveals bulging at the site. Nephrectomy is also standard procedure (figures 5.1, 5.2, 5.3).

However, in cases of rupture of the graft without thrombosis, should be attempted to suture the parenchyma and preservation of the graft (Gang S, 2009).

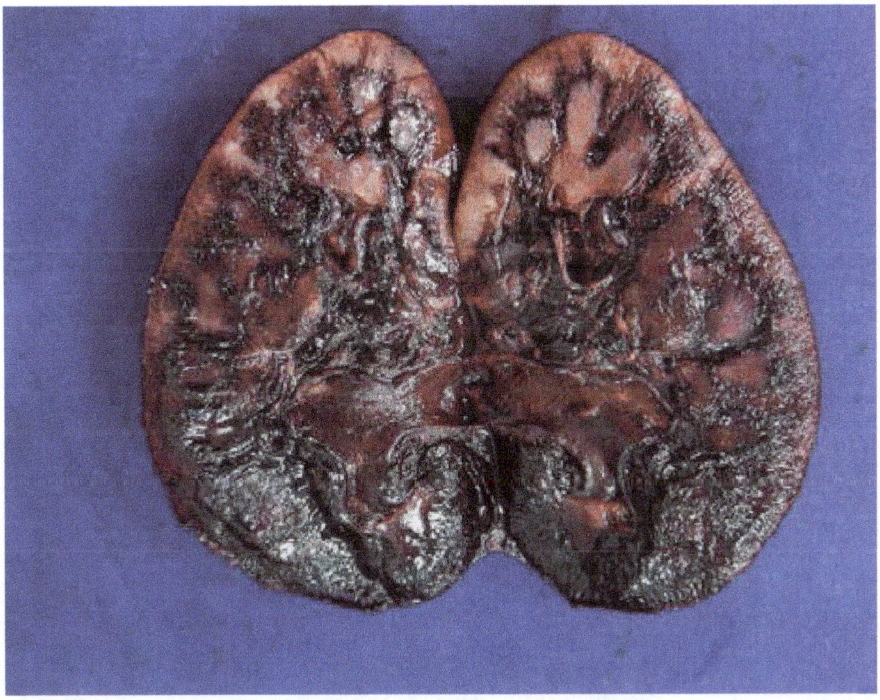

Fig. 5.1. Nephrectomy: Renal vein thrombosis.

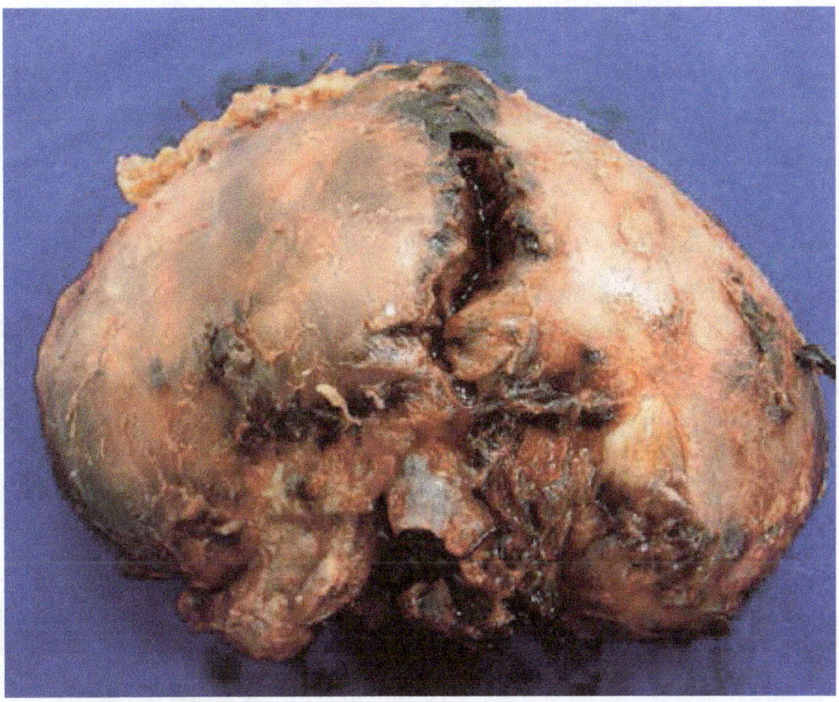

Fig. 5.2. Renal vein with thrombus inside and graft's rupture.

7. Lymphocele

Lymphocele is a lymph collection from the iliac lymphatic vessels of recipient or graft hilum that accumulates between the transplanted kidney and bladder. The average incidence of lymphocele in the literature ranges from 0.6 to 16% (Adani, Baccarani et al. 2007; Zargar-Shoshtari, Soleimani et al. 2008; Iwan-Zietek, Zietek et al. 2009). The etiology has been attributed to inadequate ligation of the delicate lymph vessels overlying the iliac vessels or present in the hilum. The method of renal uptake also appears to influence the appearance of lymphatic complications. The removal of the kidney by laparoscopy may prolong the lymphatic leak requiring drain for a longer period (Saidi, Wertheim et al. 2008). The small lymphoceles are more frequent but usually asymptomatic (Krol, Kolonko et al. 2007).
However, larger collections are manifested clinically in a few weeks to months after transplantation, bulging can occur in the surgical wound (Fig. 6.1) with or without cutaneous extravasation of lymph. In severe cases, there may be edema of lower limb ipsilateral to the graft, frequent urination due to bladder compression and ureteral obstruction leading to hydronephrosis and loss of renal graft function (Kahan and Ponticelli 2000)

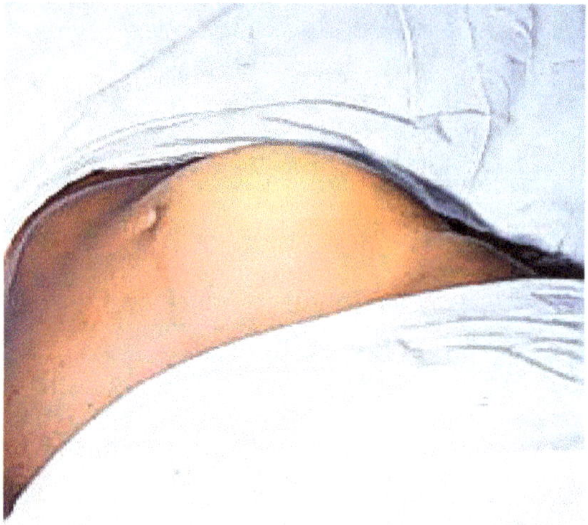

Fig. 6.1. Abdominal bulging secondary to lymphocele.

The diagnosis is confirmed by ultrasound which may show hydronephrosis, altered vascular flow by Doppler and quantify the lymphocele or the presence of other collections such as hematoma (Fig. 6.2) or urinoma (Fig. 6.3)(Krol, Kolonko et al. 2007). In cases of doubt about the etiology, a computerized axial tomography (CT) (Fig. 6.4) can be performed following puncture of the collection guided by CT or ultrasound (US) with biochemical dosages of the liquid obtained.
The treatment can be divided into expectant, puncture and drainage or surgery. As previously mentioned, small volumes of lymphocele with less than 140ml and asymptomatic, tend to resolve spontaneously without any renal graft damage. Larger collections or lymphoceles with clinical manifestations can be punctured and drained, under strictly aseptic techniques and guided by US or CT. In this case you should aim for total disappearance of the collection. If there is clinically significant recurrence, a sclerotherapy with povidone-iodine 5% ethanol or antibiotics can be performed (Chandrasekaran, Meyyappan et al. 2003; Hamza, Fischer et al. 2006; Zomorrodi and Buhluli 2007).

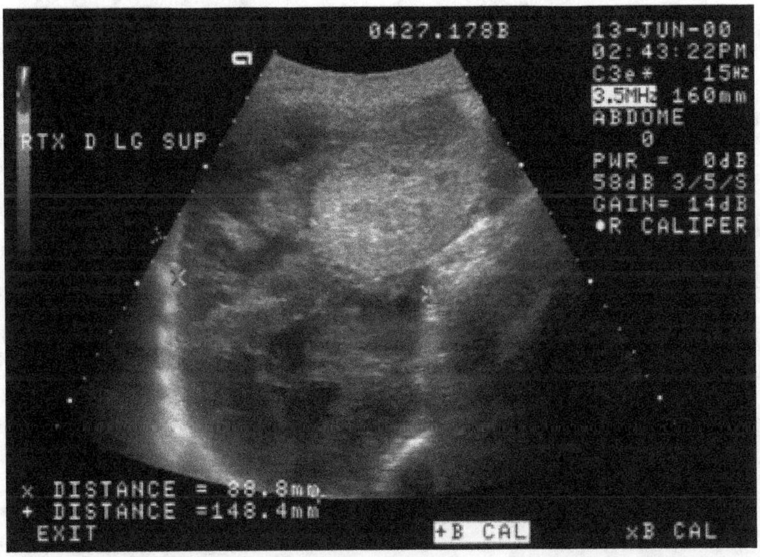

Fig. 6.2. Perinephric hematoma

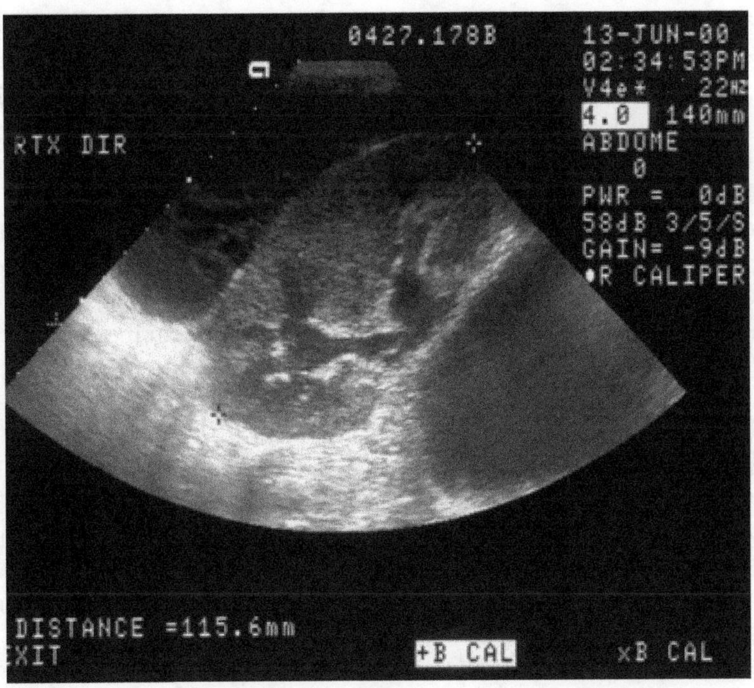

Fig. 6.3. Urinoma.

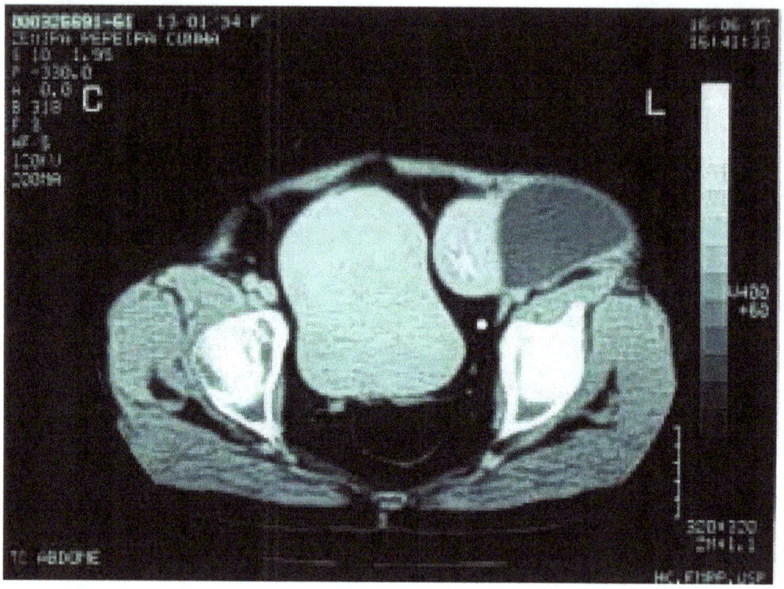

Fig. 6.4. Computerized axial tomography showing a lymphocele.

In lymphoceles larger than 500 ml, punctures, drainages and sclerotherapy are usually not effective. In cases refractory or complicated, the laparoscopic lymphocele fenestration (Marsupialization) is the procedure of choice in many centers. The laparoscopic technique reduces the risk of injury to the ureter or infection and demonstrates high rate of success. It is important to create a window sufficiently large to ensure patency of the ureter (Kahan and Ponticelli 2000).

When the location is not favorable to laparoscopy or in recurrent cases, the approach by open surgery should be performed, especially when the lymphocele is located posterior and lower to the transplanted kidney or behind the bladder (Fuller, Kang et al. 2003; Hamza, Fischer et al. 2006). In both techniques is recommended to perform the peritoneocystostomy with an oval window of at least 2.5 x 5.0 cm in width associated with interposition of short segment of omentum, allowing a good peritoneal absorption of lymphocele and avoiding internal hernias of the bowel segments (Kahan and Ponticelli 2000).

Recently was reported the treatment of recurrent and symptomatic lymphocele by inserting a Tenchoff catheter at the site of lymphocele tunneled to the abdomen, allowing the intraperitoneal drainage. This procedure offers as advantages the possibility of being performed in outpatient clinics, without general anesthesia, with good efficacy and safety, although the number of cases reported is still small (Adani, Sponza et al. 2007) (Adani, Baccarani et al. 2007).

In conclusion, the treatment of lymphoceles should begin by less invasive techniques. If there is recurrence or failure proceed to marsupialization by laparoscopy or open surgery.

8. References

Adani, G. L., U. Baccarani, et al. (2007). "Treatment of recurrent symptomatic lymphocele after kidney transplantation with intraperitoneal Tenckhoff catheter." Urology 70(4): 659-61.

Adani, G. L., M. Sponza, et al. (2007). "Intraperitoneal Tenckhoff catheter for the treatment of recurrent lymphoceles after kidney transplantation: our early experience." Transplant Proc 39(6): 1851-2.

Azhar, R. A., M. Hassanain, et al. (2010). "Successful salvage of kidney allografts threatened by ureteral stricture using pyelovesical bypass." Am J Transplant 10(6): 1414-9.

Bakir N, Sluiter WJ, Ploeg RJ. Primary renal graft thrombosis. Nephrol Dial Transplant.1996; 11:140-147.)

Baños JLG, Calabia ER, Rodrigo MHL, Martín JAP, Edreira AR, Gómez MAC, Schaan JIV, Tubet CA, Izquierdo FR, Diego RB, García RM. Aspectos quirúrgicos en los terceros y cuartos retrasplantes renales. Actas Urol Esp. 2005; 29 (2): 212-216.

Banowsky LHW. Surgical complications of renal transplantation. In: Glenn JF,ed Urologic Surgery, 4th ed. Philadelphia: JB Lippincott, 1991;252-266.

Beckmann JH, Jackobs S, Klempnauer J. Arterial reconstruction in kidney transplantation. Tx Med. 2008; 20:7-12.

Benedetti E, Troppmann C, Gillingham K, Sutherland DER, Payne W, Dunn DL, Matas AJ, Najarian JS, Gruessner RWG. Short-and long-term outcomes of kidney transplants with multiple renal arteries. Ann Surg. 1995; 221 (4):406-414.

Benoit G, Moukarzel M, Hiesse C, Verdelli G, Charpentier B, Fries D. Transplant renal artery stenosis: experience and comparative results between surgery and angioplasty.Transplant Int.1990;3:137-40.

Beyga ZT, Kahan BD: Surgical complications of kidney transplantation. J Nephrol 11:137, 1998.

Botto V, Cortese F, Baroni B, et al. Surgical complications in renal transplantation. Minerva Chir. 48(21 -22): 1341 -1346, 1993.

Bretan PN Jr, Hodge E, Streem SB, et al. Diagnosis of renal transplant fistulas. Transplant Proc 21:1962-1966, 1989.

Bruno S, Remuzzi G, Ruggenenti P. Transplant Renal Artery Stenosis. J Am Soc Nephrol. 2004; 15: 134–141.

Burgos, F. J., G. Bueno, et al. (2009). "Endourologic implants to treat complex ureteral stenosis after kidney transplantation." Transplant Proc 41(6): 2427-9.

Campbell, M. F., A. J. Wein, et al. (2007). Campbell-Walsh urology / editor-in-chief, Alan J. Wein ; editors, Louis R. Kavoussi ... [et al.]. [Philadelphia], W.B. Saunders.

Campbell SC, Streem SB, Zelch M, Hodge E, Novick AC. Percutaneous management of transplant ureteral fistulas: patient selection and long-term results. J Urol. 1993; 150:1115-1117.

Campos Freire, J., G. M. de Goes, et al. (1974). "Extravesical ureteral implantation in kidney transplantation." Urology 3(3): 304-8.

Carrasco A, Diaz C, Flores JC, Briones E, Otipka N. Late renal vein thrombosis associated with recurrence of membranous nephropathy in a renal allograft: a case report. Transplant Proc. 2008 Nov; 40(9):3259-60.

Chandrasekaran, D., R. M. Meyyappan, et al. (2003). "Instillation of povidone iodine to treat and prevent lymphocele after renal transplantation." BJU Int 91(3): 296.

Colfry AJ Jr, Schlegel JU, Lindsey ES, et al: Urological complications in renal transplantation. J Urol 112:564, 1974.

Dalgic A, Boyvat H, Karakayali G, et al: Urologic complications in 1523 renal transplantations: the Baskent University Experience. Transplant Proc 38:543, 2006.

Dreikom K. Problems of the distal ureter in renal transplantation. Urol Int. 1992;49: 76-89.

Emiroglu R, Karakayali H, Sevmis S, et al: Urologic complications in 1275 consecutive renal transplantations. Transplant Proc 33:2016, 2001.

Fathi T, Samhan M, Gawish A, Donia F, Al-Mousawi M. Renal allograft venous thrombosis is salvageable. Transplant Proc 2007 May; 39:1120-1.

Fontana, I., M. Bertocchi, et al. "Late ureteral stenosis after kidney transplantation: a single-center experience." Transplant Proc 42(4): 1174-5.

Fuller, T. F., S. M. Kang, et al. (2003). "Management of lymphoceles after renal transplantation: laparoscopic versus open drainage." J Urol 169(6): 2022-5.

Gang S, Rajapurkar M. Vascular complications following renal transplantation. JNRT. 2009; 2(1): 122 - 132.

Ghaffari S, Hakim H, Ahmadpoor P. Transplanted Renal Artery Stenosis: a Case Report and Review of Literature. J Cardiovasc Thorac Res. 2009; 1(2): 45-48.

Gibbins WS, Barr JM, Hefty TR. Complications following un-stented parallel incision extravesical ureteroneocystostomy in 1,000 kidney transplants. J Urol 148:38-40,1992.

Giustacchini P, Pisanti F, Citterio F, De Gaetano AM, Castagneto M, Nanni G. Renal vein thrombosis after renal transplantation: an important cause of graft loss. Transplant Proc. 2002; 34: 2126–2127.

Glicklich D, Tellis VA, Quinn T, Mallis M, Greenstein SM, Schechner R, et al. Comparison of captopril scan and Doppler ultrasonography as screening tests for transplant renal artery stenosis. Transplantation. 1990;49:217-8.

Hakim NS, Benedetti E, Pirenne J, et al: Complications of ureterovesical anastomosis in kidney transplant patients: the Minnesota experience. Clin Transplant 8:504, 1994.

Hamza, A., K. Fischer, et al. (2006). "Diagnostics and therapy of lymphoceles after kidney transplantation." Transplant Proc 38(3): 701-6.

Harper JD, Breda A, Leppert JT, Veale JL, Gritsch HA, Schulam PG. Experience with 750 consecutive laparoscopic donor nephrectomies—is it time to use a standardized classification of complications? J Urol. May 2010; 183, 1941-1946.

Hernández D, Rufino M, Armas S, Gonzáles A, Gutiérrez P, Barbero P, Vivancos S, Rodríguez C, de Vera JR, Torres A. Retrospective analysis of surgical complications following cadaveric kidney transplantation in the modern transplant era. Nephrol Dial Transplant. 21: 2908–2915, 2006.

Hoda MR, Greco F, Reichelt O, Heynemmann H, Fornara P. Right-sided transperitoneal hand-assisted laparoscopic donor nephrectomy: is there an issue with the renal vessels? J Endourol. 2010 Dec;24(12):1947-52.

Hoda MR, Greco F, Wagner S, Heynemmann H, Fornara P. Prospective, nonrandomized comparison between right- and left-sided hand-assisted laparoscopic donor nephrectomy. Transplant Proc. 2011; 43(1):353-356.

Hsu TH, Su LM, Ratner LE, Trock BJ, Kavoussi LR. Impact of renal artery multiplicity on outcomes of renal donors and recipients in laparoscopic donor nephrectomy. Urology. 2003; 61: 323-7.

Humar A, Matas AJ. Surgical Complications After Kidney Transplantation. Seminar in Dyalisis 2005; 18(6):505-510.

Huurman, V. A., A. G. Baranski, et al. (2008). "Transfer of ureteral carcinoma in a transplanted kidney presenting by early stenosis of the proximal ureter." Clin Transplant 22(6): 847-50.

Irtan S, Maisin A, Baudouin A, Nivoche Y, Azoulay R, Jacqz-Aigrain E, El Ghoneimi A, Aigrain Y. Renal transplantation in children: critical analysis of age related surgical complications. Pediatr Transplant. 2010 Jun; 14(4):5123-9.

Iwan-Zietek, I., Z. Zietek, et al. (2009). "Minimally invasive methods for the treatment of lymphocele after kidney transplantation." Transplant Proc 41(8): 3073-6.

Kahan, B. D. and C. Ponticelli (2000). Principles and practice of renal transplantation. [London], Martin Dunitz.

Kahan BD. Cyclosporine. N Engl J Med. 1989;321:1725-38.

Kaskarelis, I., M. Koukoulaki, et al. (2008). "Ureteral complications in renal transplant recipients successfully treated with interventional radiology." Transplant Proc 40(9): 3170-2.

Krol, R., A. Kolonko, et al. (2007). "Did volume of lymphocele after kidney transplantation determine the choice of treatment modality?" Transplant Proc 39(9): 2740-3.

Leertouwer TC, Gussenhoven EJ, Bosch JL, van Jaarsveld BC, van Dijk LC, Deinum J, et al. Stent placement for renal arterial stenosis: Where do we stand? A meta-analysis. Radiology. 2000; 216: 78–85.

Luk SH, Chan JH, Kwan TH, Tsui WC, Cheung YK, Yuen MK. Breath-hold 3D gadolinium-enhanced subtraction MRA in the detection of transplant renal artery stenosis. Clin Radiol. 1999;54:651-4.

Mazzucchi E, Souza AA, Nahas WC, Antonopoulos IM, Piovesan AC, Arap S. Surgical complications after renal transplantation in grafts with multiple arteries. Int Braz J Urol. 2005; 31 (2): 125-130.

Mazzucchi E, Souza GL, Hisano M, Antonopoulos IM, Piovesan AC, Nahas WC, Lucon AM, Srougi M. Primary reconstruction is a good option in the treatment of urinary fistula after kidney transplantation. Int Braz J Urol, 2006, 32(4):398-404.

Mundy AR, Podesta ML, Bewick M, et al: The urological complications of 1000 renal transplants. Br J Urol 53:397, 1981.

Nezami N, Tarzamni MK, H Argan, M. Doppler ultrasonographic indexes Nourifar in kidney transplant recipients. Its relationship with kidney function. Iran J Kidney Dis. 2007; (1) 2:82-87.

Penny MJ, Nankivell BJ, Disney APS. Renal graft thrombosis. Transplantation. 1994; 58: 565-569.

Poullain, J., J. M. Devevey, et al. (2010). "[Management of lithiasis of kidney transplant]." Prog Urol 20(2): 138-43.

Rengel M, Gomes da Silva G, Inchaustefgul L, Lampreave JL, Robledo R, Echenagusia A, et al. Renal artery stenosis after kidney transplantation: diagnostic and therapeutic approach. Kidney Int Suppl. 1998;54:S99-606.

Rosenthal JT. Surgical management of urological complications after kidney transplantation. Semin Urol XII(2):114-122, 1994.

Saidi, R. F., J. A. Wertheim, et al. (2008). "Impact of donor kidney recovery method on lymphatic complications in kidney transplantation." Transplant Proc 40(4): 1054-5.

Saidi R, Kawai T, Kennealey P, Tsouflas G, Elias N, Hertl M, Cosimi AB, Dicken S. C. Ko. Living donor kidney transplantation with multiple arteries. Arch Surg. 2009; 144(5):472-475.

Salehipour M, Salahi H, Jalaeian H, Bahador A, Nikeghbalian S, Barzideh E, Ariafart A, Malek-Hosseini SA. Vascular complications following 1500 consecutive living and cadaveric donor renal transplantations: a single center study. Saudi J Kidney Dis Transpl. 2009; 20(4):570-572.

Salomon L, Saporta F, Amsellem D, Hozneck A, Colombel M, Patard JJ, et al.: Results of pyeloureterostomy after ureterovesical anastomosis complications in renal transplantation. Urology, 1999; 53:908-912.

Salvatierra O Jr, Tanney D, Mak R, et al: Pediatric renal transplantation and its challenges. Transplant Rev 11:51, 1997.

Smith, K. M., A. Windsperger, et al. "Risk factors and treatment success for ureteral obstruction after pediatric renal transplantation." J Urol 183(1): 317-22.

Streem SS: Endourological management of urological complications following renal transplantation. Semin Urol 22:123, 1994.

Streen SB. Endourological management of urological complications following renal transplantation. Semin Urol XII(2):123-133, 1994.

Suaid HJ, Cassini MF, Tucci S Jr, Reis RB, Rodrigues AA Jr, Cologna AJ, Martins AC. Therapeutic option for infected urinary tract fistulas in renal transplantation. Transplant Proc. 2010 Mar; 42(2):479-482.

Thornton MJ, Thornton F, O'Callaghan J, Varghese JC, O'Brien E, Walshe J, et al. Evaluation of dynamic gadoliniumenhanced breath-hold MR angiography in the diagnosis of renal artery stenosis. AJR Am J Roentgenol.l 1999;173:1279-83.

Thrasher JB, Temple DR, Spees EK. Extravesical versus Leadbetter-Politano ureteroneocystostomy: a comparison of urological complications in 320 renal transplants. J Urol 144:1105-1109, 1990.

US Renal Data System: 1996 Annual Data Report. Bedhesta MD: National Institutes of Health, NIDDKD; 1996.

Vuruskan, H., A. Ersoy, et al. (2005). "An unusual cause of ureteral obstruction in a renal transplant recipient: ureteric aspergilloma." Transplant Proc 37(5): 2115-7.

Wilson CH, Bhatti AA, Rix DA, Soomro NA. Comparison of laparoscopic and open donor nephrectomy: UK experience. BJU Int. 2005; 95: 131-5.

Zargar MA, Shahrokh H, Fallah MMR, et al: Comparing Taguchi and anterior Lich-Gregoir ureterovesical reimplantation techniques for kidney transplantation. Transplant Proc 37:3077, 2005.

Zargar-Shoshtari, M. A., M. Soleimani, et al. (2008). "Symptomatic lymphocele after kidney transplantation: a single-center experience." Urol J 5(1): 34-6.

10

Cardiovascular Diseases in Kidney Transplantation

Roberto Marcén and Sara Jiménez
Department of Nephrology. Ramón y Cajal Hospital,
University of Alcalá de Henares, Madrid
Spain

1. Introduction

Cardiovascular diseases that include atherosclerotic diseases; coronary artery disease, cerebrovascular disease and peripheral vascular disease, and cardiac functional diseases; congestive heart failure, left ventricular hypertrophy and arrhythmias, are very common in the general population and are the first cause of mortality (Wilson &Culleton, 1998, Culleton & Wilson, 1998). Moreover, patients with chronic renal failure have an increased risk of cardiovascular disease compared with the general population, and after stratification by age and gender, cardiovascular mortality is 10 to 20 times more frequent independently of treatment; predialysis, dialysis or after kidney transplantation (Foley et al, 1998). Kidney transplantation is the best therapy of end-stage renal disease by reducing cardiovascular mortality (McDonald &Russ, 2002, Ojo et al, 2000, Wolfe et al, 1999). But even after transplantation, a recipient of 25 to 35 years of age has a 10 times higher risk of cardiovascular mortality than an individual of similar sex and gender without renal failure (Foley et al, 1998). Among the cardiovascular diseases, atherosclerotic diseases are the most frequently studied and are associated with patient outcome. Ischaemic heart disease was the cause of 53% of total mortality in a study performed in Scandinavia 15 years ago (Lindholm et al, 1995) and these findings were still prevalent in a later report (Aakhus et al, 2004). However, several authors have recently emphasized the importance of functional cardiopathies such as congestive heart failure on patient outcome (Rigatto et al, 2002).

The high incidence of cardiovacular events and mortality in renal transplant recipients has been attributed to the increased presence of traditional (Ojo, 2006) and nontraditional risk factors (Ducloux et al, 2004, De Mattos et al, 2006). As traditional risk factors do not fully explain the high cardiovascular risk it has been postulated that some of these risk factors, age, diabetes and smoking, could have a higher deleterous impact in transplant recipients than in the general population (Kasiske et al, 2000a). Other authors consider that transplant related (De Mattos et al, 2006) and nontraditional or emergent factors, hyperhomcysteinemia and inflammation, could play a predominant role in the appearance of cardiovascular events (Ducloux et al, 2004). Progressive chronic graft dysfunction and death with functioning graft are the most important causes of graft loss (Matas et al, 2002, Collins et al, 2008) and cardiovascular diseases are the leading cause of mortality in renal transplant recipients dying with a functioning graft (Pilmore et al, 2010). Consequently decreasing

cardiovascular mortality could improve patient and graft outcomes (Howard et al, 2002, Marcén et al, 2001, Morales, 2008, Vanrenterghem et al, 2008).
The present chapter reviews the cardiovascular diseases which affect renal transplant recipients and their impact on patient mortality, the risk factors associated with these complications and the therapeutical strategies to improve patient and graft outcomes.

2. Cardiovascular diseases

Renal transplant recipients are not healthy individuals. They have a past history of chronic renal failure and dialysis therapy, both having negative impact on cardiovascular risk and they present variable chronic renal failure stages. All cardiovascular diseases; atheriosclerotic and functional cardiopathies can affect transplant recipients (Table 1).

Atheroesclerotic diseases	Functional cardiopathies
Coronary artery diseases	Congestive heart failure
Cerebrovascular diseases	Left ventricular hypertrophy
Peripheral vascular diseases	Arrhythmias

Table 1. Most common cardiovascular diseases affecting transplant recipients

As in the general population, cardiovascular diseases are important causes of morbidity and mortality in renal transplant recipients. Heart diseases and cerebrovascular diseases accounted for about 35% mortality in our Unit (Figure 1).

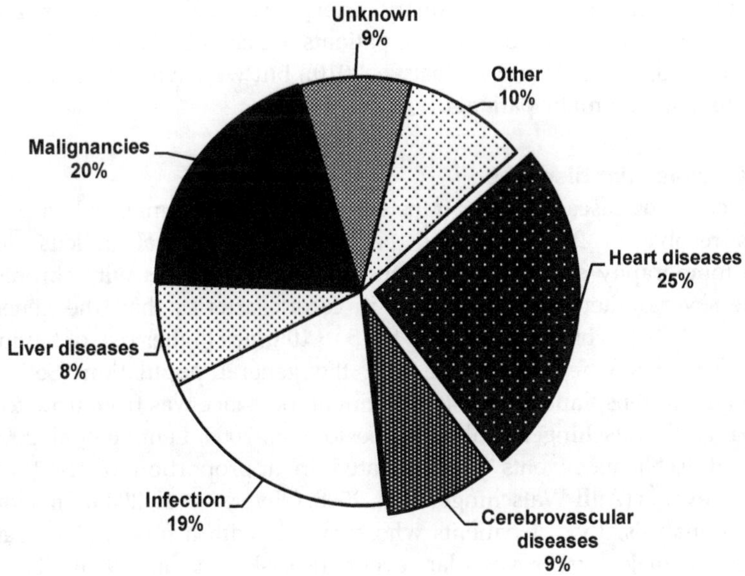

Fig. 1. Causes of mortality in 224 renal transplant recipients with functioning graft (Ramón y Cajal Hospital)

2.1 Atherosclerotic diseases

2.1.1 Coronary artery disease

Coronary artery disease is the most frequent atherosclerotic disease in the general population and a leading cause of cardiovascular mortality. It is generally admitted that coronary artery disease is between 2 and 6 times more frequent in renal transplant recipients than in the general population (Aarkhus et al, 1999, Kasiske, 1988, Lentine et al, 2005a, Marcén et al, 2006, Massy, 2001). A very high number of events occurring during the first weeks after transplantation have been attributed to surgical stress, immunosuppression and silent disease while the patient was on dialysis (Kasiske et al, 2000, 2005, Lentine et al, 2005, Marcén et al, 2006). In a retrospective study from the USA, the prevalence of coronary artery disease, defined as acute myocardial infarction, coronary revascularization procedures, or death due to coronary disease, was 23% at 15 years of follow-up and it was the cause of 18.7% of mortality (Kasiske et al, 1996). In a multicenter, retrospective study performed in Spain, the prevalence of coronary artery disease was 6.8% at 5 years (Marcén et al, 2006) and very similar findings have been reported from France (Doucloux et al, 2004), two low risk countries. Data from the United Network for Organ Sharing (UNOS) and United States Renal Data System (USRDS) registry showed that the prevalence of acute myocardial infarction was between 6% to 11 % at 3 years a 17% lower than that observed on waiting list patients (Kasiske et al, 2006, Lentine et al, 2005). Moreover, myocardial infarction has a poor prognosis and is the cause of high mortality (Herzog et al, 1998, 2000, Morales, 2008).

The diagnostic criteria and therapeutical measures must be those used in the general population and in patients with chronic renal failure (Murphy et al, 1998). As a high percentage of events occur in the first weeks or months after the procedure, efforts have to be made to prevent and treat coronary artery disease before transplantation. Several algorithms have been proposed in which patients are classified according to cardiovascular risk (Lentine et al, 2008b, Wang & Kasiske, 2010), but we have not yet the ideal diagnostic procedure for asymptomatic patients.

2.1.2 Cerebrovascular diseases

Cerebrovascular diseases include transient cerebral ischaemia, when focal neurologic symptoms resolve in 24 hours, and persistent neurological deficits documented by computed tomography or nuclear magnetic resonance. Patients with chronic renal disease have more severe atherosclerotic lesions in carotic arteries than the general population (Kennedy et al 2001). This could explain the 5 to 10 times higher risk of having ischaemic or haemorragic events when compared with the general population (Seliger et al, 2002, 2003a,b). In renal transplant recipients the annual incidence was from 0.5% to 2.3% (Abedini et al, 2009a, Aull-Watschinger et al, 2008, Cosio et al, 2005, Lentine et al, 2008a, Oliveras et al,2003), and ischaemic events predominated in a proportion of 2-3:1 compared with haemorragic events (Aull-Watschinger et al, 2008, Oliveras et al, 2003). In a long-term study, by actuarial analysis, 15% of patients who survived with a functioning graft for 15 years experienced a major crebrovascular event (Kasiske et al, 1996). The evolution of cerebrovascular diseases is poor and a mortality rate around of 50% three months after the event has been reported (Oliveras et al, 2003). In retrospective studies, cerebrovascular diseases were the cause of 5% to 8% of total mortality (Aull-Watschinger et al, 2008, Howard et al, 2002). Only the Assessment of Lescol in Renal Transplantation (ALERT) study has prospectively investigated these complications, the incidence was 8.8% during the 6.7 year follow-up period, and 21% of the cerebrovascular events, 48% of haemorragic and 8% of ischaemic, were fatal and accounted for 9.9% of total mortality (Abedini et al, 2009a).

2.1.3 Peripheral vascular disease

The incidence and clinical outcome of this complication have been seldom studied in renal transplant recipients. The diagnostic criteria include: intermitent claudication, ulceration with long-vessel disease on flow studies, amputations, by-pass or percutaneous angioplasty. The frequency reported was variable. In an old study, in which only amputation or revascularization procedures were included, the cumulative incidence was 15% at 15 years (Kasiske et al, 1996). In other studies, the incidence increased with the length of follow-up, from 2.1% at 1 year to 5.9% at 10 years (Sung et al, 2000). Data from the UNOS registry have shown a cumulative incidence of 20% in diabetic and 5% in nondiabetic patients at 3 years (Snyder et al, 2006). As the disease develops along years it is difficult to distinguish risk factors due to transplantation from those present before. The need of amputation is low about 2 to 3% (Sung et al, 2000). The disease by itself is not a cause of mortality but patients suffering from it have an increased risk of death with a functioning graft (Snyder et al, 2006, Sung et al, 2000).

3. Functional heart diseases

3.1 Congestive heart failure

Congestive heart disease is defined as dysnea plus at least two of the following characteristics; increased yugular venous pressure, basal lung rales, lung hypertension in radiography or pulmonary edema (Harnett et al, 1995). In dialysis patients, congestive heart failure is 36 times more frequent than in the general population and it is a mortality risk factor (Collins 2002, Stack &Bloemberg, 2001). Congestive heart disease has been studied less than coronary artery disease in the renal transplant population and it is associated with coronary artery disease in 30% of cases (Rigatto, 2003a,b). Its annual incidence was 3-5 times that of the general population, reached a cumulative incidence of 18.3% at 3years and was associated with poor graft function (Abbott et al, 2003b, Lentine et al, 2005, Rigatto, 2003a,b). It has a high impact on mortality, similar to that of coronary artery disease (Lentine et al, 2005).

3.2 Left ventricular hypertrophy

There are two types of left ventricular hypertrophy; concentric ventricular hypertrophy and dilatation with or without hypertrophy. The first one is associated with volume overload and the second with aortic insuficiency or severe anemia. Both types are more frequent in patients in renal failure than in the general population, reaching 20-50% in patients with chronic renal failure (Levin et al, 1996, Tucker et al, 1997) and up to 70% in those on dialysis (Foley et al, 1995, McGregor et al, 1998). Several prospective studies have shown that left ventricular hypertrophy improved during the first two years after transplantation but it was still present in about 40% of renal transplant recipients (Rigatto et al, 2000, Teruel et al, 1987). Factors related with no improvement were: age, left ventricular morphology, duration and severity of hypertension and time averaged pulse pressure (Rigatto et al, 2000). Moreover, renal transplant also improved ventricular function in most patients even in those with severe impairment (Parfrey et al 1995, Wali et al, 2005). However these findings have been recently questioned when cardiac structure was assessed by magnetic resonance

(Patel et al, 2008). Parameters of ventricular hypertrophy or impaired cardiac function were associated with increased risk of cardiovascular events and cardiovascular mortality in renal transplant recipients (Aull-Watschinger et al, 2008, McGregor et al, 2000). In a nonrandomized study, conversión from CNI to sirolimus regressed left ventricular mass thickness regardless of blood pressure changes, thus suggesting non-hemodynamic-effect mechanisms on the left ventricular mass (Paoletti et al, 2008).

3.3 Arrhythmias

Atrial fibrilation is the most common cardiac rythm disorder in the general population and in patients on dialysis (Harnett et al 1995, Zebe 2001). Data from renal transplant recipients, despite being a high risk population due to the pre-transplant history and the high prevalence of risk factors related to this complication such as hypertension and obesity, have only been recently reported. Registry studies from the USA have shown a cumulative prevalence around 7 % at 3 years (Abbott et al, 2003a, Lentine et al, 2006). Risk factors for postransplantation atrial fibrilation include older age, male gender, renal failure for hypertension, and coronary artery disease. As in the general population atrial fibrilation was associated with an increased cardiovascular mortality, up to 3 times higher than patients without the disease (Abbott et al, 2003, Lentine et al, 2006).

4. Cardiovascular risk factors

Three types of cardiovascular risk factors are generally identified in transplant recipients (Table 2). 1) Traditional risk factors are those which in the general population are associated with cardiovascular diseases, and their treatment decreases the incidence of these complications. They include; older age, hypertension, hypercholesterolemia, diabetes mellitus, tobacco smoking and obesity. Their incidence is mostly increased in advanced CKD stages (Ansell et al, 2007, Karthikeyan et al, 2004, Marcén et al, 2005). 2) Risk factors associated with the transplant; anaemia, graft dysfunction and related complications, proteinuria, and immunosuppression. Finally,3), non-traditional or emergent factors such as hyperhomocysteinemia and chronic inflammation.

Traditional risk factors	Transplant related factors	Nontraditional or emergent factors
Age Sex Hypertension Dislipidemia Diabetes Smoking Obesity	Anaemia Graft dysfunction Proteinuria Immunosuppression	Hyperhomocysteinemia Inflammation

Table 2. Cardiovascular risk factors

4.1 Traditional risk factors

4.1.1 Age and sex

Older age is a nonmodifiable cardiovascular risk factor in the general population. In renal transplant recipients it was associated with an increased risk for cardiovascular atherosclerotic diseases; ischemic heart disease, cerebrovascular disease, and peripheral vascular disease (Kasiske et al, 1996, Kasiske et al, 2006, Marcén et al, 2006, Oliveras et al, 2003, Rigatto et al, 2002, Snyder et al, 2006), and also for functional heart diseases; congestive heart failure, left ventricular hypertrophy and arrhythmias (Abbott et al, 2003, Lentine et al 2006, Rigatto et al, 2000, Rigatto et al, 2002). Male gender is a risk factor for ischemic heart disease and peripheral vascular disease (Kasiske, 1988, Rigatto et al, 2002, Kasiske et al, 2006, Marcén et al, 2006, Snyder et al, 2006) and female gender for cerebrovascular disease and congestive heart failure (Abbott et al, 2003, Lentine et al, 2008a).

4.1.2 Hypertension

It is a common complication in renal transplant recipients. Its prevalence varies between 70 and 90%. There are several causes and mechanisms of high blood pressure and many patients have several of them. A previous history of hypertension, artery graft stenosis, the own recipient kidneys, overweight, chronic graft dysfunction and immunosuppressive agents such as calcineurin inhibitors (CNIs), cyclosporine and tacrolimus, are the conditions generally associated with post-transplant hypertension (Koomans & Ligtenberg, 2001, Zhang et al, 2003). Among CNIs, cyclosporine seems to increase blood pressure more than tacrolimus (Ligtenberg et al, 2001). It has been associated with an increased risk of ischemic heart disease, congestive heart failure, left ventricular hypertrophy (Rigatto 2002) and with mortality (Kasiske et al 2004, Fernández-Fresnedo et al, 2005).

One characteristic of post-transplant hypertension is the lack of control despite treatment. In a study of 1295 patients, only 12.4% had a normal blood pressure one year after grafting and more than 95% of them were on antihypertensive therapy (Kasiske et al, 2004). Others found in their series a higher number of patients with normal blood pressure without therapy (26.0%) but they also reported that 32.0% of patients had uncontrolled blood pressure while they were on treatment (Tutone et al, 2005). Cross-sectional studies have shown that between 60 to 100% of patients according to the stage of graft failure had a blood pressure above 130/80 mm Hg and most of them were on antihypertensive therapy (Karthikeyan et al, 2004, Marcén et al, 2009a).

There are not specific blood pressure levels for renal transplant recipients and the reference values are those of the general population. As the renal transplant recipients are considered a high risk population for cardiovascular diseases, a blood pressure of 130/80 mm Hg has been recommended. Treatment includes changing life style, reducing the diet sodium intake, physical activity, low consumption of alcohol and antihypertensive agents (Choubanian et al, 2003). There are no specific antihypertensive agents to treat post-transplant hypertension and all agents can be used. The prescription has to be done taking into account the characteristic of each patient (KDIGO, 2009, Park & Luan, 2005). Most patients need to be treated with several antihypertensive agents. Studies in which angiotensin converting enzyme inhibitors or angiotensin receptor blockers have been compared with other antihypertensive agents have shown controversial results, and there are no studies in which the superiority of one agent over the others on patient survival has been definitively established (Opelz et al, 2006, Hiremath et al, 2007). There are not randomized, prospective studies that have demonstrated the beneficial effects of controlling blood pressure in renal transplant recipients, but it has been assumed that they would be similar to those obtained in the general population. However, retrospective registry studies have shown that decreasing blood pressure even several years after hypertension appearance was associated with a better patient outcome (Opelz et al, 2005).

4.1.3 Dyslipidemia

Lipid disorders are more common in renal transplant recipients than in the general population and include high levels of cholesterol and triglycerides. Also frequent are high levels of LDL-cholesterol, lipoprotein (a) and apolipoprotein B, while HDL-cholesterol can be high, normal or low. Hypercholesterolemia, total serum cholesterol above 200 mg/dl and LDL-cholesterol above 100 mg/dl, have been observed in up to 90 % of patients (Aakhus et al, 1996, Hricik et al, 1994). Several factors have been associated with hyperlipidemia; genetic predisposition, body weight gain, graft dysfunction, proteinuria, diabetes, immunosuppressive and antihypertensive agents (Massy & Kasiske, 1996).

Among immunosuppressive agents, corticosteroids, CNIs and mammalian target of rapamycin inhibitors (mTORs), sirolimus and everolimus, are those most frequently associated with hyperlipidemia. The mechanisms of corticosteroid-induced hyperlipidemia are through promoting insulin resistence and hyperinsulinism, reduction of lipoprotein lipase activity, overproduction of triglycerides and secretion of VDLD-cholesterol (Hricik et al, 1994). CNIs inhibit bile acid synthesis and binding of the drugs to the LDL-cholesterol receptor with reduction of its activity. Also a decrease in lipoprotein lipase activity and impairment of LDL-cholesterol catabolism may be involved (Moore et al, 2001). These effects seem to be more prominent with cyclosporine than with tacrolimus (Ligtenberg et al, 2001, Moore et al, 2001, Vincenti et al, 2002). mTORs are the agents with stronger hyperlipidemic effect (Kasiske et al, 2008), which is more accentuated in those patients also treated with cyclosporine than in those treated with tacrolimus (Ciancio et al, 2004). The pathogenesis of mTOR dyslipidemia is unclear. A reduced catabolism of apo B100 could be the cause of increased triglycerides and cholesterol and decreased lipoprotein lipase activity and increased free fatty acid levels may be contributing factors. Their effects are dose dependent and rapidly reversible (Kasiske et al, 2008, Webster et al, 2006).

As in the general population, hypercholesterolemia and low HDL-cholesterol levels are associated with ischemic heart disease (Kasiske, 1988 Kasiske et al, 1996, Kasiske et al, 2006, Marcén et al, 2006, Rigatto et al, 2002). The treatment of this complication may follow the recommendations given to the general population and confirmed by the transplant guidelines (KDIGO, 2009). It is important to begin with a rich diet of monosaturated fats, but diet therapy does not control hyperlipidemia and lipid-lowering agents have to be added. 3-Hydroxy-3methylglutaryl coenzyme A reductase inhibitors (statins) are the elective pharmacologic agents in hypercholesterolemic patients. Fluvastatin, pravastatin and atorvastatin seem to have a more favourable safety profile over simvastatin and lovastatin. In patients with hypertriglyceridemia, gemfibrocil is the pharmacological agent of choice. Some observational studies have shown an association between statin therapy and better patient outcome (Cosio et al, 2002a, Wiesbauer et al, 2008). However, the Assessment of Lescol in Renal Transplantation (ALERT) study did not show differences in the primary compound end point, despite a reduction of 32% in the LDL-cholesterol blood levels at 5 years follow-up, between recipients treated with fluvastatin compared with those on placebo (Holdaas et al, 2003). A later evaluation of the study showed the benefits of the treatment but only when statin therapy started in the first two years after transplantation and in low-risk recipients (Holdaas et al 2005, Jardine et al 2004). In case of statin intolerance or hyperlipidemia of difficult control, ezetimibe that blocks the cholesterol absorption in the brush border, alone or combined with statins, is an efficient and safe alternative (Buchanan et al 2006, Langone & Chuang, 2006).

4.1.4 Diabetes

In the renal transplant recipients, two types of diabetes mellitus can be distinguished, diabetes mellitus as the cause of end-stage renal disease and new onset diabetes mellitus (NODAT). The prevalence of diabetes mellitus as the cause of renal failure is variable among countries. In the USA, more than 20% of the patients on the waiting list or transplanted have diabetes mellitus as the cause of renal failure (Collins et al, 2008). The incidence of NODAT varies between 2% to 50% in the first posttransplantation year according to the criteria used in its definition (Montori et al, 2002). When the American Diabetes Association criteria were used, the incidence of NODAT at 12 months was 13% and of glucose intolerance of 33% in a study performed at the Mayo Clinic (Cosio et al, 2005). Similar findings have been observed in a prospective study from Spain (Marcén et al, 2006). As the term NODAT does not include states of impaired fasting glucose and impaired glucose tolerance which pose a cardiovascular threat similar to overt diabetes, the term transplant associated hyperglycemia (TAH) has been proposed (Crutchlow & Bloom, 2008). The most common risk factors associated with NODAT or TAH include: race, blacks or hispanics, older age, obesity, family history, hepatitis C virus infection and some immunosuppressive agents such as corticosteroids, CNIs (tacrolimus) and mTORs (Crutchlow & Bloom, 2007, Montori et al, 2002).

The effects of immunosuppresive agents on glucose metabolism have been widely reviewed (Heisel et al, 2004, Miller, 2002, Morales & Dominguez, 2006). Both CNIs, cyclosporine and tacrolimus, cause NODAT by inducing insulin resistance or by impaired insulin secretion (Hornum et al, 2010). Early trials designed to compare the efficacy and security of cyclosporine and tacrolimus, and registry data showed a higher incidence of NODAT in patients treated with tacrolimus (Kasiske et al, 2003, Mayer et al, 1997, Vincenti et al, 2002) and more recent studies have confirmed these findings (Vincenti et al 2007). Also mTORs are associated with an increased risk of NODAT (Johnston et al, 2008). These agents induce hyperglucemia by impairing insulin-mediated suppression of hepatic glucose production, by ectopic triglyceride deposition leading to insulin resistance, or by direct β cell toxicity (Crutchlow & Bloom, 2007).

Single centre and registry studies have shown the association of NODAT with acute myocardial infarction, cerebrovascular events and mortality (Cosio et al 2002b, 2005, 2008, Kasiske et al 2003, Lentine et al, 2005, 2008). The treatment has the objective of preventing the symtoms due to uncontrolled hyperglucemia and the microvascular complications as the transplant recipients develop identical complications as the nontransplanted diabetic patients (Burroughs et al, 2007). The guidelines of the American Diabetes Association and the Joint Nacional Committee on Prevention, Detection, Evaluation, and Treatment of High Blood Pressure for patients with type 2 diabetes have been recommended (Haffner SM 2003).

4.1.5 Tobacco

The effects of tobacco on the health in the general population are well known. It is a risk factor of cardiovacular diseases, malignancies and respiratory diseases (Bartecchi et al, 1994). About 25% of the renal transplant population are active smokers after transplantation (Cosio et al 1999, Kasiske & Klinger, 2000, Zitt et al, 2007). In transplant recipients, tobacco was associated with cardiovascular diseases and mortality (Kasiske & Klinger, 2000). It has been reported that the negative impact of tobacco on health disappeared after five years, and some authors emphasize that efforts have to be made to convince the patients about the benefits of avoiding smoking. There are few data about the influence of transplant on toxic habits, but some studies suggest that transplantation constituted a strong reason to give up smoking (Banas et al, 2008).

4.1.6 Obesity

Obesity is a growing health problem in the general population. Epidemiological studies have shown its association with a higher morbidity and mortality due to cardiovascular diseases (Allison et al, 1999). Transplant recipients have a tendency to gain body weight mostly in the first year after grafting. In a study performed in our Unit, the mean body weight gain in the first year was 5 kg or 8.7 % of the body weight at the time of transplantation and the percentage of obese patients increased nearly two fold, from 6.5% to 11.7% (Marcén et al, 2007). Inappropriate dietary habits, decreased physical activity, and increased appetite as a result of well-being and corticosteroid therapy are among the causes of owerweight and obesity after transplantation.

Both body weight gain and obesity (body mass index >30 kg/m2) are associated with an increased risk for NODAT, hypertension, hyperlipidemia and metabolic syndrome which are cardiovascular risk factors (Armstrong et al, 2005, El-Agroudy et al 2004). The effects of weight gain and obesity on graft and patient outcome are controversial. Some authors do not find that the complication has any impact on patient mortality (Chang et al 2007, Marcén at al, 2007, Massarweh et al, 2005). However, other studies and registry data have shown their negative impact on patient survival due to an increased cardiovascular and infectious mortality (Aalten et al, 2006, El-Agroudy et al 2004, Meier-Kriesche et al, 2002). In our opinion, controlling weight gain and weight reduction in patients with marked obesity seems to be a goal to improve well-being and outcomes in renal transplant recipients.

4.2 Risk factors associated with transplantation

4.2.1 Anaemia

Post-transplant anaemia is a common complication that has only been recently studied and considered. Its prevalence depends greatly on the definition criteria and the time post-transplant. Nowadays, there is a trend toward the use of the World Health Organization criteria which define anaemia as serum haemoglobin less than 12 g/dl in women and less than 13 g/dl in men. The prevalence of anaemia is about 90% during the first posttransplant weeks and decreases to 25% to 35% at 12 months and remains stable or slightly increases thereafter (Kamar et al, 2008, Vanrenterghem et al, 2003, Yorgin et al, 2002). In cross-sectional studies the prevalence of anaemia reached more than one third of patients and it was severe, serum haemoglobin below 11 g/dl, in about 10% (Karthikeyan et al, 2004, Marcen et al, 2009a, Molnar et al, 2007, Vanrenterghem et al, 2003). The origen of anaemia is multifactorial and graft function is the most important factor (Shah et al, 2006, Vanrenterghem et al, 2003, Yorgin et al, 2002). However, it does not completely explain post-transplant anaemia, as renal transplant recipients have more severe anaemia for each chronic renal disease stage when compared with nontransplantation subjects (Chadban et al, 2007). Several immunosuppressive agents such as azathioprine, mycophenolate mofetil (MMF), enteric coated mycophenolic acid (EC-MPA) and mTORs may cause anemia due to bone marrow toxicity or to disorders on iron homeostasis (Augustine et al, 2004, Fishbane et al, 2009, Vanrenterghem et al, 2003, Wang et al, 2004). The combination of MMF or EC-MPA with mTORs is specially toxic for the bone marrow (Hricik, 2003, Rigatto, 2006). Other

medications as angiotensin converting enzyme inhibitors and angiotensin receptor blockers are known to cause anaemia and should be cautiously used.
Recent studies have shown an association between anaemia and graft survival, cardiovascular diseases and mortality. Post-transplant anaemia seems to be a risk factor of congestive heart failure and of left ventricular hypertrophy but not of ischaemic heart disease (Borrow et al, 2008, Rigatto et al, 2002, 2003b). In addition, anaemia has been associated with increased mortality in some studies (Chhabra et al, 2008, Imoagene-Oyedeji et al, 2006, Kamar et al, 2008, Molnar et al, 2007) but not in others (Winkelmayer et al, 2006). The treatment of anaemia must follow the recommendations given for patients with chronic kidney disease in the Kidney Disease Outcomes Quality Initiative (KDOQI) guidelines (KDIGO, 2009). Iron supplementation and erythropoiesis stimulant agents should be administered to maintain serum haemoglobin between 11 and 12 g/dl.

4.2.2 Graft dysfunction

Renal function measured by the estimated glomerular filtration rate (eGFR) is a cardiovascular risk factor in the general population (Go et al, 2004). An important number of renal transplant recipients have different stages of renal failure (Figure 2), and at least two thirds have chronic renal failure defined by an eGFR below 60 ml/min/1.73m2 (Ansell et al, 2007, Karthikeyan et al, 2004, Marcén et al, 2005). As cardiovascular diseases are the leading cause of renal transplant recipient mortality, it seems logical to think in the existence of some links between premature cardiovascular death and poor graft function. Registry and prospective studies have demonstrated a correlation betwen serum creatinine and cardiovascular events or cardiovascular mortality (Fellstrom et al, 2005, Meier-Kriescheet al, 2003, Pilmore et al, 2010, Soveri et al, 2006). However, for other authors the increased cardiovascular risk of patients with poor graft function is mostly due to the effects of hypertension and anaemia than to graft failure itself (Rigatto et al, 2002). Moreover, uncontrolled hyperparathyroidism mostly in recipients with poor graft function may be a risk factor for progression of coronary artery calcification (Mazzaferro et al, 2009). The treatment of renal dysfunction includes the control of hypertension and dyslipidemias (Arias et al, 2005, Opelz et a, 2005, Wiesbauer et al, 2008) as well as the use of non-nephrotoxic immunosuppressive agents as MMF, EC-MPA and belatacept and dose reduction or withdrawal of CNIs.
The prevalence of proteinuria in the renal transplant recipients is between 7.5 and 45% (Knoll, 2009). It is a risk factor of progressive renal function loss and of cardiovascular disease in nontransplantation patients. Retrospective studies have reported that proteinuria is an important predictor of cardiovascular events and mortality in renal transplant recipients (Fernandez-Fresnedo et al, 2002, Roodnat 2001). It is important to note that proteinuria is frequently associated with graft dysfunction, hypertension and obesity and the effects of proteinuria on cardiovascular events could be mediated by these conditions or viceversa. Treatment of proteinuria includes control of hypertension, maintaning blood pressure levels below 120/80 mm Hg, of dyslipidemias and of overweigth, and avoiding immunosuppressive agents associated with proteinuria as mTORs (Amer & Cosio, 2009). Angiotensin converting enzime inhibitors and angiotensin receptor blockers are the elective agents of treatment of hypertension in patients with proteinuria because of their antiproteinuric effects. However, these agents can deteriorate graft function and increase the severity of anaemia, both cardiovascular risk factors as well. Moreover, there are no definitive studies which support the effectiveness of this treatment.

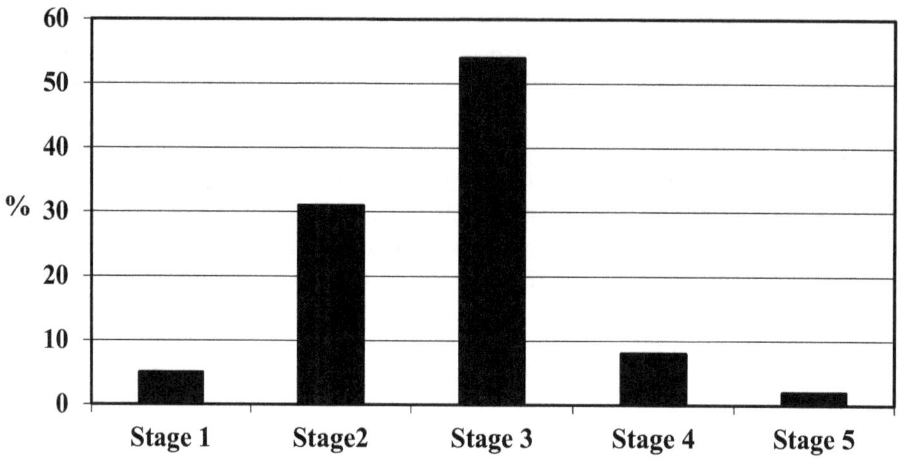

Fig. 2. Distribution of chronic kidney disease stages at 12 months in 447 renal transplant recipients (Ramón y Cajal Hospital)

4.2.3 Immunosuppression

The effects of immunosuppressive agents in cardiovascular risk factors have been previously reviewed (Miller, 2002, Marcén, 2009b, Morales & Dominguez-Gil, 2006). In addition, the impact of these agents on each cardiovascular risk factor has already been described. Corticosteroids and CNIs are the agents with worst cardiovascular risk profile, increasing the incidence and severity of traditional risk factors such as hypertension, hyperlipidemia, diabetes and obesity. CNIs also are nephrotoxic and cause graft function impairment. mTORs increase the risk of anaemia, hyperlipidemia, diabetes and proteinuria (Webster et al, 2006, Schena et al, 2009). MMF and EC-MPA may increase the risk of anaemia but have no impact in the other cardiovascular risk factors. Combinations of CNIs with MMF and EC-MPA or with mTOR allow corticosteroid withdrawal without harm. On the other hand, MMF and EC-MPA and mTORs alone or in combination can be used for CNI dose reduction or withdrawal. All these strategies have been shown to be effective in improving cardiovascular risk but there are no prospective studies in which this improvement is followed by a lower incidence of cardiovascular events or mortality (Schena et al, 2009). Among the new immunosuppressive agents, belatacept improved short-term cardiovascular risk profile and graft function when compared with cyclosporine (Vincenti et al, 2010, Durrbach et al 2010). However, phase II trials with tasocitinib have shown no improvement in hyperlipidemia and blood pressure when compared with patients who received tacrolimus (Busque et al, 2009).

4.3 Emergent risk factors

4.3.1 Hyperhomocysteinemia

Homocystein is a sulfur amino acid produced in all cells, and hyperhomocysteinemia has been considered a cardiovascular risk factor in the general population. Hyperhomocysteinemia is present in around 60% to 70% of renal transplant recipients. Homocystein levels are related with graft function, folic acid levels, serum albumin, age, and treatment with CNIs (Bostom et al, 1999, Ducloux et al, 2000, Friedman et al, 2002). The impact of homocystein levels on cardiovascular events is controversial. Some authors found an association between the homocystein levels and cardiovascular diseases (Ducloux et al, 2000, 2004) and a prospective study has shown that homocystein levels above 12 µmol/l were associated with 2.44 times increased mortality (Winkelmayer et al, 2005). Other authors have not found this association (Hagen et al, 2001). The treatment consists in the administration of folic acid supplements (5 mg/day) even with normal folic acid levels (Fernandez-Miranda et al, 2000). The efficacy of this therapy in the prevention of cardiovascular events has been examined in the Folic Acid for Vascular Outcome Reduction in Transplantation (FAVORIT). This trial should contribute to answer this question (Bostom et al, 2009).

4.3.2 Inflammation

C-reactive protein (CRP) is an acute phase marker of inflammation. It is produced by the liver under control of several citokines. In the general population, C-reactive protein is associated with obesity and poor renal function (Stuveling et al, 2003). It is also a negative predictor of acute myocardial infarction, cerebrovascular disease and cardiovascular mortality (Ridker et al, 1997). In renal transplant recipients, its levels are associated with graft function, waist circumference and smoking (Van Ree et al, 2005). The association between graft function and C-reactive protein levels could be explained by the situation of chronic low-grade inflammation, by being a marker of graft-mediated immune response or by a decreased renal excretion. As in the general population, it has been considered a risk factor of cardiovascular disease and mortality (Ducloux et al 2004, Winkelmayer et al 2004). Data from the ALERT study have confirmed the previous findings, baseline levels of CRP as well as of IL-6, another inflammation marker, were independently associated with major cardiovascular events and all-cause mortality (Abedini et al, 2009b). Results from a retrospective study have shown an association between MMF therapy and less inflammation than other immunosuppressive agents (Wong et al, 2007).

5. Therapeutical strategies

The management of each particular cardiovascular disease in renal transplant recipients should be similar to that used in the general population. In addition, clinical trials have demonstrated that cardiovascular events and cardiovascular mortality have been reduced by controlling blood glucose, lipid levels and blood pressure in the general population. As interventional studies are lacking in the transplant population, it seems reasonable to extrapolate these findings to transplant recipients. However, transplant recipients present differences from the general population, one of them is the high incidence of graft dysfunction. Preserving graft function has to be a goal in the management of transplant recipients and this could be partly accomplished by controlling the traditional cardiovascular risk factors and by a prudent use of immunosuppressive agents. CNIs minimization or withdrawal may be individually considered. Additional interventions such as treatment of anaemia with erytropoyesis stimulating agents could help in the prevention of cardiovascular diseases but the optimal haemoglobin threshold has to be determined. The benefits of lowering homocysteine levels have not been proved. In addition, long-term interventional studies should be performed in order to improve graft and patient outcomes (Table 3).

Control of cardiovascular risk factors	Preserving graft function	Treating emergent factors
Blood pressure Dislipidemias Diabetes Smoking Obesity Anaemia	Minimization/avoidance of CNIs Control of proteinuria	Folic acid supplements Aspirin

Table 3. Prevention and treatment of cardiovascular diseases after transplantation.

6. Summary

Cardiovascular diseases are common after transplantation. Coronary vascular disease, cerebrovascular disease and congestive heart failure are the diseases most commonly associated with mortality. The increased incidence of cardiovascular events could be partly explained by the high prevalence of traditional risk factors which are not adequately controlled and by the presence of renal dysfunction. Pretransplant evaluation of candidates, control of traditional risk factors and preservation of graft function should be the measures taken to improve patient outcome. The control of traditional risk factors has been effective in the reduction of cardiovascular events in the general population and there are no reasons to believe that it does not work in the transplant population. In addition, adequate control of traditional risk factors could preserve progression of graft failure. A prudent use of immunosuppressive agents could also help to improve the cardiovascular risk profile and graft function. The benefits of additional interventions need to be proved.

7. References

Aakhus, S., Dahl, K. & Widerøe, TE. (1863). Hyperlipidaemia in renal transplant patients. *J Intern Med*. Vol.239, No.5, (May 1996), pp.407-415. ISSN: 0954-6820.

Aakhus, S., Dahl, K. & Wideroe, TE. (1986). Cardiovascular morbidity and risk factors in renal transplant patients. *Nephrol Dial Transplant*. Vol. 14, No.3, (March 1999) pp.648-654. ISSN: 0931-0509.

Aakhus, S., Dahl, K. & Wideroe, TE. (1987). Cardiovascular disease in stable renal transplant patients in Norway: morbidity and mortality during a 5-yr follow-up. *Clin Transplant*. Vol. 18, No.5, (October 2004), pp.596-604. ISSN: 0902-0063.

Aalten, J., Christiaans, MA., de Fijter, H., Hené, R., van der Heijde, JH., Roodnat. J., Surachno, J. & Hoitsma, A. (1988). The influence of obesity on short- and long-term graft and patient survival after renal transplantation. *Transplant Int*. Vol.19, No.11 (November 2006), PP. 901-907. ISSN.0934-0874.

Abbott, KC., Reynols, JC., Taylor, AJ. & Agodoa, LY. (2001). Hospitalized atrial fibrillation after renal transplantation in the United States. *Am J Transplant* . Vol. 3, No.4, (June 2003a), pp.471-476. ISSN: 1600-6135.

Abbott, KC., Yuan, CM., Taylor, AJ., Cruess, DF. & Agodoa, LY. (1990). Early renal insufficiency and hospitalized heart disease after renal transplantation in the era of modern immunosuppression. *J Am Soc Nephrol* Vol.14, No.9, (November 2003b), pp.2358-2365, ISSN: 1046-6673.

Abedini, S., Holme, I., Fellstrom, B., Jardine, A., Cole, E., Maes, B. & Holdaas, H. on behalf of the ALERT study group. (1963). Cerebrovascular events in renal transplant recipients. *Transplantation*. Vol.87, No.1, (January 2009a), pp.112-7. ISSN: 0041-1337.

Abedini, S., Holme, I., März, W., Weihrauch, G., Fellstróm, B., Jardine, A., Cole, E., Maes, B., Neumayer, H-H., Gronhagen-Riska, C., Ambühl, P. & Holdaas, H on behalf of the ALERT study group. (2006). Inflammation in renal transplantation. *Clin J Am Soc Nephrol* Vol.4, No.7, (July 2009b), pp. 1246-1254. ISSN: 1555-9041.

Allison, DB., Fontaine, KR., Manson, JE., Stevens, J. & Vantallie, TB. (1883). Annual deaths attibutable to obesity in the United States. *JAMA* Vol.282, No.16, (October 1999), pp.1530-1538, ISSN. 0098-7484.

Amer, H. & Cosio, FG. (1990). Significance and management of proteinuria in kidney transplant recipients. *J Am Soc Nephrol.* Vol.20, No.12, (December 2009), pp. 2490-2492, ISSN: 1046-6673.

Ansell, D., Udayarej, UP., Steenkamp, R. & Dudley, CRK. (2001). Chronic renal failure in kidney transplant recipients. Do they receive optimum care?: data from the UK renal registry. *Am J Transplant* Vol.7, No.5, (May 2007), pp.1167-1176. ISSN:1600-6135.

Arias, M., Fernández-Fresnedo, G., Rodrigo, E., Ruiz, JC., González-Cotorruelo, J. & Gómez-Alamillo, C. (1972). Non-Immunologic intervention in chronic allograft nephropathy. *Kidney Int* Vol.99 (December 2005), pp.S118-S123, ISSN: 0085-2538.

Armstrong, KA., Campbell, SB., Hawley, CM., Nicol. DL., Johnson, DW. & Isbel, NM. (2001). Obesity is associated with worsening cardiovascular risk factor profiles and proteinuria progression in renal transplant recipients *Am J Transplant* . Vol.5, No.11, (November 2005), pp.2710-2718, ISSN.1600-6135.

Augustine, JJ., Knauss, TC., Schulak, JA., Bodziak, KA., Siegel, C. & Hricik, DE. (2001). Comparative effects of sirolimus and mycophenolate mofetil on erythropoiesis in kidney transplant patients. *Am J Transplant*. Vol.4, No.12, (December 2004), pp.2001-2006, ISSN.1600-6135.

Aull-Watschinger, S., Konstantin, H., Demetriou, D., Schillinger, M., Habicht, A., Hörl, WH. & Watschinger, B. (1986). Pre-transplant predictors of cerebrovascular events after kidney transplantation. *Nephrol Dial Transplant* Vol. 23, No. 4 (April 2008), pp. 1429-1435, ISSN: 0931-0509.

Banas, MC., Banas, B., Wolf, J., Hoffman, U., Krüger, B., Böger, CA., Orth, SR. & Krämer, BK. (1986). Smoking behaviour of patients before and after renal transplantation. *Nephrol Dial Transplant* Vol.23, No.4, (April 2008), pp.1442-1446, ISSN.0931-0509.

Bartecchi, CE., MacKenzie, TD. & Schrier, RW. (1812). The human cost of tobacco use (first of two parts). *New Engl J Med.* Vol.330, No.13 (March 1994), pp.907-912, ISSN. 0028-4793.

Borrows, R., Loucaidou, M., Chusney, G., Borrows, S., Tromp, JV., Cairns, T., Griffith, M., Hakim, N., McLean, A., Palmer, A., Papalois, V. & Taube, D. (1986). Anaemia and congestive heart failure early post-renal transplantation. *Nephrol Dial Transplant.* Vol.23, No.5, (May 2008), pp.3:1728-1734, ISSN.0931-0509.

Bostom, AG., Gohh, RY., Beaulieu, AJ., Han, H., Jacques, PF., Selhub, J., Dworkin, L. & Rosenberg, IH. (1963). Determinants of fasting plasma total homocysteine levels among chronic stable renal transplant recipients. *Transplantation*. Vol.68, No.2, (July 1999), pp.257-261, ISSN: 0041-1337.

Bostom, AG., Carpenter, MA., Hunsicker, L., Jacques, PF., Kusek, JW., Levey, AS., McKenney, JL., Mercier, RY., Pfeffer, MA. & Selhub, J. (1981). Baseline characteristics of participants in the folic acid for vascular outcome reduction in transplantation (FAVORIT) trial. *Am J Kidney Dis.* Vol.53, No.1, (January 2009), pp.121-128, ISSN: 0272-6386.

Buchanan, C., Smith, L, Corbett, J., Nelson, E. & Shihab F. (2001). A retrospective analysid of ezetimibe treatment in renal transplant recipients. *Am J Trasplant* Vol.6, No.4, (April 2006), pp.770-774, ISSN: 1600-6135.

Burroughs, TE., Swindle, J., Takemoto, S., Lentine, KL., Machnicki, G., Irish, WD., Brennan, DC. & Schnitzler, MA. (1963). Diabetic complications associated with new-onset diabetes mellitus in renal transplant recipients. *Transplantation* Vol.83, No.8 (April 2007), pp.1027-1034, ISSN. 0041-1337.

Busque, S., Leventhal, J., Brennan, DC., Steinberg, S., Klintmalm, G., Shah, T., Mulgaonkar, S., Bromberg, JS., Vincenti, F., Harharan, S., Slakey, D., Peddi, VR., Fisher, RA., Lawendy, N., Wang, C. & Chan, G. (2001). Calcineurin-inhibitor-free immunosuppression based on the JAK inhibitor CP-690,550: a pilot study in the novo kidney allograft recipients. *Am J Transplant.* Vol.9, No.8 (August 2009), pp.1936-1945, ISSN: 1600-6135.

Chadban, SJ., Baines, L., Polkingghome, K., Jefferys, A., Dogra, S., Kanganas, C., Irish, A., Eris, J. & Walker, R. (1981). Anemia after kidney transplantation is not completely explained by reduced kidney function. *Am J Kidney Dis.* Vol.49, No.2, (February 2007), pp.301-309, ISSN.0272-6386.

Chhabra, D., Grafals, M., Skaro, AI., Parker, M. & Gallon, L. (2006). Impact of anemia after renal transplantation on patient and graft survival and on rate of acute rejection. *Clin J Am Soc Nephrol.* Vol.3, No.4, (July 2008), pp.1168-1174, ISSN.1555- 9041.

Chang, SH., Coates, PT. & McDonald, SP. (1963). Effects of body mass index at transplant on outcomes of kidney transplantation. *Transplantation.* Vol.84, No.8, (October 2007), pp.981-987, ISSN. 0041-1337.

Chobanian, AV., Bakris, GL., Black, HR., Cushman, WC., Green, LA., Izzo, JL. Jones, DW., Materson, BJ., Oparil, S., Wright, JT. & Roccella, EJ. (1883). Seventh report of the joint national comittee on prevention, detection, evaluation, and treatment of high blood pressure. The JNC 7 report. *JAMA.* Vol. 289, No.19, (December 2003), pp.2560-2572, ISSN: 0098-7484.

Ciancio, G., Burke, GW., Gaynor, JJ., Mattiazzi, A., Roth, D., Kupin, W., Nicolas, M., Ruiz, P., Rosen, A. & Miller, J. (1963). A randomized long-term trial of tacrolimus/sirolimus versus tacrolimus/mycophenolate mofetil, versus cyclosporine (NEORAL)/ sirolimus in renal transplantation II. Survival, function, and protocol compliance at 1 year. *Transplantation* Vol.77, No.2, (January 2004), pp.252-258, ISSN: 0041-1337.

Collins AJ. (1972). Impact of congestive heart failure and other cardiac diseases on patients outcomes. *Kidney Int.* Suppl 81 (October 2002), pp.S3-7, ISSN: 0085-2538.

Collins, AJ., Foley, RN., Herzog, C., Chavers, BM., Gilbertson, D., Ishani, A., Kasiske, BL., Liu, J., Mau, LW., McBean, M., Murray, A., St Peter, W., Guo, H., Li, Q., Li, S., Li, S., Peng, Y., Qiu, Y., Roberts, T., Skeans, M., Snyder, J., Solid, C., Wang, C., Weinhandl, E., Zaun, D., Arko, C., Chen, SC., Dalleska, F., Daniels, F., Dunning, S., Ebben, J., Frazier, E., Hanzlik, C., Johnson, R., Sheets, D., Wang, X., Forrest, B., Constantini, E., Everson, S., Eggers, PW. & Agodoa L. (2008). (1981). Excerpts from the United States Renal Data System 2007 annual data report. *Am J Kidney Dis.* Vol. 51, 1 Suppl 1, (January 2008), pp.S1-320, ISSN: 0272-6386.

Cosio, FG., Falkenhaim, MF., Pesavento, TE., Yim, S., Alamir, A., Henry, ML. & Ferguson, RM. (1987). Patient survival after renal transplantation.II. The impact of smoking . *Clin Transplant* Vol.13, No.4, (August 1999), pp.336-341. ISSN. 0902-0063.

Cosio, FG., Pesavento, TE., Pelletier, RP., Henry, M., Ferguson, RM., Kim, S. & Lemeshow, S. (1981). Patient survival after renal transplantation III: the effects of statins, *Am J Kidney Dis* Vol.40, No.3, (September 2002a), pp.638-643. ISSN. 0272-6386.

Cosio, FG., Pesavento, TE., Kim, S., Osei, K., Henry, M. & Ferguson, RM. (1972). Patient survival after renal transplantation:IV. Impact of post-transplant diabetes. *Kidney Int.* Vol.62, No.4 (October 2002b), pp. 1440-1446. ISSN. 0085-2538.

Cosio, FG., Kudva, Y., van der Velde, M., Larson, TS., Textor, SC., Griffin, MD. & Stegall, MD. (1972) New onset hyperglycemia and diabetes are associated with increased cardiovascular risk after kidney transplantation. *Kidney Int* . Vol.67, No.6, (June 2005), pp. 2415-2421. ISSN: 0085-2538.

Cosio, FG., Hickson, LJ., Griffin, MD., Stegall, MD. & Kudva, Y. (2001). Patient survival and cardiovascular risk after kidney transplantation: the challenge of diabetes. *Am J Transplant* Vol.8, No.3, (March 2008), pp.593-599, ISSN. 1600-6135.

Crutchlow MF & Bloom RD. (2006). Transplant-associated hyperglycemia:a new look at an old problem. *Clin J Am Soc Nephrol* Vol.2, No.2, (March 2007), pp.343-355, ISSN: 1555-9041

Culleton, BF. & Wilson, PWF. (1990). Cardiovascular disease: risk factors, secular trends, and therapeutic guidelines. *J Am Soc Nephrol.* Vol.9, 12 suppl, (December 1998), pp:S5-S15, ISSN: 1046-6673.

De Mattos, AM., Prather, J., Olyaei, AJ., Shibagaki, Y., Keith, DS., Mori, M., Norman, DJ. et Becker, T. (1972). Cardiovascular events following renal transplantation: role of traditional and transplant-specific risk factors. *Kidney Int.* Vol. 70, No. 4, (August 2006), pp.757-764, ISSN: 0085-2538.

Ducloux, D., Motte, G., Challier, B., Gibey, R. & Chalopin, JM. (1990). Serum total homocysteine and cardiovascular ocurrence in chronic stable renal transplant recipients: a prospective study. *J Am Soc Nephrol.* Vol.11, No.1, (January 2000), pp.134- 137, ISSN: 1046-6673.

Ducloux, D., Kazory, A. & Chalopin, JM. (1972). Predicting coronary heart disease in renal transplant recipients: a prospective study. *Kidney Int* . Vol. 66, No.1, (July 2004), pp.441-447, ISSN: 0085-2538.

Durrbach, A., Pestana, JM., Pearson, T., Vincenti, F., García, CD., Campistol, J., Rial, MdeC., Florman, S., Block, A., Di Russo, G., Xing, J., Garg, P. & Grinyo, J. (2001). A phase III study of belatacept versus cyclosporine in kidney transplants from extended criteria donors (BENEFIT-EXT study). *Am J Transplant.* Vol.10, No.3, (March 2010), pp.547-557, ISSN: 1600- 6135.

El-Agroudy, AE., Wafa, EW., Greith, OE., El-Dein, ABS. & Ghoneim, MA. (1963). Weight gain after renal transplantation is a risk factor for patient and graft outcome. *Transplantation.* Vol15, No.77, (May 2004), pp.1381-1385. ISSN.0041-1337.

Fellström, B., Jardine, AG., Soveri, I., Cole, E., Neumayer, HH., Maes, B., Gimpelewicz, C. & Holdaas, H. (1963). Renal dysfunction as a risk factor for mortality and cardiovascular disease in renal transplantation: experience from the Assessment of Lescol in Renal Transplant trial. *Transplantation* Vol.79; No.7, (August 2005), pp. 1160-1163, ISSN: 0041-1337.

Fernández-Fresnedo, G., Escallada, R., Rodrigo, E., De Francisco, AL., Cotorruelo, JG., Sanz De Castro, S., Zubimendi, JA., Ruiz, JC. & Arias, M. (1963). The risk of cardiovascular disease associated with proteinuria in renal transplant patients. *Transplantation*. Vol.76, No.8, (April 2002), pp.1345-1348, ISSN: 0041-1337.

Fernández-Fresnedo, G., Escallada, R., Martin de Francisco, AL., Ruiz, JC., Rodrigo, E., Sanz de Castro, S., GonzalezCotorruelo, .J & Arias, M. (2001). Association between pulse pressure and cardiovascular disease in renal transplant patients. Am J Transplant Vol.5, No.2, (February, 2005), pp.394-398, ISSN: 1600-6135.

Fernandez-Miranda, C., Gómez, P., Díaz-Rubio, P., Estenoz, J., Carillo, JL., Andrés, A. & Morales, JM. (1987). Plasma homocysteine levels in renal transplanted patients on cyclosporine or tacrolimus therapy: effect of treatment with folic acid. *Clin Transplant*. Vol.14, No.2, (April 2000), pp.110-114, ISSN: 0902-0063.

Fishbane, S., Cohen, DJ., Coyne, DW., Djamali, A., Singh, AK. & Wish, JB. (1972). Posttransplant anemia: the role of sirolimus. *Kidney Int* . Vol.76, No.4, (August 2009), pp.376-382, ISSN.0085-2538.

Foley, RN., Parfrey, PS., Harnett, JD., Kent, GM., Murray, DC. & Barré, PE. (1990). The prognostic importance of left ventricular geometry in uremic cardiomyopathy. *J Am Soc Nephrol*. Vol.5, No.12, (June 1995), pp. 2024-2031, ISSN: 1046-6673.

Foley, RN. Parfrey, PS. & Sarnak, MJ (1981). Clinical epidemiology of cardiovascular disease in chronic renal disease. *Am J Kidney Dis*. Vol.32, No.5, suppl.3, (November 1998), pp.S112-S119, ISSN: 0272-6386.

Friedman, AN., Rosenberg, IH., Selhub, J., Levey, AS. & Bostom, AG. (2001). Hyperhomocysteinemia in renal transplant recipients. *Am J Trasnsplant* . Vol.2, No.4, (April 2002), pp.308-313, ISSN: 1600-6135.

Go, AS., Chertow, GM., Fan, D., McCulloch, CE. & Hsu, C. (1812). Chronic kidney disease and the risks of death, cardiovascular events, and hospitalization. *N Engl J Med* Vol.351; No.13, (September 2004), pp.1296-1305, ISSN: 0028-4793.

Haffner, SM. (1978). Management of dyslipidemia in adults with diabetes. *Diabetes Care* Vol26, Suppl 1, (January 2003), pp.S83- S86. ISSN. 0149-5992.

Hagen, W., Födinger, M., Heinz, G., Buchmayer, H., Hörl, WH. & Sunder-Plassman, G. (1972). Effect of MTHFR genotypes and hyperhomocysteinemia on patient and graft survival in kidney transplant recipients. *Kidney Int* . Vol.78, (February 2001), pp.S253-S257, ISSN: 0085-2538.

Harnett, JD., Foley, RN., Kent, GM., Barre, PE., Murray, D. & Parfrey, PS. (1972). Congestive heart failure in dialysis patients: prevalence, incidence, prognosis and risk factors. *Kidney Int* . Vol.47, No.3, (March 1995), pp.884-890, ISSN: 0085-2538.

Heisel O, Heisel R, Balshaw R & Keown P. (2001). New onset diabetes mellitus in patients receiving calcineurin inhibitors: a systematic review and meta-analysis. *Am J Transplant* Vol.4, No.4, (April 2004), pp.583-595, ISSN: 1600-6135.

Herzog, CA., Ma, JZ & Collins AJ (1812). Poor long-term survival after acute myocardial infarction among patients on long-term dialysis. *N Enl J Med*. Vol. 339, No.12, (September 1998), pp. 799-805, ISSN: 0028-4793.

Herzog, CA., Ma, JZ. & Collins, AJ. (1981). Long term survival of renal transplant recipients in the United States after acute myocardial infarction. *Am J Kidney Dis*. Vol. 36, No. 1, (July 2000), pp.145-153, ISSN: 0272-6386.

Hiremath, S., Ferguson, D., Doucette, S., Mulay, AV. & Knoll, GA. (2001). Renin angiotensin system blockade in kidney transplantation: a systematic review of the evidence. *Am J Transplant*. Vol.7, No.10, (October 2007), pp. 2350-2360, ISSN: 1600-6135.

Holdaas, H., Fellström, B., Jardina, AG., Holme, I., Nyberg, G., Fauchald, P., Frönhagen-Riska, C., Madsen, S., Neumayer, H-H., Cole, E., Maes, B., Ambühl, P., Olsson,

AG., Haertmann, A., Solbu, DO. & Pedersen, TR. on behalf of the Assessment of Lescol in renal transplantation (ALERT) Study Investigators. (1823). Effect of fluvastatin on cardiac outcomes in renal transplant recipients: a multicentre, randomised, placebo-controlled trial. *Lancet* Vol.361, No.9374, (June 2003), pp:2024-2031, ISSN: 0140-6736.

Holdaas, H., Fellström, B., Jardine, AG. Nyberg, G., Grönhagen-Riska, C., Madsen, S., Neumayer, HH., Cole, E., Maes, B., Ambühl, P., Logan, JO., Staffler, B. & Gimpelewicz, C.(1986). Beneficial effect of early initiation of lipid-lowering therapy following renal transplantation. *Nephrol Dial Transplant* Vol.20, No.5, (May 2005), pp.974-980, ISSN: 0931-0509.

Hornum M, Jorgensen KA, Hansen JM, Nielsen FT, Christensen KB, Mathiesen ER &Feldt-Rasmussen B. (1990). New-onset diabetes mellitus after kidney transplantation in Denmark. *Clin J Am Soc Nephrol* Vol.5, No.4, (April, 2010), pp.709-716, ISSN. 1555-9041.

Howard, RJ., Patton, PR., Reed, AI., Hemming, AW., Van der Werf, WJ., Pfaff, WW., Srinivas, TR. & Scornik JC. (1963). The changing causes of graft loss and death after kidney transplantation. *Transplantation.* Vol. 73, No. 12, (April 2002), pp.1923-1928, ISSN: 0041-1337.

Hricik, DE. (1981). Posttransplant hyperlipidemia: the treatment dilemma. *Am J Kidney Dis.* Vol.23, No.5, (May 1994), pp.766-771, ISSN: 0272-6386.

Hricik, DE. (2001). Anemia after kidney transplantation-is the incidence increasing?. *Am J Transplant.* Vol.3, No.7, (July 2003), pp.771-772, ISSN.1600-6135.

Imoagene-Oyedeji, AE., Rosas, SE., Doyle, AM., Goral, S. & Bloom, RD. (1990). Posttransplantation anemia at 12 months in kidney recipients treated with mycophenolate mofetil: risk factors and implications for mortality. *J Am Soc Nephrol.* Vol.17, No.11, (November 2006), pp.3240-7, ISSN.1046-6673.

Jardine, AG., Holdaas, H., Fellström, B., Cole, E., Nyberg, G., Grönhagen-Riska, C., Madsen, S., Neumayer, HH., Maes, B., Ambühl, P., Olsson, AG., Holme, I., Fauchald, P., Gimpelwicz, C. & Pedersen, TR. (2001). Fluvastatin prevents cardiac death and myocardial infarction in renal transplant recipients: Pos-hoc subgroup analyses of the ALERT study. *Am J Transplant* Vol4, No.6 (June 2004), pp.988-995, ISSN: 1600-6135.

Johnston, O., Rose, CL., Webster, AC. & Gill, JS. (1990). Sirolimus is associated with new-onset diabetes in kidney transplant recipients. *J Am Soc Nephrol* Vol.19, No.7, (July 2008), pp.1411-1418, ISSN.1046-6673.

Kamar, N. & Rostaing, L. (1963). Negative impact of one-year anemia on long-term patient and graft survival in kidney transplant patients receiving calcineurin inhibitors and mycophenolate mofetil. *Transplantation.* Vol.85, No.8, (April 2008), pp.1120-1124, ISSN.0041-1337.

Karthikeyan, V., Karpinski, J., Nair, RC. & Knol,l G. (2001). The burden of chronic kidney disease in renal transplant recipients. *Am J Transplant.* Vol.4, No.2, (February 2004), pp.262-269. ISSN.1600-6135.

Kasiske, BL. (1946). Risk factors fos accelerated atheroesclerosis in renal transplant recipients. *Am J Med.* Vol. 84, No. 6, (January 1988), pp. 985-992, ISSN: 0002-9343.

Kasiske, BL., Guijarro, C., Massy, ZA., Wiederkehr, MR. & Ma, JZ. (1990). Cardiovascular disease after renal transplantation. *J Am Soc Nephrol.* Vol.7, No. 1, (January 1996), pp.158-165, ISSN: 1046-6673.

Kasiske, BL., Chakkera, HA & Roel J. (1990). Explained and unexplained ischemic heart disease risk after renal transplantation. *J Am Soc Nephrol.* Vol. 11 No. 11, (September 2000a) pp. 1735-1743. ISSN. 1046-6673.

Kasiske, BL. & Klinger, D. (1990). Cigarrette smoking in renal transplant recipients. *J Am Soc Nephrol* Vol.11, No.4, (April 2000b), pp. 753-759. ISSN. 1046-6673.

Kasiske, BL., Synder, JJ., Gilberston, D. & Matas, AJ. (2001). Diabetes mellitus after kidney transplantation in the United States. *Am J Transplant* Vol.3, No.2, (February 2003), pp.178-185, ISSN.1600-6135.

Kasiske, BL., Anjum, S., Shah, R., Skogen, J., Kandaswamy, C., Danielson, B., O'Shaughnessy, EA., Dahl, DC., Silkensen, JR., Sahadevan, M. & Snyder, JJ. (1981). Hypertension after kidney transplantation. *Am J Kidney Dis* Vol.43, No.6, (April 2004), pp. 1071-1081, ISSN: 0272-6386.

Kasiske, BL., Malik, MA. & Herzog, CA. (1963). Risk-stratified screening for ischemic heart disease in kidney transplant candidates. *Transplantation.* Vol. 80, No. 6, (September 2005), pp. 815-20. ISSN: 0041-1337.

Kasiske, BL., Maclean, JR. & Snyder JJ. (1990). Acute myocardial infarction and kidney transplantation. *J Am Soc Nephrol.* Vol. 17, No.3, (March 2006), pp. 900-907, ISSN: 1046-6673.

Kasiske, BL., de Mattos, A., Flechneer, SM., Gallon, L., Meier-Kriesche, H-U., Weir, MR. & Wilkinson, A. (2001). Mammalian target of rapamycin inhibitor dyslipidemia in kidney transplant recipients. *Am J Transplant* Vol.8, No7, (July 2008), pp. 1384-1392, ISSN: 1600-6135.

KDIGO clinical practice guideline for the care of kidney transplant recipients. (2001). *Am J Transplant.* Vol.9, Suppl 3 (November 2009), pp.S1-155. ISSN.1600-6135.

Kennedy, R., Case, C., Fathi, R., Johnson, D., Isbel, N. & Marwick, TH. (1946). Does renal failure cause an atherosclerotic milieu in patients with end-stage renal disease? *Am J Med.* Vol.110, No.3, (February 2001), pp.:198-204, ISSN: 0002-9343.

Knoll, GA. (1981). Proteinuria in kidney transplant recipients: prevalence, prognosis and evidence-based management. *Am J Kidney Dis.* Vol.54, No.6 (December 2009), pp.1131-1144, ISSN: 0272-6386.

Koomans, HE. & Ligtenberg, G. (1963). Mechanism and consequences of arterial hypertension after renal transplantation. *Transplantation* Vol.72, 6 Suppl, (September 2001), pp.S9-S12, ISSN: 0041-1337.

Langone, AJ. & Chuang, P. (1963). Ezetimibe in renal transplant patients with hyperlipidemia resistant to HMG-CoA reductase inhibitors. *Transplantation* Vol.81, No.5, (March 2006), pp.804-807, ISSN: 0041-1337.

Lentine, KL., Brennan, DC. & Schnitzler, MA. (1990). Incidence and predictors of myocardial infarction after kidney transplantation. *J Am Soc Nephrol.* Vol. 16, No. 2, (February 2005), pp.496-506. ISSN. 1046-6673.

Lentine, KL., Schnitzler, MA., Abbott, KC., Li. L., Burroughs, TE., Irish, W. & Brennan, DC. (1981). De novo congestive heart failure after kidney transplantation: a common condition with poor prognostic implications. *Am J Kidney Dis* Vol.46, No.4, (October 2005), pp.720-733, ISSN. 0272-6386.

Lentine, KL., Schnitzler, MA., Abbott, KC. Li, L., Xiao, H., Burroughs, TE., Takemoto, SK., Willoughby, LM., Gavard, JA. & Brennan, DC. (2006). Incidence, predictors, and associated outcomes of atrial fibrillation after kidney transplantation. *Clin J Am Soc Nephrol* Vol.1, No.2, (March 2006), pp.288-296, ISSN: 1555-9041.

Lentine, KL., Rocca Rey, LA., Kolli, S., Bacchi. G., Schnitzler, MA., Abbott, KC., Xiao, H. & Brennan, DC. (2006). Variations in the risk for cerebrovascular events after kidney transplant compared with experience on the waiting list and after graft failure. *Clin J Am Soc Nephrol* Vol. 3, No.4, (July 2008a), pp. 1090-1101. ISSN. 1555-9041.

Lentine, KL., Schnitzler, MA., Brennan, DC., Snyder, JJ., Hauptman, PJ., Abbott, KC., Axelrod, D., Salvalaggio, PR. & Kasiske, B. (2006). Cardiac evaluation before kidney transplantation: a practice patterns analysis in Medicare-insured dialysis patients. *Clin J Am Soc Nephrol.* Vol.3, No.4, (April 2008b), pp. 1115-24. ISSN. 1555-9041.

Levin, A., Singer, J., Thompson, CR., Ross, H. & Lewis, M. (1981). Prevalent left ventricular hypertrophy in the predialysis population : identifying opportunities for intervention. *Am J Kidney Dis* . Vol.27, No.3, (March 1996), pp. 347-354, ISSN: 0272-6386.

Ligtenberg, G., Hene, RJ., Blankestijn, PJ. & Koemans, HA (1990). Cardiovascular risk factors in renal transplant recipients: cyclosporin A versus tacrolimus. *J Am Soc Nephrol* Vol.12, No.2, (February 2001), pp.368-373, ISSN: 1046-6673..

Lindholm, A., Albrechtsen, D., Frodin, L., Tufveson, G., Persson, NH. & Lundgran, G. (1963). Ischemic heart disease-major cause of death and graft loss alter transplantation in Scandinavia. *Transplantation.* Vol. 60, No. 5, (September 1995), pp.451-457, ISSN: 0041-1337.

Marcén, R., Pascual, J., Teruel, JL. Villafruela. JJ., Rivera, ME., Mampaso, F., Burgos, FJ. & Ortuño, J. (1963). Outcome of cadaveric renal transplant patients treated for 10 years with cyclosporine. Is chronic allograft nephropathy the major cause of graft loss?. *Transplantation.* Vol.72, No.1, (July 2001), pp.57-62, ISSN: 0041-1337.

Marcén, R., Pascual, J., Tenorio, M., Ocaña, J., Teruel, JL., Villafruela, JJ., Fernández, M., Burgos & FJ., Ortuño, J. (1969). Chronic kidney disease in renal transplant recipients. *Transplant Proc.* Vol.37, No.9, (November 2005), pp.3718-3720, ISSN:0041- 1345.

Marcén, R., Morales, JM., del Castillo, D., Campistol, JM., Serón, D., Valdés, F., Anaya, F., Andrés, A., Arias, M., Bustamante, J., Capdevila, L., Escuin, F., Gil-Vernet, S., González-Molina, M., Lampreave, I., Oppenheimer, F., & Pallardó, L., for the Spanish Renal Forum. (1969). Posttransplant diabetes mellitus in renal allograft recipients: a prospective multicenter study at 2 years. *Transplant Proc* Vol.38, No.10, (December 2006), pp:3530-3532. ISSN: 0041-1345.

Marcén, R., Morales, JM., Arias, M., Fernández-Juarez, G., Fernández-Fresnedo, G., Ahdrés, A., Rodrigo, E., Pascual, J., Dominguez, B. & Ortuño, J. (1990). Ischemic heart disease after renal transplantation in patients on cyclosporine in Spain. *J Am Soc Nephrol.* Vol.17, 12 Suppl 3, (December 2006), pp.S286-S290, ISSN: 1046-6673.

Marcén, R., Fernández, A., Pascual, J., Teruel, JL., Villafruela, JJ., Rodríguez, N., Martins, J., Burgos, FJ. & Ortuño, J. (1969). High body mass index and posttransplant weigth gain are not risk factors for kidney graft and patient outcomes. *Transplant Proc* . Vol.39, No.7, (September 2007), pp.:2205-2207, ISSN. 0041-1345.

Marcén, R., del Castillo, D., Capdevila, L., Fernandez-Fresnedo, G., Rodrigo, E., Cantarell, C., Fernandez-Rodriguez, A., Lópes- Silva, MO., Camps, J., Aljama, P., Ortuño, J. & Arias, M. (1963). Achieving chronic kidney disease treatment targets in renal transplant recipients: results from a cross-sectional study in Spain. *Transplantation* Vol. 87, No.9, (May 2009a), pp. 1340-1346. ISSN.0041-1337.

Marcén, R. (1971). Immunosuppressive drugs in kidney transplantation. Impact on patient survival, and incidence of cardiovascular disease, malignancy and infection. *Drugs*. Vol.69, No.16, (November 2009b), pp. 2227-2243. ISSN.0012- 6667.

Massarweh, NN., Clayton, JL., Mangum, CA., Florman, SS. & Slakey, DP. (1963). High body mass index and short-and long- term renal allograft survival in adults. *Transplantation*. Vol.80, No.10, (November 2005), pp.1430-1434, ISSN. 0041-1337.

Massy, ZA. (1963). Hyperlipidemia and cardiovascular disease after organ transplantation. *Transplantation*. Vol.72, suppl.6, (September 2001), pp.S13-S15, ISSN: 0041-1337.

Massy, ZA. & Kasiske, BL. (1990). Post-transplant hyperlipidemia: mechanism and management. *J Am Soc Nephrol*. Vol.7, No.7, (July 1996), pp.971-977, ISSN: 1046-6673.

Matas, AJ., Humar, A., Gillingham, KJ., Payne, WD., Gruessner, RWG., Kandaswamy, R., Dunn, DL., Najasrian, JS. & Sutherland, DER. (1972). Five preventable causes of kidney graft loss in the 1990s: A single-center analysis. *Kidney Int* Vol. 62, No. 2, (August 2002), pp.704-714, ISSN: 0085-2538.

Mayer, AD., Dmitrewski, J., Squifflet, JP., Besse, T., Grabensee, B., Klein, B., Eigler, FW., Heemann, U., Pichlmayr, R., Behrend, M., Vanrenterghem, Y., Donck, J., van Hooff, J., Christiaans, M., Morales, JM., Andres, A., Johnson, RW., Short, C., Buchholz, B., Rehmert, N., Land, W., Schleibner, S., Forsythe, JL., Talbot, D., & Pohanka, E., (1963). Multicenter randomized trial comparing tacrolimus (FK506) and cyclosporine in the prevention of renal allograft rejection. A report of the European tacrolimus multicenter renal study group. *Transplantation* Vol.64, No.3 (August 1997), pp.436-443, ISSN. 0041-1337.

Mazzaferro, S., Pascquali, M., Taggi, F., Baldinelli, M., Conte, C., Muci, ML., Pirozzi, N., Carbone, I., Francone, M. & Pugliese, F. (2006). Progression of coronary artery calcification in renal transplantation and the role of secondary hyperparathyroidism and inflammation. *Clin J Am Soc Nephrol* Vol.4, No.3 (March 2009), pp.685-690, ISSN: 1555-9041.

McDonald, SP. & Russ, GR. (1986). Survival of recipients of cadaveric kidney transplants compared with those receiving dialysis treatment in Australia an New Zealand 1991-2001. *Nephrol Dial Transplant*. Vol.17, No.12, (December 2002) pp.2212-2219, ISSN: 0931-0509.

McGregor, E., Jardine, AG., Murray, LS., Dargie, HJ., Rodger, RS., Junor, BJ., McMillan, MA. & Briggs JD. (1986). Pre-operative echocardiographic abnormalities and adverse outcome following renal transplantation. *Nephrol Dial Transplant*. Vol.13, No.6, (June 1998), pp.1499-505, ISSN: 0931-0509

McGregor, E., Steward, G., Rodger, SC. & Jardine AG. (1986). Early echocardiographic changes and survival following transplantation. *Nephrol Dial Transplant*. Vol.15, No.1, (January 2000), pp.93-93, ISSN: 0931-0509.

Meier-Kriesche, HU., Vaghela, M., Thambuganipalle, R., Friedman, G., Jacobs, M. & Kaplan, B. (163). The effect of body mass index on long-term renal allograft. *Transplantation*. Vol.68, No.9, (November 1999), pp.1294-1297, ISSN: 0041-1337.

Meier-Kriesche, HU., Arndorfer, JA. & Kaplan, B. (1963). The impact of body mass index on renal transplant outcomes: a significant independent risk factor for graft failure and patient death. *Transplantation*. Vol.73, No.1, (January 2002), pp.70-74, ISSN.0041-1337.

Meier-Kriesche, HU., Baliga, R. & Kaplan, B. (1963). Decreased renal function is a strong risk factor for cardiovascular death after renal transplantation. *Transplantation* Vol.75, No.8 (April 2003), pp.1291-1205, ISSN: 0041-1337.

Miller LW. (2001). Cardiovascular toxicities of immunosuppressive agents. *Am J Transplant.* Vol.2, No.9, (October 2002), pp.807- 818, ISSN: 1600-6135.

Molnar, MZ., Czira, M., Ambrus, C., Kovacs, AC., Pap, J., Remport, A., Szeifer, L. & Mucsi, I. (2001). Anemia is associated with mortality in kidney-transplanted patients- a prospective cohort study. *Am J Transplant.* Vol.7, No.4, (April 2007), pp. 818-824, ISSN.1600-6135.

Montori, VM., Basu, A., Erwin, PJ., Velosa, JA., Gabriel, SE.& Kudva, YC.(1978). Posttransplantation diabetes. A systematic review of the literature. *Diabetes Care* Vol. 25, No.3, (March, 2002), pp.538-592, ISSN: 0149-5992.

Moore, R., Hernandez, D. & Valantine, H. (1990). Calcineurin inhibitors and post-transplant hyperlipidaemias. *Drugs Saf* Vol.24, No.10, (2001), pp.755-766.

Morales, JM. & Dominguez-Gil, B. (1990). Impact of tacrolimus and mycophenolate mofetil combination on cardiovascular risk profile after transplantation. *J Am Soc Nephrol* Vol.17, 12 Suppl 3, (December 2006), pp.S296-S303, ISSN: 1046-6673.

Morales, JM., Marcén, R., Andrés, A., González- Molina, M., del Castillo, D., Cabello, M., Capdevila, L., Campistol, JM., Oppenheimer, F., Serón, D., Gil-Vernet, S., Lampreave, I., Valdés, F., Anaya, F., Escuin, F., Arias, M., Pallardó, L. & Bustamente J. (1972). Renal transplantation in the moderm immunosuppresive era in Spain: four-year results from a multicenter database focus on post-transplant cardiovascular disease. *Kidney Int Suppl.* Vol.111, (December 2008), pp. S94-S99, ISSN: 0085-2538.

Murphy, SW., Foley, RN. & Parfrey, PS. (1981). Screening and treatment for cardiovascular disease in patients with chronic renal disease. *Am J Kidney Dis.* Vol.32, 5 Suppl 3, (November 1998), pp.S184-S199, ISSN: 0272-6386..

Ojo, AO., Hanson, JA., Wolfe, RA., Leichtman, AB., Agodoa, LY. & Port FK. (1972). Long-term survival in renal transplant recipients with graft function. *Kidney Int* . Vol. 57, No.1, (January 2000), pp. 307-313, ISSN: 0085-2538.

Ojo, AO. (1963). Cardiovascular complications after renal transplantation and their prevention. *Transplantation.* Vol.82, No.5, (September 2006), pp.603-611, ISSN: 0041-1337.

Oliveras, A., Roquer, J., Puig, JM., Rodriguez, A., Mir, M., Orfila, A., Masramon, J. & Loveras, J. (1987). Stroke in renal transplant recipients: epidemiology, predictive risk factors and outcome. *Clin Transplant* Vol. 17, No.1, (February 2003), pp.1-8, ISSN:0902-0063.

Opelz, G., Döhler, B. for the Collaborative Transplant Study. (2001). Improved long-term outcomes after renal transplantation associated with blood pressue control. *Am J Transplant.* . Vol.5, No.11, (November 2005), pp.2725-2731, ISSN: 1600.6135.

Opelz, G., Zeier, M., Laux, G., Morath, C. & Döhler, B. (1990). No improvement of patients or graft survival in transplant recipients treated with angiotensin-converting enzyme inhibitors or angiotensin II type 1 receptor blockers: a collaborative transplant study report. *J Am Soc Nephrol* . Vol.17, No.11, (November 2006), pp.3257-3262, ISSN: 1046-6673.

Paoletti, E., Amidore, M., Cassottana, P., Gherzi, M., Marsano, L. & Cannella, G. (1981). Effects of sirolimus on left ventricular hypertrophy in kidney transplant recipients:

a 1-year nonrandomized controlled trial. *Am J Kidney Dis* . Vol.52, No.2, (August 2008), pp.324-330, ISSN: 0272-6386.

Parfrey, PS., Harnett, JD., Foley, RN., Kent, GM., Murray, DC., Barre, PE. & Guttmann. RD. (1963). Impact of renal transplantation on uremic cardiomyopathy. *Transplantation* . Vol. 60. No. 9, (November 1995), pp. 908-914, ISSN: 0041- 1337.

Park, JM. & Luan, FL. (1990). Management of hypertension in solid-organ transplantation. *Prog Transplant*. Vol.15, No.1, (March 2005), pp. 17-22, ISSN: 1526-9248.

Patel, RK., Mark, PB., Jonhston, N., McGregor, E., Dargie, H. &, Jardine AG. (2006). Renal transplantation is not associated with regression of left ventricular hypertrophy: a magnetic resonance study. *Clin J Am Soc Nephrol* . Vol.3, No.6, (November 2008), pp.1807-1811, ISSN: 1555-9041.

Pilmore, H., Dent, H., Chang, S., McDonald, SP. & Chadban SJ. (1963). Reduction in cardiovascular death after kidney transplantation. *Transplantation*. Vol. 89, No. 7, (April 2010), pp.851-857. ISSN: 0041-1337.

Ridker, PM., Cushman, M., Stampfer, MJ., Tracy, RP. & Hennekens, CH. (1812). Inflammation , aspirin, and the risk of cardiovascular disease in apparently healthy men. *N Engl J Med* . Vol.336, No.14, (April 1997), pp.973-979, ISSN: 0028-4793.

Rigatto, C., Foley, RN., Kent, GM., Guttman, R. & Parfrey, PS. (1963). Long-term changes in left ventricular hypertrophy after renal transplantation. *Transplantation* . Vol.70, No.4, (August 2000), pp. 570-575, ISSN: 0041-1337.

Rigatto, C., Parfrey, P., Foley, R., Negrijn, C., Tribula, C. & Jeffey J. (1990). Congestive heart failure in renal transplant recipients: risk factors, outcomes, and relationship with ischemic heart disease. *J Am Soc Nephrol* . Vol.13, No.4, (April 2002), pp. 1084-1090. ISSN.1046-6673.

Rigatto, C. (1990). Clinical epidemiology of cardiac disease in renal transplant recipients. *Semi in Dial* Vol.16, No.2, (March-April 2003a), pp. 106-110, ISSN: 1525-139X.

Rigatto, C., Foley, R., Jeffery, J., Negrijn, C., Tribula, C. & Parfrey P. (1990). Electrocardiographic left ventricular hypertrophy in renal transplant recipients: prognostic value and impact of blood pressure and anemia. *J Am Soc Nephrol* Vol. 14. No. 2, (February 2003b), pp.462-468. ISSN.1046-6673.

Rigatto, C. (2001). Anemia, renal transplantation and the anemia paradox. *Semin Nephrol*. Vol.26, No.4, (July 2006), pp.307- *312*.ISSN 0270-9295.

Roodnat, JI., Muldr, PGH., Rischen-Vos, J., van Riemsdijk, IC., van Gelder, T., Zietse R., Izermans, JN. & Weimar, W. (1963). Proteinuria after renal transplantation affects not only graft survival but also patient survival. *Transplantation*. Vol.72, No.3, (August 2001), pp.438-444, ISSN: 0041-1337.

Schena, FP., Pascoe, MD., Aberu, J., del Carmen, Rial, M., Oberbauer, R., Brennan, DC., Campistol, JM., Racusen, L., Polinsky, MS., Goldberg-Alberts, R., Li, H., Scarola, J. & Neylan, JF. for the sirolimus CONVERT trial study group. (1963). Conversion from calcineurin inhibitors to sirolimus maintenance therapy in renal allograft recipients: 24-months efficacy and safety results from the CONVERT trial. *Transplantation*. Vol.87, No.2 (January 2009), pp.233-242, ISSN: 0041-1337.

Seliger, SL., Weiss, NS., Gillen, DL., Kestenbaum, B., Ball, A., Sherrard, DJ. & Stehman-Breen, CO. (1972). HMG-CoA reductase inhibitors are associated with reduced mortality in ESRD patients. *Kidney Int*. Vol.61, No.1, (January 2002), pp.297-304, ISSN:0085-2538.

Seliger, SL., Gillen, DL., Longstreth, WT., Kestenbaum, B. & Stehman-Breen CO. (1972). Elevated risk of stroke among patients with end-stage renal disease. *Kidney Int.* Vol. 64, No.2, (August 2003), pp.603-609, ISSN:0085-2538.

Seliger, SL., Gillen, DL., Tirschwell, D., Wasse, H., Kestenbaum, BR. & Stehman-Breen CO. (1990). Risk factors for incident stroke among patients with end-stage renal disease. *J Am Soc Nephrol* Vol. 14, No.10 (October 2003), pp.2623-2631, ISSN: 1046-6673.

Shah, N., Al-Khoury, S., Afzali, B., Covic, A., Roche, A., Msarsh, J., Macdougall, IC. & Goldsmirhm DJA. (1963). Posttransplantation anemia in adult renal allograft recipients: prevalence and predictors. *Transplantation* Vol.81, No.8 (April 2006), pp.1112-1118, ISSN.0041-1337.

Snyder, JJ., Kasiske, BL. & Mac Lean, R. (1990). Peripheral arterial disease and renal transplantation. *J Am Soc Nephrol* Vol.17, No.7, (July 2006), pp.2056-2068, ISSN: 1046-6673.

Soveri, I., Holdaas, H., Jardine, A., Gimpelewicz, C., Staffler, B. & Fellström, B. (1986). Renal transplant dysfunction-importance quantified in comparison with traditional risk factors for cardiovascular disease and mortality. *Nephrol Dial Transplant* Vol.21, No.8, (August 2006), pp.2282-2289. ISSN:0931-0509.

Stack, AG. & Bloembergen, WE. (1981). A cross-sectional study of the prevalence and clinical correlates of congestive heart failure among incident U.S. dialysis patients. *Am J Kidney Dis* Vol. 38, No. 5, (November 2001), pp. 992-1000, ISSN: 0272- 6386.

Stuveling, EM., Hillege, HL., Bakker, SJ., Gans, RO., De Jong, PE. & de Zeeuw, D. (1972). C-reactive protein is associated with renal function abnormalities in a non-diabetic population. *Kidney Int* . Vol.63, No.2, (February 2003), pp.654-661, ISSN: 0085-2538.

Sung, RS., Althoen, M., Howell, TA. & Merion, RM. (1963). Peripheral vascular occlusive disease in renal transplant recipients: risk factors and impact on kidney allograft survival. *Transplantation.* Vol.70, No.7, (October 2000), pp. 1049-1054, ISSN: 0041-1337.

Teruel, JL., Rodriguez Padial, L., Quereda, C., Yuste, P., Marcen, R. & Ortuño, J. (1963). Regression of left ventricular hypertrophy after renal transplantation. A prospective study. *Transplantation.* Vol.43, No.2, (February 1987), pp.307-309, ISSN: 0041-1337

Tucker, B., Fabbian, F., Giles, M., Thuraisingham, RC., Raine, AE. & Baker LR. (1997). Left ventricular hypertrophy and ambulatory blood pressure monitoring in chronic renal failure. *Nephrol Dial Transplant* Vol.12, No.4, (April 1997), pp. 724-728, ISSN: 0272-6376.

Tutone, VK., Mark, PB., Steward, GA., Tan, CC., Geddes, CC. & Jardine AG. (1987). Hypertension, antihypertensive agents and outcomes following renal transplantation. *Clin Transplant* Vol.19, No. 2, (April 2005), pp.181-192, ISSN: 0902-0063.

Van Ree, RM., de Vries, APJ., Oterdoom ,LH., The, TH., Gansevoort, RT., van der Heide, JJH., van Son, WJ., Ploeg, RJ., de Jong, PE., Gans, ROB. & Bakker, SJL. (1986).Abdominal obesity and smoking are important determinants of C-reactive protein in renal transplant recipients. *Nephrol Dial Transplant* . Vol.20, No.11 (November 2005), pp.2524-2531, ISSN: 0931-0509.

Vanrenterghem, Y., Ponticelli, C., Morales, JM., Abramowicz, D., Baboolal, K., Eklund, B., Kliem, V., Legendre, C., Morais Sarmento, AL. & Vincenti, F. (2001). Prevalence and management of anemia in renal transplant recipients: a European survey. *Am J Transplant*. Vol.3, No.7, (July 2003), pp.835-845, ISSN.1600-6135.

Vanrenterghem, YFC., Claes, K., Montagnino, G., Fieuws, S., Maes, B., Villa, M. & Ponticelli, C. (1963). Risk factors for cardiovascular events after successful renal transplantation. *Transplantation*. Vol. 85, No.2, (January 2008), pp. 209-216, ISSN: 0041-1337.

Vincenti, F., Jensik, SC., Filo, RS., Millar, J. & Pirsch, J. (1963). A long-term comparison of tacrolimus (FK506) and cyclosporine in kidney transplantation: evidence for improved allograft survival at five years. *Transplantation* Vol.73, No.5 (March 2005), pp. 775-782. ISSN. 0041-1337.

Vincenti, F., Friman, S., Scheuermann, E., Rostaing, L., Jenssen, T., Campistol, JM., Uchida, K.., Pescovitz, MD., Marchetti, P., Tuncer, M., Citterio, F., Wiecek, A., Chadban, S., El-Shahawy, M., Budde, K. & Goto, N. on behalf of the DIRECT investigators. (2001). Results of an international, randomised trial comparing glucose metabolism disorders and outcome with cyclosporine versus tacrolimus. *Am J Transpl* Vol.7, No.6, (June 2007), pp. 1506-1514, ISSN.1600-6135.

Vincenti, F., Charpentier, B., Vanrenterghen, Y., Rostaing, L., Bresnahan, B., Darji, P., Massari, P., Mondragon-Ramirez, GA., Agarwal, M., Di Russo, G., Lin, CS., Garg, P. & Larsen, CP. (2001). A phase III study of belatacept-based immunosuppression regimens versus cyclosporine in renal transplant recipients (BENEFIT study). *Am J Transplant*. Vol.10, No.3, (March 2010), pp.535-546, ISSN: 1600-6135.

Wali, RK., Wang, GS., Gottlieb, SS., Bellumkonda, L., Hansalia, R., Ramos, E., Drachenberg, C., Papadimitriou, J., Brisco, MA., Blahut, S., Fink, JC., Fisher, ML., Bartlett, ST. & Weir MR. (1983). Effect of kidney transplantation on left ventricular systolic dysfunction and congestive heart failure in patients with end-stage renal disease. *J Am Coll Cardiol*, Vol. 45, No.7 (April 2005), pp.1051-1060, ISSN: 0735-1097.

Wang, K., Zhang, H., Li, Y., Wei, Q., Li, H., Yang, Y. & Lu, Y. (1969). Safety of mycophenolate mofetil versus azathioprine in renal transplantation: a systematic review. *Transplant Proc*. Vol.36, No7, (September 2004), pp.2068-2070, ISSN.0041-1345.

Wang, JH. & Kasiske, BL. (1992). Screening and management of pretransplant cardiovascular disease. *Curr Opin Nephrol Hypertens*. Vol.19, No.6, (November 2010), pp.586-591, ISSN: 1473-6543.

Webster, AC., Lee, VWS., Chapman, JR. & Craig, JC. (1963). Target of rapamycin inhibitors (sirolimus and everolimus) for primary immunosuppression of kidney transplant recipients; a systemsatic review meta-analysis of randomized trials. *Transplantation* Vol.81, No.9, (May 2006), pp. 1234-1248, ISSN: 0041-1337.

Wiesbauer, F., Heinze, G., Mitterbauer, C., Harnoncourt, F., Hörl, WH. & Oberbauer, R. (1990). Statin use is associated with prolonged survival of renal transplant recipients. *J Am Soc Nephrol* Vol.19, No.11, (November 2008), pp. 2211-2218, ISSN: 1046-6673.

Wilson, PWF. & Culleton, BF. (19981). Epidemiology of cardiovascular disease in the United States. *A J Kidney Dis*. Vol 32, No5, suppl 3. (November 1998), pp.S56-S65, ISSN: 0272-6386.

Winkelmayer, WC., Lorenz, M., Kramar, R., Fodinger, M., Hörl, WH. & Sunder-Plassmann, G. (2001). C-reactive protein and body mass index independently predict mortality in kidney transplant recipients. *Am J Transplant*. Vol.4, No.7, (July 2004), pp.1148-1154, ISSN: 1600-6135.

Winkelmayer, WC., Kramar, R., Curhan, GC., Chandraker, A., Endler, G., Födinger, M., Hörl, WH. & Sunder Plassmann, G. (1990). Fasting plasma total homocysteine levels and mortality and allograaft loss in kidney transplant recipients: a prospective study. *J Am Soc Nephrol* . Vol.16, No.1, (January 2005), pp.255-260, ISSN: 1046-6673.

Winkelmayer, WC., Chandraker, A., Brookhart, MA., Kramar, R. & Sunder-Plassmann, G. (1986). A prospective stydy of anaemia and long-term outcomes in kidney transplant recipients. *Nephrol Dial Transplant.* Vol.21, No.12, (December 2006), pp.3559-3566, ISSN.0931-0509.

Wolfe, RA., Ashby, VB., Milford, EL., Ojo, AO., Ettenger, RE., Agodoa, LY., Held, PJ. & Port, FK. (1812). Comparison of mortality in all patients on dialysis, patients on dialysis awaiting transplantation, and recipients of a first cadaveric transplant. *N Engl J Med.* Vol. 341, No.23 (December 1999), pp.1725-1730, ISSN: 0028-4793.

Wong, BM., Huang, M., Zaltzman, JS. & Prasad, GV. (1963). Mycophenolate mofetil and C-reactive protein in renal transplant recipients. *Transplantation.* Vol.83, No.1, (January 2007), pp.48-53, ISSN: 0041 1337.

Yorgin, PD., Scandling, JD., Belson, A., Sanchez, J., Alexander, SR. & Andreoni, KA. (2001). Late post-transplant anemia in adult renal transplant recipients. An under-recognized problem? *Am J Transplant.* Vol.2, No.5, (May 2002), pp.429-435, ISSN.1600-6135.

Zhang, R., Leslie, B., Boudreaux, JP., Frey, D. & Reisin E. (1827). Hypertension after kidney transplantation: impact, pathogenesis and therapy. Am J Med Sci Vol: 325, No.4, (April 2003), pp.202-208, ISSN: 1538-2990.

Zebe H. (1986). Atrial fibrillation in dialysis patients. *Nephrol Dial Transplant.* Vol. 16, No.5, (June 2001), pp. 765-8, ISSN: 0931- 0509.

Zitt, N., Kollerits, B., Neyer, U., Mark, W., Heininger, D., Mayer, G., Kronenberg, F., & Lhotta, K. (1986). Cigarette smoking and chronic allograft nephropathy. *Nephrol Dial Transplant.* Vol.22, No.10, (October 2007), pp.3034-3034, ISSN. 0931-0509

Permissions

All chapters in this book were first published by InTech Open; hereby published with permission under the Creative Commons Attribution License or equivalent. Every chapter published in this book has been scrutinized by our experts. Their significance has been extensively debated. The topics covered herein carry significant findings which will fuel the growth of the discipline. They may even be implemented as practical applications or may be referred to as a beginning point for another development.

The contributors of this book come from diverse backgrounds, making this book a truly international effort. This book will bring forth new frontiers with its revolutionizing research information and detailed analysis of the nascent developments around the world.

We would like to thank all the contributing authors for lending their expertise to make the book truly unique. They have played a crucial role in the development of this book. Without their invaluable contributions this book wouldn't have been possible. They have made vital efforts to compile up to date information on the varied aspects of this subject to make this book a valuable addition to the collection of many professionals and students.

This book was conceptualized with the vision of imparting up-to-date information and advanced data in this field. To ensure the same, a matchless editorial board was set up. Every individual on the board went through rigorous rounds of assessment to prove their worth. After which they invested a large part of their time researching and compiling the most relevant data for our readers.

The editorial board has been involved in producing this book since its inception. They have spent rigorous hours researching and exploring the diverse topics which have resulted in the successful publishing of this book. They have passed on their knowledge of decades through this book. To expedite this challenging task, the publisher supported the team at every step. A small team of assistant editors was also appointed to further simplify the editing procedure and attain best results for the readers.

Apart from the editorial board, the designing team has also invested a significant amount of their time in understanding the subject and creating the most relevant covers. They scrutinized every image to scout for the most suitable representation of the subject and create an appropriate cover for the book.

The publishing team has been an ardent support to the editorial, designing and production team. Their endless efforts to recruit the best for this project, has resulted in the accomplishment of this book. They are a veteran in the field of academics and their pool of knowledge is as vast as their experience in printing. Their expertise and guidance has proved useful at every step. Their uncompromising quality standards have made this book an exceptional effort. Their encouragement from time to time has been an inspiration for everyone.

The publisher and the editorial board hope that this book will prove to be a valuable piece of knowledge for researchers, students, practitioners and scholars across the globe.

List of Contributors

Ehtuish Ehtuish
Surgery Department Tripoli Central Hospital & National Organ Transplantation Program, Libya

Yasser Haggag and Imran Ahmad
Guy's and St Thomas NHS Foundation Trust, UK

Squifflet Jean-Paul
University of Liege, Belgium

Hung Do Nguyen and Rebecca Croke
Sir Charles Gairdner Hospital, Department of Renal Medicine, Western Australia, Australia

Kenneth Yong and Wai H Lim
Sir Charles Gairdner Hospital, Department of Renal Medicine, Western Australia, Australia
University of Western Australia, Western Australia, Australia

Shih-Chieh Jeff Chueh and Bashir R. Sankari
Glickman Urological and Kidney Institute, Cleveland Clinic and Cleveland Clinic Lerner College of Medicine, OH, USA

Ole Øyen
Oslo University Hospital Rikshospitalet, Clinic for Specialised Medicine and Surgery, Norway

Alex Chang and Susan Hou
Loyola University Medical Center, Department of Medicine, Division of Nephrology and Hypertension, USA

Holly Kramer
Loyola University Medical Center, Department of Medicine, Division of Nephrology and Hypertension, USA
Department of Preventive Medicine and Epidemiology, USA

Levent B. Kıdak
Izmir Bozyaka Training and Research Hospital, Hospital and Health Care Institutions Management, Deputy of Head Physician, Izmir, Turkey

Marcelo Ferreira Cassini, Murilo Ferreira de Andrade and Silvio Tucci Junior
Ribeirão Preto Medical School, São Paulo University, Brazil

Roberto Marcén and Sara Jiménez
Department of Nephrology, Ramón y Cajal Hospital, University of Alcalá de Henares, Madrid, Spain

Index

www.ingramcontent.com/pod-product-compliance
Lightning Source LLC
LaVergne TN
LVHW062233200926
848484LV00006B/1527
* 9 7 9 8 8 8 7 4 0 1 4 8 5 *